Nursing
Leadership

Nursing Leadership

A Concise Encyclopedia

EDITOR-IN-CHIEF
HARRIET R. FELDMAN, PhD, RN, FAAN

ASSOCIATE EDITORS
MARILYN JAFFE-RUIZ, EdD, RN
MARGARET L. McCLURE, RN, EdD, FAAN
MARTHA J. GREENBERG, PhD, RN
THOMAS D. SMITH, MS, RN, CNAA, BC
M. JANICE NELSON, EdD, RN
ANGELA BARRON McBRIDE, PhD, RN FAAN
G. RUMAY ALEXANDER, EdD, RN

SPRINGER PUBLISHING COMPANY
New York

Springer Publishing Company, LLC
11 West 42nd Street
New York, NY 10036
www.springerpub.com

Acquisitions Editor: Sally J. Barhydt
Production Editor: Shana Meyer
Cover design: Joanne E. Honigman
Composition: Aptara Inc.

08 09 10 11 / 5 4 3 2 1

Library of Congress Cataloging-in-Publication Data

Nursing leadership : a concise encyclopedia / editor-in-chief, Harriet R. Feldman ; associate editors, Martha J. Greenberg . . . [et al.].
    p. ; cm.
    Includes bibliographical references and index.
    ISBN 978-0-8261-0258-4 (hardback)
  1. Nursing—Administration—Encyclopedias. 2. Nurse administrators—Encyclopedias. I. Feldman, Harriet R.
    [DNLM: 1. Leadership—Encyclopedias—English. 2. Nursing, Supervisory—Encyclopedias—English. 3. Nurse Administrators—Encyclopedias—English. WY 13 N9738 2008]

  RT89.N7943 2008
  610.7303—dc22

2007037206

Printed in the United States of America by Bang Printing.

Leadership skills develop over a lifetime, so I would like to publicly thank some of the important people in my life who gave me the support over the years to accomplish all that I have:

To my parents, Florence and Mickey Martin, their faith and unconditional love guided me toward success;

To my husband, Ron Feldman, you always challenge me to think in alternative ways;

To my mentors, especially Drs. Madeline Schwaid and June S. Rothberg, for gently showing me the way so I could grow as a professional and person.

—*Harriet*

Contents

List of Entries

Editors' Bios

Harriet R. Feldman, PhD, RN, FAAN, is professor and Dean of the Lienhard School of Nursing at Pace University (1993–Present) and Interim Dean of the Pace University School of Education (2006–2008). Dr. Feldman has held administrative, teaching, and clinical positions for more than 40 years. She was also editor of two nursing journals; *Scholarly Inquiry for Nursing Practice: An International Journal* and *Nursing Leadership Forum*. Three of her books have received American Journal of Nursing Book of the Year Awards: 2001 (*Nurses in the Political Arena: The Public Face of Nursing,* co-authored with Dr. Sandra B. Lewenson), 2005 (*Educating Nurses for Leadership,* co-edited with Dr. Martha J. Greenberg), and 2007 (*Teaching and Learning Evidence-Based Practice: A Guide for Educators,* co-edited with Dr. Rona F. Levin). Other books by Dr. Feldman include *Strategies for Nursing Leadership* (2001), *Nursing Leaders Speak Out* (2001), and *The Nursing Shortage: Strategies for Recruitment and Retention in Clinical Practice and Education* (2003). She has more than 80 refereed journal articles and editorials to her credit. Dr. Feldman holds the following appointments: Chair (Vice Chair, 2007) of the Board of Commissioners of the Commission on Collegiate Nursing Education and member of the Health Advisory Committee to Representative Nita Lowey. She is a Fellow of the American Academy of Nursing and a Fellow of the New York Academy of Medicine.

Marilyn Jaffe-Ruiz, EdD, RN, is professor of nursing at the Lienhard School of Nursing, Pace University, New York City, New York. Her areas of specialization include leadership, education, psychiatric mental health nursing, cultural competence, and siblings and families of the intellectually disabled. She teaches at both the graduate and undergraduate levels. Dr. Jaffe-Ruiz served as Pace University's Chief Academic Officer with the title of Provost and Executive Vice President for Academic Affairs from 1998 to 2003. Formerly, she was Vice Provost and, before that, Dean of the Lienhard School of Nursing at Pace, a position that she held for 7 years. Dr. Jaffe-Ruiz has held faculty positions at Pace University and Columbia University. In 2001, Dr. Jaffe-Ruiz was inducted into the Teachers College Nursing Hall of Fame and made an honorary member of the Golden Key International Honor Society at Pace University. In 2006, she received the Dr. Martin Luther King Social Justice Award, and in 2002 she received the Diversity Leadership Award at Pace University. She received the Anne Krauss Volunteer of the Year Award from the New York City Chapter of the Association for the Help of Retarded Children (AHRC) in May 2007.

Margaret L. McClure, RN, EdD, FAAN, is a professor at New York University, where she holds appointments in both the School of Medicine and the College of Nursing. For almost 20 years, she was the chief nursing officer at New York University Medical Center, where she also served as the chief operating officer and hospital administrator. A prolific writer and lecturer, Dr. McClure is internationally recognized as a nursing leader. Her best-known contribution to the literature is *Magnet Hospitals: Attraction and Retention of Professional Nurses,* which she coauthored under the auspices of the American Academy of Nursing. In 2002, she completed a compilation of all the work that has been done to date regarding this subject, titled *Magnet Hospitals Revisited.*

Martha J. Greenberg, PhD, RN, is Associate Professor at the Lienhard School of Nursing at Pace University in Pleasantville, New York. She has served in leadership roles as chairperson of the 4-year Baccalaureate Nursing Program from 1995 to 2000 and 2007–Present. She teaches didactic and clinical nursing leadership and management courses in the undergraduate nursing programs and complementary healing and holistic nursing courses in both the undergraduate and graduate programs. Dr. Greenberg maintains a clinical practice in medical-surgical nursing and serves on a variety of community boards and task forces in Westchester County, New York. Her areas of research interest are humor and complementary health and healing practices.

Thomas D. Smith, MS, RN, CNAA, BC, is Chief Nursing Officer and Senior Vice President, Patient Care Services at Cambridge Health Alliance, which is a public, academic integrated delivery system serving Cambridge and Somerville, Massachusetts, as well as seven adjacent communities in the metro-north region of Boston. From 1996 to 2005, he was Senior Vice President for Nursing at The Mount Sinai Hospital in New York City, the first full-service hospital in Manhattan to receive the Magnet Award for nursing excellence. In addition, he currently serves as Senior Advisor at the New York University College of Nursing. Mr. Smith is the recipient of numerous awards, including the Grace E. Davidson Award for contributions to the education of nursing students at New York University College of Nursing and the Anne Kibrick Award for excellence in nursing leadership at the University of Massachusetts, Boston. He is a member of the Board of Trustees of the Foundation of the National Student Nurses Association, and he is currently serving as a member of the Commission on Collegiate Nursing Education (CCNE).

M. Janice Nelson, EdD, RN, is professor and dean emerita of the College of Nursing, Upstate Medical University of the State University of New York at Syracuse. She currently serves as a trustee on the Board of Directors of the Foundation of the New York State Nurses, Inc. In addition to teaching and administrative roles, over the past 25 years Dr. Nelson served as president and board member of the Central Counties Professional Nurses Association and president and board member of Nurses Educational Funds, Inc. She was active on the Board of Directors of the Central New York Visiting Nurse Association as well as the Syracuse Home Association—a multilevel retirement community. Nelson is recipient of a number of awards including induction into the Nursing Hall of Fame at Teachers College, Columbia University, and recognition for Distinguished Achievement in Nursing Education from the Nursing Education Alumni Association of Teachers College, Columbia University; she was recognized as a Distinguished Alumna from Daeman College in Buffalo, New York.

Angela Barron McBride, PhD, RN, FAAN, is Distinguished Professor-University Dean Emerita at Indiana University School of Nursing. She is on the board of Clarian Health, the largest hospital network in Indiana and chairs their Committee on Quality and Patient Safety. Known for her contributions to women's mental health, she served as president of Sigma Theta Tau International (1987–1989) during the building of their International Center for Nursing Scholarship, and of the American Academy of Nursing (1993–1995). Elected in 1995 to the Institute of Medicine, Dr. McBride was named a "Living Legend" by the American Academy of Nursing in 2006.

G. Rumay Alexander, EdD, RN, is associate professor and the Director of the Office of Multicultural Affairs in the School of Nursing at the University of North Carolina-Chapel Hill, and has over 25 years of experience in the areas of cultural diversity, public policy, advocacy, strategic planning, and workforce issues. At a national level, she has served as a Commissioner on the American Hospital Association's Workforce Commission, the Board of the American Organization of Nurse Executives, the National Quality Forum Nursing Care Performance Measures' Steering Committee, and the American Hospital Association's Leadership Circle of Eliminating Racial and Ethnic Disparities in Health Care.

Contributors

Nancy R. Adams, RN, MSN, FAAN
Former Major General
19th Chief, Army Nurse Corps
Fort Lauderdale, Florida

Linda H. Aiken, PhD, RN, FAAN
University of Pennsylvania
School of Nursing
Philadelphia, Pennsylvania

G. Rumay Alexander, EdD, RN
School of Nursing
University of North Carolina
Chapel Hill, North Carolina

Karen A. Ballard, MA, RN
Nurse Consultant
New York, New York

Cecilia R. Barron, PhD, RN
University of Nebraska Medical
   Center
College of Nursing
Omaha, Nebraska

Marie Boltz, PhD, APRN-BC
The Hartford Institute for
   Geriatric Nursing
New York University College of
   Nursing
New York, New York

Susan Bowar-Ferres, PhD, RN, CNAA, BC
NYU Hospitals Center
New York, New York

Patricia Flatley Brennan, PhD, RN, FAAN
School of Nursing and College of
   Engineering
University of Wisconsin-Madison
Madison, Wisconsin

Ingrid E. Brodin, RN, MS
Cambridge Health Alliance
Cambridge, Massachusetts

Jo Ann Brooks, DNS, RN, FAAN, FCCP
Clarian Healthcare Partners, Inc.
Indianapolis, Indiana

Marion E. Broome, PhD, RN, FAAN
Indiana University School of Nursing
Indianapolis, Indiana

Billye J. Brown, EdD, RN(R), FAAN
The University of Texas at Austin School of Nursing
Austin, Texas

Peter I. Buerhaus, PhD, RN, FAAN
Vanderbilt University School of Nursing
Nashville, Tennessee

Ann T. Bures, RN, MA, CHCR
University of Maryland Medical Center
Baltimore, Maryland

Jennifer Paup Butlin, EdD
Commission on Collegiate Nursing Education
Washington, District of Columbia

Elizabeth Capezuti, PhD, RN, FAAN
The Hartford Institute for Geriatric Nursing
New York University College of Nursing
New York, New York

Sean Clarke, RN, PhD, CRNP
University of Pennsylvania School of Nursing
Philadelphia, Pennsylvania

Christine Coughlin, EdD, RN
Adelphi University
School of Nursing
Garden City, New York

Judith DeBlasio, RN, MSN
Lienhard School of Nursing
Pace University
Pleasantville, New York

Joanne Disch, PhD, RN, FAAN
University of Minnesota School of Nursing
Minneapolis, Minnesota

Marianne Ditomassi, RN, MSN, MBA
Massachusetts General Hospital
Boston, Massachusetts

Jane Dolan, RN, MSN
Lienhard School of Nursing
Pace University
Pleasantville, New York

Gloria F. Donnelly, PhD, RN, FAAN
College of Nursing and Health Professions
Drexel University
Philadelphia, Pennsylvania

Jeffrey N. Doucette, MS, RN, CEN, CHE, CNAA, BC
Duke University Medical Center
Durham, North Carolina

Kathleen Dracup, DNSc, FNP, RN, FAAN
School of Nursing
University of California
San Francisco, California

Rhetaugh Graves Dumas, PhD, RN, FAAN
University of Michigan
Ann Arbor, Michigan

Patricia R. Ebright, DNS, CNS, RN
Indiana University School of Nursing
Indianapolis, Indiana

David N. Ekstrom, PhD, RN
Lienhard School of Nursing
Pace University
New York, New York

Jeanette Ives Erickson, RN, MS
Massachusetts General Hospital
Boston, Massachusetts

Claire M. Fagin, PhD, RN, FAAN
University of Pennsylvania School of Nursing
Philadelphia, Pennsylvania

Dolores Fazzino, RN, MSN, C-FNP, CRNFA
Consultant
Encinitas, California

Harriet R. Feldman, PhD, RN, FAAN
Lienhard School of Nursing
Pace University
Pleasantville, New York

Joyce J. Fitzpatrick, PhD, RN, FAAN
Frances Payne Bolton School of Nursing
Case Western Reserve University
Cleveland, Ohio

Terry Fulmer, PhD, RN, FAAN
New York University
New York, New York

Lillee Smith Gelinas, MSN, RN, FAAN
VHA Inc.
Irving, Texas

Diane M. Gengo, MS, APRN, BC
Cambridge Health Alliance
Cambridge, Massachusetts

Millicent Gorham, MBA
National Black Nurses Association
Silver Spring, Maryland

Martha J. Greenberg, PhD, RN
Lienhard School of Nursing
Pace University
Pleasantville, New York

Dina Greenfield, BS, RN
Lienhard School of Nursing
Pace University
New York, New York

Mary T. Quinn Griffin, PhD, RN
Frances Payne Bolton School of Nursing
Case Western Reserve University
Cleveland, Ohio

Judith Haber, PhD, APRN, BC, FAAN
New York University
New York, New York

Karen Toby Haghenbeck, PhD, RN, FNP
Lienhard School of Nursing
Pace University
Pleasantville, New York

Edward J. Halloran, RN, MPH, PhD, FAAN
School of Nursing
University of North Carolina
Chapel Hill, North Carolina

Judith A. Halstead, DNS, RN
Indiana University School of
    Nursing
Indianapolis, Indiana

Wylecia Wiggs Harris, MBA, CAE
Center for American Nurses
Silver Spring, Maryland

**Martha L. Henderson, MSN,
    MDiv, DMin, APRN**
University of North Carolina
Chapel Hill, North Carolina

**Ada Sue Hinshaw, PhD, RN,
    FAAN**
University of Michigan School of
    Nursing
Ann Arbor, Michigan

**Nancy Hollingsworth, RN, MSN,
    MBA**
Saint Agnes Medical Center
Fresno, California

**William L. Holzemer, RN, PhD,
    FAAN**
School of Nursing
University of California
San Francisco, California

Lauren M. Huber, BSN, RN
Montefiore Hospital
Bronx, New York

**Michael E. Impollonia, RN,
    MSN, CNA, BC**
The Mount Sinai Hospital
New York, New York

Marilyn Jaffe-Ruiz, EdD, RN
Lienhard School of Nursing
Pace University
New York, New York

**Carrie Houser James, MSN, RN,
    CNA, BC, CCE**
Center for American Nurses
Silver Spring, Maryland

**Stacy Hutton Johnson, RN,
    MS/MBA**
Nursing Director Bigelow 11
Massachusetts General
    Hospital
Boston, Massachusetts

**Cheryl Bland Jones, PhD, RN,
    FAAN**
School of Nursing
University of North Carolina
Chapel Hill, North Carolina

**Dorothy A. Jones, EdD, RNC,
    FAAN**
Massachusetts General
    Hospital
Center for Nursing Research
Boston, Massachusetts

Dayle Joseph, EdD, RN
University of Rhode Island
Kingston, Rhode Island

**David M. Keepnews, PhD, JD,
    RN, FAAN**
Adelphi University
School of Nursing
Garden City, New York

**Shaké Ketefian, EdD, RN,
    FAAN**
University of Michigan School of
    Nursing
Ann Arbor, Michigan

Susan P. Kossman, PhD, RN
Illinois State University
Normal, Illinois

Karren Kowalski, PhD, RN, FAAN
Colorado Center for Nursing
  Excellence
Denver, Colorado

Karen W. Laufer, RN, MA, CPN
The Mount Sinai Hospital
New York, New York

Kim L. Carnahan Lewis, MN, ARNP
Positive Outlook Associates, LLC
Vancouver, Washington

Bettye Davis Lewis, EdD, RN, FAAN
National Black Nurses Association
Silver Spring, Maryland

Linda L. Lindeke, PhD, RN, CNP
University of Minnesota School of
  Nursing
Minneapolis, Minnesota

Diane Mancino, EdD, RN, CAE
National Student Nurses
  Association
Brooklyn, New York

Milisa Manojlovich, PhD, RN, CCRN
University of Michigan School of
  Nursing
Ann Arbor, Michigan

Pam Maraldo, PhD, RN, FAAN
Girls Incorporated, New York City
New York, New York

Angela Barron McBride, PhD, RN, FAAN
Indiana University School of
  Nursing
Indianapolis, Indiana

Margaret L. McClure, PhD, RN, FAAN
New York University
New York, New York

Mary Ann McGinley, PhD, RN
Thomas Jefferson University
  Hospitals
Philadelphia, Pennsylvania

Bernadette Mazurek Melnyk, PhD, RN, CPNP/NPP, FAAN, FNAP
College of Nursing & Healthcare
  Innovation
Arizona State University
Phoenix, Arizona

Vickie L. Milazzo, RN, MSN, JD
Vickie Milazzo Institute
Houston, Texas

Ronda Mintz-Binder, MN, RN
University of Texas
Arlington, Texas

Deena A. Nardi, PhD, APN, CNS, FAAN
University of St. Francis
American Academy of Nursing
Joliet, Illinois

M. Janice Nelson, EdD, RN
State University of New York
Upstate Medical University
College of Nursing
Syracuse, New York

Barbara L. Nichols, DHL, MS, RN, FAAN
Commission on Graduates of
  Foreign Nursing Schools
Philadelphia, Pennsylvania

Stephanie J. Offord, BA, BSN, RN
New York, New York

Kathleen R. Parisien, RN, MA
The Mount Sinai Hospital
New York, New York

Bro. Ignatius Perkins, OP, DNSc, MA, Ed, RN, FAAN
Dominican Friars Health Care
  Ministry of New York
New York, New York

Daniel J. Pesut, PhD, APRN, BC, FAAN
Indiana University School of
  Nursing
Indianapolis, Indiana

Denise Peterson, RN, BA
Cambridge Health Alliance
Cambridge, Massachusetts

Tim Porter-O'Grady, EdD, APRN, FAAN
College of Nursing
Arizona State University
Phoenix, Arizona

Lyn M. Puhek, RN, MSN, CNS
National University, Department
  of Nursing
La Jolla, California

Kathryn Gardner Rapala, JD, RN
Purdue University School of
  Nursing
West Lafayette, Indiana

Cindy A. Reilly, BSN, RN
Quality and Performance
  Improvement
Cambridge Health Alliance
Cambridge, Massachusetts

Hila Richardson, DrPH, RN, FAAN
New York University
New York, New York

Carol A. Romano, PhD, RN, FAAN
National Institutes of Health
  Clinical Center
Bethesda, Maryland

Marlene M. Rosenkoetter, PhD, RN, FAAN
Medical College of Georgia
American Academy of Nursing
Augusta, Georgia

Lisa Sacco, APRN-BC, MSN
Comprehensive Health Center
San Diego, California

Charlotte Seckman, MSN, RN, BC
Department of Clinical Research
  Informatics
National Institutes of Health
  Clinical Center
Bethesda, Maryland

Gloria R. Smith, RN, MPH, MA, PhD, FAAN, Hon. FRCN
WK Kellogg Foundation
Battle Creek, Michigan

Thomas D. Smith, MS, RN, CNAA, BC
Patient Care Services
Cambridge Health Alliance
Cambridge, Massachusetts

Patricia L. Starck, DSN, RN, FAAN
University of Texas Health Science
  Center at Houston
Houston, Texas

Lillian Gatlin Stokes, PhD, RN, FAAN
Indiana University School of Nursing
Indianapolis, Indiana

Pamela Austin Thompson, RN, MS, FAAN
American Organization of Nurse Executives
Washington, DC

Marion Burns Tuck, PhD, RN
Department of Nursing
Thomas Jefferson University Hospitals
Philadelphia, Pennsylvania

Theresa M. Valiga, EdD, RN, FAAN
National League for Nursing
New York, New York

Judy L. Vallarelli, MS, RN, APRN, BC
NES Associates, LTD
Yorktown Heights, New York

Tener Goodwin Veenema, PhD, MPH, MS, CPNP
Center for Disaster Medicine and Emergency Preparedness
University of Rochester
Rochester, New York

Katherine Vestal, RN, PhD, FAAN, FACHE
Work Innovations LLC
Lake Leelanau, Michigan

Maria L. Vezina, EdD, RN
The Mount Sinai Hospital
New York, New York

Meredith Wallace, PhD, APRN
Yale University
School of Nursing
New Haven, Connecticut

Anne W. Wojner-Alexandrov, PhD, RN, CCRN, FAAN
College of Nursing & Healthcare Innovation
Arizona State University
Phoenix, Arizona

Barbara Zittel, PhD, RN
New York State Boards for Nursing and Respiratory Therapy
Albany, New York

Eileen H. Zungolo, EdD, RN, CNE, FAAN
School of Nursing
Duquesne University
Pittsburgh, Pennsylvania

Foreword

Tomorrow's leaders will be those with a taste for paradox,
a talent for organizational ambiguity,
and the capacity to hold new and dissimilar
ideas comfortably in their minds.
They will lead by conviction, not by power.
(Harlan Cleveland)

Today's health care leaders are sorely challenged by increasing consumer demands, contradictory priorities, rapidly shifting incentives, insufficient resources, and a dysfunctional health care system. By contrast, health care leaders have been blessed by increasing consumer involvement, technological possibilities, a passionate engagement by students entering health care, and a national awakening to the idea that health care must be a priority. Although these blessings are also challenges, they provide the impetus for transforming our current health care system into one that is truly driven by the needs of patients and families; health care must be holistic, personalized, convenient, effective, and efficient.

Being a leader in health care today is often about *taking people on a journey on which nobody wants to go*. It involves change, replacement, loss, and growth. It is also about engaging people on a journey that can be co-created as we go along. No one has to have all of the answers; we just have to know what the goal is and to explore the options for getting there. Leadership in this environment requires three things:

* An understanding of the context in which health care is delivered
* A compelling vision, or perhaps merely an idea, of how things "could be better"
* An ability to connect with others and move from "here" to "there"

Leaders are those who are able to tolerate ambiguity and paradox while maintaining a clear focus on the goal and creating positive spaces for all to participate.

Nursing Leadership: A Concise Encyclopedia is an important reference for all leaders and future leaders in health care. The 150+ entries, written by acknowledged luminaries in the nursing field who have both experience in and wisdom about health care, are organized around nine themes. Five of the themes embrace the most salient theories of management and leadership, including the characteristics and skills required of leaders in today's complex health care system. Entries are varied and are based on the assumption that nurse clinicians, academics, and researchers share many of the same challenges but also have to adapt their leadership styles and visions to suit the unique challenges demanded by different roles and institutional missions. The nursing shortage, which is acute and different from all others in its intensity, has been greatly affecting practice and academia dramatically. Thus, consideration of what is required by leaders and managers in both settings is timely.

The movement of the health care system toward greater accountability to the public it serves is reflected in the remaining four themes: professional standards, health care delivery standards and health policy, quality outcomes, and informatics and technology. All of the most important professional organizations in health care are described in this text, and readers will find that these organizations play a key role in determining how best to define successful outcomes, while protecting the public from adverse consequences of care. Novices will find these listings particularly helpful, because many organizations have overlapping aims and share similar missions. Leaders in nursing today experience the impact of professional organizations, and it is important that they be involved in all aspects of the discussion leading to new regulations. Active participation in health policy is not a choice for nurse leaders; it is a mandate.

We are delighted to introduce this text to a new generation of readers. The challenges in nursing, as well as in health care, have never been greater. The need for resources such as this text is profound.

Joanne Disch, PhD, RN, FAAN
Professor and Lillehei Chair in Nursing Leadership
Director, Katharine J. Densford International Center
for Nursing Leadership
School of Nursing
University of Minnesota

Kathleen Dracup, DNSc, FNP, RN, FAAN
Dean and Chair of Nursing Education
School of Nursing
University of California, San Francisco

Preface

Nursing Leadership: A Concise Encyclopedia grew out of a long-standing and enduring commitment to describe and define the concept and field of nursing leadership. In a number of past publications, including articles, editorials, and books, as well as in presentations around the world, I have tried to share that commitment. The *Encyclopedia* presents another venue to provide students, faculty, nurse managers, executives, and others with a concise resource for information about the range of knowledge and roles encompassed by the term *nursing leadership*. Included are descriptions of the contributions of key nursing leaders, the knowledge base and traits of leadership, skills and models on which leadership is based, the regulatory environment of health care, the range of practice settings and roles, and the design of quality outcomes. Nine themes were developed, around which the entries were organized: Characteristics of Leaders; Management and Executive Skills; Theories and Models of Management and Leadership; Major Leaders in Nursing; Professional Standards; Health Care Delivery Standards and Health Policy; Leadership in Practice, Education, and Research; Quality Outcomes; and Informatics and Technology. The associate editors and I hope that you will use this reference guide and the practical skills and references of each entry to further develop your understanding of what leaders and aspiring leaders need to know to be successful. Along with the seven associate editors, Dr. Marilyn Jaffe-Ruiz, Dr. Margaret McClure, Dr. Martha J. Greenberg, Mr. Thomas Smith, Dr. M. Janice Nelson, Dr. Angela Barron McBride, and Dr. Rumay Alexander, there were many contributors who were invited to write entries because of their expertise in one or more areas. So we have the benefit in the *Encyclopedia* of the experience and expertise of dozens of nursing leaders. Assembling this wonderful group is just part of the story. The staff at Springer Publishing Company, with whom I have been associated for more than 20 years, and especially Sally Barhydt, provided great support to the publication.

In the 2005 fable, "Our Iceberg is Melting," by John Kotter and Holger Rathgeber, a penguin colony is faced with a dilemma—the melting iceberg, which threatens their home. They need to find a solution quickly, and the fable takes the reader through the change process to guide us in a "world that just keeps moving faster and faster." Informal and formal leaders teach us important lessons about the art and science of leadership, for example, working effectively in groups, persuading others, communicating and advancing one's vision, dealing with naysayers, and celebrating success. Similar to the penguins, who in the process of solving their dilemma learned to think and feel differently, I am confident that the many topics and resources of the *Encyclopedia* will enhance your leadership skills and opportunities to be successful.

Harriet R. Feldman, PhD, RN, FAAN
Editor-in-Chief

A

Academic Leadership

ACADEMIC LEADERSHIP is an anomaly, and should be. Academic leadership is most like leadership of an orchestra rather than a corporation, and should be. Academic leaders, colleagues among colleagues, lead by persuasion rather than mandate. Academic leadership focuses on building excellence, and rewards competition for excellence rather than rewarding competition for personal gratification or pleasing the leader. Academic leadership shows by vision and example that individual differences and personality quirks can be accommodated and even embraced so long as productivity and quest for excellence is maintained.

What does that quest for excellence include and how does the academic leader, essentially without the power of the corporate leader, achieve this? The academic leader "... may be judged by the extent to which she influences and supports the faculty in individual and school development...." The academic leader "must have sufficient ego strengths to recognize that building leaders and sharing leadership does not in any way diminish [her] prestige..." (Fagin, 2000). Reaching for excellence is not a finite process. But no part of it can be achieved without an atmosphere of openness and trust and rewarding excellence in the shared value system of the group. The academic leader moves the discipline forward and represents the institution in the best way possible. Faculty want their leader to represent them to the administration, help them achieve their full rights and respect, present the discipline in the most reputable way possible, and be able to engage in the broad campus and alumni arenas in a way that brings positive attention to nursing. The academic leader must be a superb role model of the values espoused, must be able to mentor others, must recognize instances of success, and may manipulate the organizational structure and resources to support goal achievement. Along the way, a certain degree of ambiguity is inevitable. For some leaders, that is an easy call; for others, it is more uncomfortable.

Ambiguity is a trait that some find difficult to accept; however, for the academic leader, ambiguity is not a negative. It has its place in that it gives the leader time to evaluate situations and to change one's own opinions as experience dictates. The faculty member who finds ambiguity intolerable is one who needs to be encouraged to think creatively and to tolerate differences of opinion. Being unwilling to accept or to demonstrate ambiguity may result in rigidity, which is anathema to leadership in academia or anywhere. By contrast, academic leadership requires strength and fortitude as well as strategy to accomplish institutional goals, which may not be popular with all faculty. The academic leader's ability to balance these traits is best demonstrated in the reverse by those with a rigid belief in "consensus," which in some cases defies the entire notion of leadership.

"Teaching and research are the main missions of universities and a suitable system of governance should, therefore, make these activities as efficient as possible." Rosovsky's (1990) view of governance is crucial for academic leaders to understand fully. Students are the business of universities and need to be attended to with interest and dedication by faculty who are appointed to tenure holding positions. Although research is vital for advancement of the discipline, it is not an either/or situation. In the quest for new knowledge, the transfer of that knowledge to the next generation is the *sine qua non* of the fully credentialed faculty member. Attention to research alone is possible if one is employed by a research institute at which the staff may work with postdoctoral trainees and the like, but in an academic institution faculty research must be reconciled with dedication to building future leaders and practitioners. The academic leader must have the vision—defined here as an awareness of current trends and future needs of the profession and health care system—the strategic approach, and the personal skills to make this holistic role possible. In academia, students are the principal business that keeps an institution going and growing.

But in academia as well as other venues, there seems to be an absence of transformational leaders "who not only respond to their institutional challenges but also speak for their professions and for the public they serve" (Fagin, 2000). The Institute of Medicine (2004) described transformational leadership as benefiting the leader and the led because it is a process by which both are stimulated to achieve their preferred future. Vision alone does not accomplish the vital tasks of leadership in academia or any other venue. The leader must have the ability to refine and refocus problems and pose a variety of scenarios and solutions. This component of leadership has been described by Foote and Cottrell (1955) as "interpersonal competence." Interpersonal competence is the skill or set of abilities allowing an individual to shape the responses he gets from others. Clearly, this is a developmental ability because self-knowledge and experience are necessary to predict the impact of one's own actions on another and having a large and varied repertoire of possible lines of action and appropriate tactics.

Peter Senge's (1990) definition of a learning organization helps to focus the academic mission. "A learning organization . . . is continually expanding its capacity to create its future. For such an organization, it is not enough merely to survive. 'Survival learning' . . . is important. . . . But for a learning organization . . . [it] must be joined by 'generative learning,' learning that enhances our capacity to create." Leaders in academia are the resource for the future since their primary goals should be building the discipline and developing the next generation of leaders. Leaders can be made, not born.

CLAIRE M. FAGIN

REFERENCES

Fagin, C. M. (1983). The dean and faculty development. In M. E. Conway & O. Andruskiw (Eds.), *Administrative theory and practice*. East Norwalk, CT: Appleton, Century, Crofts.

Fagin, C. M. (2000). *Essays on nursing leadership*. New York: Springer Publishing.

Foote, N., & Cottrell, L. (1955). *Identity and interpersonal competence*. Chicago: University of Chicago Press.

Institute of Medicine. (2004). *Keeping patients safe: Transforming the work environment of nurses*. Washington, DC: National Academies Press.

Rosovsky, H. (1990). *The university: An owner's manual*. New York: W. W. Norton & Company.

Senge, P. M. (1990). *The fifth discipline*. New York: Doubleday.

Accreditation in
Nursing Education

ACCREDITATION IN HIGHER EDUCATION is both general (as in regional accreditation) and specialized (as in nursing education, law, business, and other disciplines). General accreditation is under the purview of the Council for Higher Education Accreditation (CHEA). "A national advocate and institutional voice for self-regulation of academic quality through accreditation, CHEA is an association of 3,000 degree-granting colleges and universities and recognizes 60 institutional and programmatic accrediting organizations" (Council for Higher Education Accreditation, 2007). There are eight regional accrediting bodies for universities and colleges (Council for Higher Education Directories, 2007). Specialized accreditation in nursing education is a process by which the quality of educational programs is ensured (Bourke & Ihrke, 2005). Nursing education programs voluntarily choose to participate in the accreditation process as one means of publicly demonstrating that program outcomes meet educational standards that have been established by the profession. There are two major evaluative components to the accreditation process—an extensive self-study conducted by the faculty of the program and an accompanying peer review process conducted on-site by external reviewers.

6

Although accreditation is considered to be a voluntary process, there are many benefits to nursing programs participating in the process. In addition to providing an opportunity to evaluate the quality of program outcomes and develop plans for continuous quality improvement, accreditation can be a recruiting factor in attracting qualified students and faculty, affect a program's eligibility to receive external funding and students' ability to receive financial aid, and also influence graduates' ability to enroll in subsequent nursing education programs (Iwasiw, Goldenberg, & Andrusyszyn, 2005). For these reasons, most nursing programs choose to pursue accreditation.

Two national professional nursing organizations currently accredit nursing education programs. The National League for Nursing Accrediting Commission (NLNAC) accredits all nursing programs including licensed practical (vocational) nursing, diploma, Associate's degree, baccalaureate, and Master's degree programs. The Commission on Collegiate Nursing Education (CCNE) accredits baccalaureate, Master's degree, and Doctor of Nursing Practice degree programs. Research-focused doctoral programs (PhD, EdD, DNS, DNSc) are not currently subject to accreditation by the professional nursing accrediting organizations. Educational programs can choose to be accredited by either organization; some programs choose to be accredited by both.

The accreditation process provides a thorough evaluative review of all components of the education program with an emphasis on program outcomes. Substantive program elements that are usually reviewed include outcomes related to: curriculum; institutional, and program governance; fiscal and institutional resources; instructional learning resources; student support services; qualifications of faculty and students; faculty and student accomplishments; and existence of a program evaluation plan that guides faculty decision making. It is important that faculty have a clear understanding of the accreditation standards that guide the implementation of their nursing program. The accreditation standards that have been established by NLNAC can be found at the following Web site: http://www.nlnac.org/home.htm. The accreditation standards that have been established by CCNE can be found at the following Web site: http://www.aacn.nche.edu/Accreditation/index.htm.

The process by which a nursing program achieves accreditation is similar for both NLNAC and CCNE. Before receiving an on-site visit from external reviewers, the program faculty prepare and the chief program officer (e.g., chair, dean) submit a written self-study report that addresses each accreditation standard. This self-study provides faculty with an opportunity to identify program strengths and areas for improvement, and to cite evidence that supports the faculty's findings. After submission of the self-study report, the program receives an on-site visit from a team of peer reviewers, who validate the findings reported in the self-study and review additional data provided by the program during the visit. Following the on-site visit, the team of reviewers prepares a report of their findings, which is submitted to the agency for a decision on the accreditation status of the program. It is not the responsibility of the external reviewers to make recommendations regarding the accreditation status of the program.

Programs that meet all standards receive accreditation for the full number of years (8 years for NLNAC, 5 years for first-time CCNE applicants, and 10 years continuing applicants for CCNE), after which they will need to seek reaccreditation. Programs that do not fully meet all standards may receive accreditation for a limited number of years before they must undergo another visit; it is also possible that a program will be denied accreditation. Programs that receive a limited accreditation term or are denied accreditation are given a report of the standards not met and the improvements that need to be made before the program will again be eligible to seek accreditation. The accreditation status of educational programs is publicly reported by the accrediting agency.

JUDITH A. HALSTEAD

REFERENCES

Bourke, M. P., & Ihrke, B. A. (2005). The evaluation process: An overview. In D. M. Billings & J. A. Halstead (Eds.), *Teaching in nursing: A guide for faculty* (2nd ed., pp. 443–464). St. Louis, MO: Elsevier Saunders.

Council for Higher Education Accreditation. (2007). *Accreditation serving the public interest*. Retrieved August 15, 2007, from http://www.chea.org/pdf/chea_glance_2006.pdf

Council for Higher Education Directories. (2007). *Directories: Regional accrediting organizations 2006–2007*. Retrieved August 15, 2007, from http://www.chea.org/Directories/regional.asp

Iwasiw, C., Goldenberg, D., & Andrusyszyn, M. (2005). Planning curriculum evaluation. In *Curriculum development in nursing education* (pp. 221–242). Sudbury, MA: Jones and Bartlett.

Accreditation in Nursing Practice

ACCREDITATION IN THE PRACTICE setting is a formal process of recognition or conformance to standards that are intended to reflect quality and safety in health care settings. Health care organizations in many countries throughout the world voluntarily participate in the accreditation process to demonstrate to the public their accountability to continuously improve the quality and safety of their care. Accreditation is often required for a health care institution or program to be eligible for third party insurance payment for rendered patient care services. Although there are many organizations that provide accreditation of health care systems, the most well-known and comprehensive is the Joint Commission (previously known as the Joint Commission on Accreditation of Healthcare Organizations, or JCAHO). This organization will be described in this entry as an exemplar for accreditation in the practice setting. Other accrediting organizations that also provide valuable information dependant on the health care setting or program are the Commission on Accreditation of Rehabilitation Facilities (CARF), Community Health Accreditation Program (CHAP), Utilization Review Accreditation Committee (URAC), and Accreditation Commission for Healthcare (ACHC).

9

Organized health care improvement efforts began with the work of Dr. Ernest Codman, who in 1910 introduced the concept of an "end result system." This system would track each hospitalized patient to determine if treatment was effective. If treatment was not deemed to be effective, hospital personnel would explore the reasons and implement a new process for improvement. A colleague of Dr. Codman's, Franklin Martin, MD, founded the American College of Surgeons (ACS), which then brought the concept of "end result" to another level. The ACS developed "minimum standards" which were subsequently required for review and assessment when on-site inspections of hospitals for accreditation by the ACS began in 1918.

By 1950, over 3,200 hospitals participated in the inspections, which were intended to promote improvements in care. As a result of these improvements, the American Medical Association, American College of Physicians, Canadian Medical Association, and the American Hospital Association joined forces with the ACS to create the Joint Commission on Accreditation of Hospitals (JCAH) in 1951. JCAH developed standards of performance for a variety of patient care settings, including acute and long-term care, ambulatory care, mental health, laboratory and pathology services, and hospice care. The "minimum standard" threshold developed by ACS was modified and enhanced by JCAH to promote performance that exceeded basic requirements.

In 1987, The Joint Commission on Accreditation of Hospitals changed their name to the Joint Commission on Accreditation of Healthcare Organizations (JCAHO). This reorganization set the climate for change and further refocused their expectations of institutions seeking accreditation. Health care organizations were required to show comprehensive and continuous improvement efforts through outcome and process metrics that demonstrated performance exemplifying safe and reliable care. JCAHO announced in 2002 the Shared Visions—New Pathways initiative, which was focused on critical systems to improve and ensure the safety and quality of patient care. A 24/7/365 readiness campaign was established with unannounced surveys. The Joint Commission currently performs accreditation surveys through the use of a "tracer" methodology for assessment. The on-site surveyors assess the delivery of services throughout episodes of care, observing the patient as she or he touches multiple providers and processes. This format allows for the assessment of the continuity, quality, safety, and patient centeredness of care in a longitudinal fashion.

Organizations measure their performance over time through the collection and analysis of data, demonstrating accountability and commitment to continuous high performance. Because of mandated reporting requirements, the public is able to visit multiple Internet sites to view, compare and subsequently select the organization or provider that achieves the best performance. Accreditation is one mechanism to promote adherence to standards in the practice setting. Survey readiness has become an integral part of the daily operations of health care organizations, and has resulted in measurable improvements in patient care delivery.

CINDY A. REILLY

WEB REFERENCES

Accreditation Commission for Health Care (ACHC), www.achc.org

American College of Physicians (ACP), www.acponline.org

American College of Surgeons (ACS), www.facs.org

American Hospital Association (AHA), www.aha.org

American Medical Association (AMA), www.assn.org

American Nursing Association (ANA), www.ana.org

Centers for Medicare & Medicaid Services (CMS), www.cms.hhs.gov

Commission on Accreditation of Rehabilitation Facilities (CARF), www.carf.org

Community Health Accreditation Program (CHAP), www.chapinc.org

National League for Nursing (NLN), www.nln.org

The Joint Commission on Accreditation of Healthcare Organizations (JCAHO), www.jcaho.org

Utilization Review Accreditation Committee (URAC), www.urac.org

Advance Directives Within the Context of Advance Care Planning

ADVANCE DIRECTIVES (ADs) are legal documents signed by individuals with decision-making capacity to direct health professionals and loved ones about their treatment wishes. ADs are applicable only when a person is terminally or critically ill or has advanced dementia and is unable to make informed decisions or is in a persistent vegetative state. They are most effective when part of advance care planning. There are two primary kinds of AD documents. First is the living will, a statement that says, essentially, "If I am terminally and irreversibly ill, or in a persistent vegetative state, I do not want my life prolonged by extraordinary means." In some states, a living will includes specific options, such as, no cardiopulmonary resuscitation attempt in the case of a respiratory or cardiac arrest; no ventilator support; or no tube feeding or artificial hydration. The living will may be a handwritten, personalized directive rather than a formal state-generated form.

The second primary kind of advance directive document is the health care proxy, or durable power of attorney for health care (DPOAHC), in which an individual appoints someone to speak for him/herself

13

*Advance
Directives
Within the
Context of
Advance Care
Planning*

regarding medical treatment when the person cannot make his or her decisions. DPOAHC is to be distinguished from the "power of attorney," which is a legal representative chosen to make business decisions. The "responsible other" on admitting documents of some institutions, such as nursing homes, usually refers to a family member or the person responsible for payment. If a person has a DPOAHC, the designee's legal authority supersedes a family member's authority regarding medical decisions. A DPOAHC is particularly important when the patient desires that a partner who is not a spouse become his/her legal spokesperson. The family should be informed of this arrangement and invited to be part of the decision-making process if possible. Although most states have some form of both AD documents, some have one or the other. The documents of each state can be downloaded free online with accompanying information regarding notarization and witnesses if required (National Hospice and Palliative Care Organization, 2004).

The Patient Self-Determination Act of 1990 is a national law requiring that any institution that accepts federal funds must ask every newly admitted patient or his/her representative if she/he has an advance directive and obtain it for the record. They also must educate patients and the community about their rights. ADs are most effective when they are a part of conversations in which an advocate for the patient's wishes emerges (Singer, Martin, & Kelner, 1999).

Advance care planning (ACP) is a dynamic process of preparing for death, and is the appropriate context for facilitating completion of advance directives. The ACP process entails an individual making a plan for a comfortable death in keeping with his/her values. It involves introspection about what is important in living and in dying as well as discussion with loved ones about one's end-of-life wishes, specifically regarding medical treatment and care issues. Hammes and Rooney (1998) found that advance directives within an ACP process enabled 96% of those with ADs to experience deaths consistent with their wishes. Most individuals are fearful of the dying process, but not death itself. In a study by Henderson (1990), subjects' death anxiety decreased significantly by their having the opportunity to be specific about life-sustaining treatments they wanted to forego. Addenda to advance directives, such as Five Wishes (Aging with Dignity, 1996) or an Advance Care Planning Worksheet (Henderson, 2003), enable patients to document in detail their wishes for treatment and care.

Although completion of ADs should be part of routine health care, there are specific times in which ACP becomes urgent, such as destabilization of a chronic disease or the diagnosis of a terminal illness. There are also ways, discussed elsewhere, to introduce the subject of end-of-life decision making and guide the conversation (Henderson, 2004; UNC Program on Aging, 2003). When decisions are made, it is essential that

14

ADVANCE
DIRECTIVES
WITHIN THE
CONTEXT OF
ADVANCE CARE
PLANNING

these be documented, discussed, and distributed to health care providers and loved ones.

Based on a patient's values and wishes, in an ACP discussion it is helpful for patients to state their preference of four basic options: (1) "I want to remain in my place of residence with comfort care as the goal and hospice care if possible"; (2) "If necessary to achieve comfort, I would go to the hospital briefly for symptom relief, then return to my usual place of residence for comfort care"; (3) "If it is unclear whether or not I could respond to a trial of therapy, including life support, I would like to have this trial, but stop the treatment in a few days if it is not working"; (4) "I would like all measures provided to keep me alive as long as possible, regardless of the discomfort this may entail" (Henderson, 2003). The medical team can then make treatment suggestions based on the patient's preference.

Nurses are key to helping patients become aware of their need for ACP and acting as effective advocates. According to professional nursing standards, the nurse has an ethical responsibility to help patients realize their right to self-determination (American Nurses Association, 1997). End-of-life decision making, however, may be influenced by cultural norms. For example, many Hispanics and Asians would prefer that the family or the eldest male make such decisions, implying that a nurse needs to inquire who the patient wants to make important decisions for him/her. Advance care planning not only can make possible a comfortable death according to patient wishes, but it also can relieve the family of the burden of decision making. Instead of a possible crisis, the time of dying can be one of gentle closure, when a person has had "quality" time, said good-byes, and left a good memory for loved ones.

MARTHA L. HENDERSON

REFERENCES

Aging with Dignity. (1996). *Five wishes.* Retrieved September 9, 2006, from http://www.agingwithdignity.org/5wishes.html

American Nurses Association. (1997). *Scope and standards of the advance practice registered nurse.* Washington, DC: National Academies Press.

Hammes, B. J., & Rooney, B. L. (1998). Death and end-of-life planning in one midwestern community. *Archives of Internal Medicine, 158*(4), 383–390.

Henderson, M. L. (1990). Beyond the living will. *Gerontologist, 30*(4), 480–485.

Henderson, M. L. (2003). *Advance care planning worksheet.* Retrieved September 9, 2006, from http://viper.med.unc.edu/acp/pdfs/blank_patient_acp_worksheet.pdf

Henderson, M. L. (2004). Nuts and bolts of advance care planning. *The American Journal for Nurse Practitioners, 8*(9), 41–52.

National Hospice and Palliative Care Organization. (2004). *State-specific advance directives from Caring Information through National Hospice and Palliative Care Organization.* Retrieved September 9, 2006, from http://www.caringinfo.org/i4a/pages/Index.cfm?pageid=3425

Singer, P. A., Martin, D. K., & Kelner, M. (1999). Quality end-of-life care: Patients' perspectives. *Journal of the American Medical Association, 281*(2), 163–168.

University of North Carolina, Program on Aging. (2003). *Advance care planning educational module.* Retrieved September 9, 2006, from http://viper.med.unc.edu/acp

Advanced Practice Registered Nurses

T HE ADVANCED PRACTICE REGISTERED NURSE (APRN) is a registered nurse who has met advanced educational and clinical practice
requirements beyond baccalaureate nursing education. APRNs, or
advanced practice nurses (APNs) as they are sometimes called, include
clinical nurse specialists (CNSs), certified registered nurse anesthetists
(CRNAs), certified nurse midwives (CNMs), and nurse practitioners (NPs).
State nurse practice acts delineate what APRNs can do, and vary widely
among states.

CLINICAL NURSE SPECIALISTS

T HE ROOTS OF THE clinical nurse specialist movement started in the
1880s with psychiatric nursing and the origins of the reform movement initiated earlier by the Quakers, protesting the brutal treatment of
the insane (D'Antonio, 1991; Hamric, Spross, & Hanson, 2005). A training
program for psychiatric nurses was established in 1880 at McLean Hospital in Massachusetts, with the first Master's program in psychiatry started
decades later by Hildegarde Peplau at Rutgers University in 1955. With the

16

passage of the 1964 Nurse Training Act, a proliferation of programs to prepare these APRNs occurred and clinical nurse specialization emerged as a major force (Hamric et al., 2005). In the late 1960s and 1970s, specialty nursing organizations, such as the American Association of Critical-Care Nurses and the Oncology Nursing Society, were established to meet the educational needs of nurses at the entry and advanced levels. Today, the CNS is a registered nurse with (1) an earned graduate degree with a clinical concentration and (2) a practice base focused on patients and their families. When available, professional certification for practice at an advanced level is desirable; however, for some areas of clinical specialization, certification exams have not yet been developed (Hamric et al., 2005). Most CNSs practice in the hospital, although increasingly they may be practicing in the community or independently. Because of their depth of knowledge and expertise in a clinical area, they are often responsible for developing protocols, standards, and guidelines for the care of a particular patient population, and for fostering healthy work environments for staff (Disch, Walton, & Barnsteiner, 2001). A major challenge facing CNSs is defining and documenting their outcomes since much of their influence stems from improving quality through enhancing the care environment and practice of others.

CERTIFIED REGISTERED NURSE ANESTHETISTS

T HE ORIGINS OF modern nurse anesthesia also can be traced to the late 1800s. The practice of nurses giving anesthesia was so common that in her 1893 textbook entitled *Nursing: Its Principles and Practices for Hospital and Private Use,* Isabel Adams Hampton Robb included a chapter on the administration of anesthesia (Bankert, 1989). A Certified Registered Nurse Anesthetist (CRNA) is a registered nurse who is educationally prepared at the Master's level to provide anesthesia and anesthesia-related services in collaboration with other health care professionals. To become a CRNA, a nurse anesthesia graduate must successfully complete the National Certification Examination. CRNAs may practice in care team settings with anesthesiologists, or independently, especially in rural areas. CRNAs are the sole anesthesia providers for approximately 50% of hospital surgeries and more than 65% in rural hospitals (American Association of Nurse Anesthetists [AANA], 2007). Based on data from the AANA 2005 Practice Profile, CRNAs administer approximately 27 million anesthetics in the U.S. each year. In rural America, CRNAs are the primary anesthesia care providers. With CRNAs providing high-quality, safe anesthesia care, rural health facilities in medically underserved areas are able to offer obstetrical, surgical and trauma stabilization services (AANA, 2007). Leaders in AANA and CRNA educators are working together to increase the number of educational programs to ensure that the supply of nurse anesthetists keeps pace with the demand. At the same time, CRNA educators and practitioners alike are debating the merits of requiring doctoral preparation for entry level into practice. Another issue facing the specialty is the resistance by some physicians and hospitals to allow them to practice to their full scope; in many states, legal action has been taken.

MIDWIFERY

N URSE-MIDWIFERY began in 1925 when Mary Breckinridge, an RN who received midwifery education in England, brought the British model of nurse-midwifery to the United States. The first nurse-midwifery education program began in 1932 in New York City. Today, certified nurse-midwives (CNMs) are individuals educated in the two disciplines of nursing and midwifery and certified nationally. Because they are educated in two distinct disciplines, nurse-midwives are unique among APRNs. The scope of nurse-midwifery practice includes prenatal care, labor and birth, well-woman gynecologic care, and basic primary care. The American College of Nurse Midwives (ACNM) defines Core Competencies for Basic Midwifery Practice, Standards for the Practice of Midwifery, a Code of Ethics, and a Philosophy statement. National accreditation of nurse-midwifery programs by the ACNM Division of Accreditation began in the 1970s. Graduates of accredited programs are eligible for certification by the American Midwifery Certification Board. A direct entry (nonnursing) midwifery option, utilizing the same accreditation and certification mechanisms, including some prerequisite courses, began in 1997 in New York State, resulting in the certified midwife (CM) credential. Other midwives (sometimes called lay, home-birth, or direct entry midwives) practicing primarily in home birth settings are increasingly recognized by state licensing agencies and third-party payers (M. Avery, personal communication, September 5, 2006). Education varies from more formal to apprentice-type education and can include accreditation and certification. Current issues are equitable reimbursement for CNMs/CMs under Medicaid regulations, the rising cesarean section rate, and lack of health insurance for underserved women and their families.

NURSE PRACTITIONERS

T HE FIRST NURSE PRACTITIONER (NP) role was developed in 1965 by Loretta Ford, PhD, RN, and Henry Silver, MD, as a demonstration project at the University of Colorado. The stated goal was to "determine the safety, efficacy, and quality of a new mode of nursing practice designed to improve health care to children and families and to develop a new nursing role" (Ford & Silver, 1967, p. 43). The focus was on health promotion, illness prevention and increasing access to care. Envisioned originally as providing care for children and their families, the role became so successful that it was soon adopted for other specialties (adult, family, gerontology, neonatal) and, increasingly, in other settings, such as clinics, critical care units (Kleinpell, 2005), and more recently, even supermarkets (Trossman, 2005). Wherever they are employed, NPs usually perform direct patient care, including comprehensive assessments to promote health and prevent illness and injury. They are skilled in differential diagnoses, develop holistic health and disease management plans, and deliver care that is personalized, cost-effective, and timely. Numerous studies have reported positive NP care outcomes for patients, families, and communities (Brown & Grimes, 1995; Burl, Bonner, Rao, & Khan, 1998; Horrocks, Anderson, & Salisbury, 2002; Mundinger et al., 2000; Sarkissian & Wennberg, 1999).

COMMON ISSUES FOR APRNs

F ROM AN EVOLUTIONARY standpoint, APRNs have moved from an uncertain beginning to mainstream acceptance by many as a skilled health care professional with tremendous career opportunities in today's health care environment. With increased visibility and independent practice options, however, APRNs also predictably face several challenges that must be successfully tackled if sustained growth is to be achieved. First, confusion about the full scope of the role and lack of support still persists in many communities and organizations, and not only from physicians (Lindeke & Jukkala, 2003). Nurse colleagues and administrators also can pose a challenge to fully understanding and accepting the role. Second, the nature of the relationship between physicians and APRNs continues to be rocky in many settings. An increasing number of physicians are staunch supporters of and partners with APRNs since they appreciate the benefits of APRN colleagues with complementary areas of knowledge and expertise—but many are not. Even though legally sanctioned, APRNs are often prevented from practicing interdependently and independently in congruence with their full scopes of practice. This affects not only the APRN but also the public who is prevented access to a capable, cost-effective health care provider. Third, concerns about adequate reimbursement and malpractice coverage for APRNs are increasing nationally, just as they are for physicians who must, at times, incur a significant financial burden to practice. Fourth, changes in the educational requirements to become an APRN (i.e., moving toward doctoral preparation) have been proposed and are being hotly debated within the profession as the recommended start date of 2015 looms for a Doctor of Nursing Practice degree (American Association of Colleges of Nursing, 2006). A related issue is the imminent nursing faculty shortage—and the fact that finding enough qualified faculty to teach today's cohort of APRN students is already a challenge, much less meeting the increased demand that is on the horizon. The APRN can seek positions in education and service to meet the dual challenges of nursing faculty and nursing shortages.

JOANNE DISCH
LINDA L. LINDEKE

See Also
Faculty Shortages in Registered Nurses Preparatory Programs

REFERENCES

American Association of Colleges of Nursing. (2006). *Doctor of nursing practice.* Retrieved September 10, 2006, from http://www.aacn.nche.edu/DNP/index.htm

American Association of Nurse Anesthetists. (2007). *Certified registered nurse anesthetists at a glance.* Retrieved August 12, 2007, from http://www.aana.com/aboutaana.aspx?ucNavMenu_TSMenuTargetID=179&ucNavMenu_TSMenuTargetType=4&ucNavMenu_TSMenuID=6&id=265

Bankert, M. (1989). *Watchful care, a history of America's nurse anesthetists.* New York: Continuum.

Brown, S. A., & Grimes, D. E. (1995). A meta-analysis of nurse practitioners and nurse midwives in primary care. *Nursing Research, 44*(6), 332–339.

Burl, J. B., Bonner, A., Rao, M., & Khan, A. M. (1998). Geriatric nurse practitioners in long-term care: Demonstration of effectiveness in managed care. *Journal of the American Geriatrics Society, 46*(4), 506–510.

Council on Accreditation of Nurse Anesthesia Educational Programs. (2004). *Standards for accreditation of nurse anesthesia educational program.* Park Ridge, IL: American Association of Nurse Anesthetists.

D'Antonio, P. (1991). Staff needs and patient care: Seclusion and restraint in a nineteenth-century insane asylum. *Transactions and Studies of the College of Physicians of Philadelphia, 13*(4), 411–423.

Disch, J., Walton, M., & Barnsteiner, J. H. (2001). The role of the clinical nurse specialist in creating a healthy work environment. *AACN Clinical Issues: Advanced Practice in Acute and Critical Care, 12*(3), 345–355.

Ford, L. D., & Silver, H. K. (1967). Expanded role of the nurse in child care. *Nursing Outlook, 15,* 43–45.

Hamric, A. B., Spross, J. A., & Hanson, C. M. (2005). *Advanced practice nursing* (3rd ed.). St. Louis, MO: Elsevier Saunders.

Horrocks, S., Anderson, E., & Salisbury, C. (2002). Systematic review of whether nurse practitioners working in primary care can provide equivalent care to doctors. *British Medical Journal, 324*(7341), 819–823.

Kleinpell, R. (2005). Acute care nurse practitioner practice: Results of a 5-year longitudinal study. *American Journal of Critical-Care, 14*(3), 211–219.

Lindeke, L., & Jukkala, A. (2003). *Rural nurse practitioner practice in Minnesota: Barriers and strategies for success.* Minneapolis, MN: Collaborative Rural Nurse Practitioner Project.

Lindeke, L., Zwygart-Stauffacher, M., Avery, M., & Fagerlund K. (2006). Overview of advanced practice nursing. In M. P. Mirr Jansen & M. Zwygart-Stauffacher (Eds.), *Advanced practice nursing: Core concepts for professional role development* (3rd ed.). New York: Springer Publishing.

Mundinger, M. O., Kane, R. L., Lenz, E. R., Totten, A. M., Tsai, W. Y., Cleary, P. D., et al. (2000). Primary care outcomes in patients treated by nurse practitioners or physicians: A randomized trial. *Journal of the American Medical Association, 283*(1), 59–68.

Sarkissian, S., & Wennberg, R. (1999). Effects of acute care nurse practitioner role on epilepsy monitoring outcomes. *Outcomes Management for Nursing Practice, 3*(4), 161–166.

Trossman, S. (2005, May/June). One-stop shopping—and some help for that strep throat. *The American Nurse, 37*(3), 1, 6.

Advocacy

NURSING HAS A LONG and distinguished history of advocacy from the trenches of Crimea to the halls of the U.S. Congress. Past-American Nurses Association President Dorothy Cornelius once observed: "There is a great recognition of the need for nursing to speak with one voice on social issues in the areas of poverty, malnutrition, hunger and discrimination, all of which profoundly affect the health and well-being of the people of this country.... Nursing is the conscience of the health care system" (van Betten & Moriarty, 2004, p. 145). Nurses advocate in their daily nursing practice on behalf of patients and their families—they track down the physician for a change in pain medication, work with the social worker to find a "safe haven" for an abused mother, and request more nursing staff. This is the everyday advocacy that nurses do so well. Increasingly, nurses have taken their advocacy skills into the political arena, promoting grassroots and legislative support and political activity to advance nursing's agenda for health care reform and for the future of the profession (American Nurses Association, 1995, 2002).

KAREN A. BALLARD

See Also
Center for Nursing Advocacy

REFERENCES

American Nurses Association. (1995). *Nursing's agenda for health care reform.* Washington, DC: Author.

American Nurses Association. (2002). *Nursing's agenda for the future.* Washington, DC: Author.

van Betten, P. T., & Moriarty, M. (2004). *Nursing illuminations: A book of days.* Chicago: Mosby.

Affirmative Action

AFFIRMATIVE ACTION is about equal opportunity and the use of policies to pave the way for all citizens of the United States to have the chance to be successful. Its purpose is to overcome the history of the subordination and segregation of certain groups of people in our society. President John F. Kennedy first used the term in the early 1960s. On March 6, 1961, he issued Executive Order 10925, which created the Committee on Equal Employment Opportunity and mandated that projects financed with federal funds "take affirmative action" to ensure that hiring and employment practices were free of racial bias. President Lyndon B. Johnson took further action on July 2, 1964, and signed the most sweeping civil rights legislation since Reconstruction, the Civil Rights Act of 1964, which prohibited discrimination of all kinds based on race, color, religion, or national origin.

The underlying foundation of the affirmative action concept is that unless positive action is undertaken to overcome the systemic institutional forms of exclusion and discrimination, benign neutral employment practices will perpetuate the status quo indefinitely. The objective is to have equal employment opportunity as a sustaining and permanent feature of the workplace. In an eloquent speech delivered to the graduating class at Howard University on June 4, 1965, President Johnson framed the concept underlying affirmative action, asserting that civil rights laws alone are not enough to remedy discrimination:

> *"You do not wipe away the scars of centuries by saying: 'now, you are free to go where you want, do as you desire, and choose the leaders you please.' You do not take a man who for years has been hobbled by chains, liberate him, bring him to the starting line of a race, saying, 'you are free to compete with all the others,' and still justly believe you have been completely fair. . . . This is the next and more profound stage of the battle for civil rights. We seek not just freedom but opportunity-not just legal equity but human ability-not just equality as a right and a theory, but equality as a fact and a result."*

Another move was made by President Johnson in September 24, 1965, when he issued Executive Order 11246, which requires government contractors to "take affirmative action" toward prospective minority employees in all aspects of hiring and employment. Contractors must take specific measures to ensure equality in hiring and must document these efforts. On October 13, 1967, the order was amended to cover discrimination on the basis of gender. President Richard M. Nixon implemented goals and timetables to expand the affirmative action executive order. During the presidency of Gerald R. Ford, the Rehabilitation Act of 1973 and the Vietnam Era Veterans Readjustment Act of 1974 were enacted. These acts guaranteed that federal contractors would have affirmative action programs established for recruiting and hiring people with disabilities and Vietnam veterans. The Age Discrimination Act of 1975 also was enacted during Ford's presidency. This act barred discrimination in hiring or firing of older persons.

President Bill Clinton articulated four standards of fairness for all affirmative action programs approximately 40 years after the concept's initial debut:

1. no quotas in theory or practice;
2. no illegal discrimination of any kind;
3. no preference for people who are not qualified for any job or other opportunity; and
4. as soon as a program has succeeded, it must be retired. Any program that does not meet these four principles should be eliminated or reformed to meet them.

The scrutiny regarding privileges to some and discrimination eventually permeated two other main sectors of people's lives: education and health care. Accusations were hurled of reversed discrimination by the majority and that unfair preference toward less qualified minority applicants were displacing and subsequently causing qualified majority college applicants to be rejected for admission. The first significant challenges to affirmative action in educational admissions practices came in the 1970s with the *University of California Regents vs. Bakke.* This case officially set the parameters for admissions practices in higher education for almost 25 years. At that time, the Supreme Court, in a 5-to-4 decision, upheld the right of universities to use race as one of the many admission factors to be considered as a part of a holistic review; however, it specifically prohibited the use of quotas or separate admissions tracks.

Proposition 209 in California (1996), Initiative 200 in the state of Washington (1998 and reaffirmed in 2004), and the *Hopwood* case (vs. University of Texas, 2001) were other significant anti–affirmative action cases, which basically prohibited consideration of race, religion, sex, color, ethnicity, or national origin as criteria for admission. Student body diversity was not considered a feature of "compelling interest" and therefore not a basis for consideration in admission criteria. Other states followed suit, namely, Washington and Florida. Since the year 2000, the University of Michigan has been center stage on this issue and in the most important affirmative action decision since the 1978 *Bakke* case, the Supreme Court (5–4) upheld the University's Law School's policy, ruling that race can be one of many factors considered by colleges when selecting their students. The Supreme Court went on to rule (6–3) that a formulaic approach utilizing a point system at the undergraduate level had to be modified because it did not provide the "individualized consideration" of applicants deemed necessary in previous Supreme Court decisions on the matter.

Having equal access to good health care is critical to having equal opportunity to success. In terms of health care, evidence abounds that there has been inequity in hiring and firing practices as well as in the delivery of health outcomes typically referred to as health disparities. On March 25, 1966, at the Second National Convention of the Medical Committee for Human Rights in Chicago, Illinois, Dr. Martin Luther King Jr. said, "Of all the forms of inequality, injustice in healthcare is the most shocking and inhumane" (*Kentucky Citizen/Congressional Hearing,* 2006). The health care system was not invulnerable to the same forces found outside its walls. Their far-reaching effects are at the roots of many of the factors previously mentioned.

With the publication of the Institute of Medicine (IOM; 2002) report *Unequal Treatment* health disparities finally were brought from the dark into the light and has become the topic and focus of many research studies, discussions, and target actions. The IOM landmark report, *Unequal Treatment: Confronting Racial and Ethnic Disparities in Health Care,* cited a host of contributing factors housed both within the knowledge, skills, and attitudes of individual health care providers, and within the structure and processes of the health care system. Many have posited that increasing minority representation in the health provider workforce is the most effective place to start to rectify the situation. Having employment allows one to make a living, pay for needed services, be able to obtain education, and access health care. The major obstacles to achieving that goal lie in the domains of employment and education, right where affirmative action policies and concepts had its beginnings. Yet the debate for such policies and actions continues.

G. RUMAY ALEXANDER

REFERENCES

Brunner, B. (n.d.). *Timeline of affirmative action milestones.* Retrieved November 10, 2006, from http://www.infoplease.com/spot/affirmativetimeline 1.html

Institute of Medicine, Committee on Understanding and Eliminating Racial and Ethnic Disparities in Health Care, Board on Health Sciences Policy. (2002). *Unequal treatment: Confronting racial and ethnic disparities in health care.* Washington, DC: National Academies Press.

Kentucky Citizen/Congressional Hearing. (2006). *Hearings archives/2006 KY.* Retrieved August 10, 2007, from http://www.healthcare-now.org/hearings_archives_ky2006.html

University of Wisconsin-Stevens Point, Equity & Affirmative Action Office. (2005). *Frequently asked questions.* Retrieved November 10, 2006, from http://www.uwsp.edu/equity/faq.htm

Agency for Healthcare Research and Quality (AHRQ)

THE AGENCY FOR HEALTHCARE RESEARCH AND QUALITY (AHRQ) is a division of the U.S. Department of Health and Human Services and is located in Rockville, Maryland. The AHRQ strives to improve all aspects of health care for Americans by supporting research and partnerships within health systems (AHRQ, 2005). AHRQ is classified as a U.S. Public Health Service Agency and was created in 1989. AHRQ has three primary goals: (a) advance clinical practice, (b) increase health care availability and cost effective delivery of health options to the public, and (c) maintain communication with the legislature to encourage optimal quality, usage and cost containment of health care services (AHRQ, 2005). Therefore, specific grants are made available to encourage a competitive proposal process that underscores the priority goals of this organization. AHRQ provides notice regarding the highest priorities for each application year along with consistent updates of the research priorities throughout each year. Grants are available in the following global categories: *clinical information,* such as evidence-based practice, outcomes and effectiveness, and technology; *specific populations,* such as women, children, minorities, elderly, disabled, and inner-city; *public health preparedness* within the areas of bioterrorism and safety and quality of health care; and *quality and patient safety,* which focuses on health information technology, medical errors, quality improvement, and communication with consumers (AHRQ, 2006).

RONDA MINTZ-BINDER

REFERENCES

Agency for Healthcare Research and Quality. (2005). *Special emphasis notice: Research priorities for the Agency for Healthcare Research and Quality.* Retrieved July 6, 2006, from http://grants.nih.gov/grants/guide/notice-files/NOT-HS-06-032.html

Agency for Healthcare Research and Quality. (2006). *Homepage.* Retrieved July 6, 2006, from http://www.ahrq.gov

Alcott, Louisa May

LOUISA MAY ALCOTT was born in Germantown, Pennsylvania, on November 29, 1832. She died in Boston, Massachusetts, on March 6, 1888. A noted transcendentalist and author, Alcott was educated chiefly by her father, but she also enjoyed instruction from family friends such as Henry David Thoreau, Ralph Waldo Emerson, Nathaniel Hawthorne, and Margaret Fuller. Because of issues surrounding her family's poverty, Alcott was very young when she began earning an income as a seamstress, domestic help, governess, teacher, and writer. When approximately 28 years of age, Alcott began writing for the *Atlantic Monthly*. At age 30, she served as an untrained nurse in the Union Hospital at Georgetown, DC for 6 weeks. It was this experience that permeated her letters home, which were edited and published in the *Commonwealth* and collected as *Hospital Sketches* in 1863 (Eiselein & Phillips, 2001; Stern, 1950). It was these publications that gained Louisa May Alcott critical recognition as a writer. Alcott is well known for her overwhelmingly successful publications such as *Little Women, Little Men, Eight Cousins,* and *An Old Fashioned Girl,* to name a few.

Alcott continued to write throughout her life, but her health worsened as she aged due to the effects of mercury poisoning and typhoid, which she had contracted during her service in the American Civil War.

M. JANICE NELSON

REFERENCES

Eiselein, G., & Phillips, A. K. (2001). *The Louisa May Alcott encyclopedia.* [Online]. Retrieved August 10, 2007, from http://www.questia.com/reader/action/readchecked?docid=102141637

Stern, M. B. (1950). *Louisa May Alcott.* [Online]. Retrieved August 10, 2007, from http://www.questia.com/reader/print

Shealy, D. (Ed.). (2005). *Alcott in her own time: A biographical chronicle of her life, drawn from recollections, interviews, and memoirs by family, friends, and associates.* Iowa City: University of Iowa Press.

American Academy
of Nursing

THE **AMERICAN ACADEMY OF NURSING** **(AAN)** is a subsidiary of
the American Nurses Association (ANA). The mission of the AAN is
to serve the public and the nursing profession by advancing health
policy and practice through the generation, synthesis, and dissemination of nursing knowledge (http://www.aan.net.org). Established in 1973
under the aegis of the ANA, membership is by invitation. Applicants
must be sponsored by two Fellows in good standing with the Academy
and must be a current member of the ANA or an ANA constituent. In
addition, criteria for membership include: evidence of outstanding contributions that have made an impact on nursing practice at the national
level and evidence of potential to continue contributions to nursing and
the Academy.

As of 2006, the Academy was comprised of approximately 1,600 Fellows of the American Academy of Nursing (FAAN). Fellows are recognized nursing leaders in education, management, practice, and research.
Fellows work with other leaders in health care on expert panels, the
Institute of Medicine, American Nurses Foundation, AAN Scholar-in-
Residence Program, and the facilitation of appointments to policy positions. Fellows come together annually to address crucial health issues

and to identify research and policy initiatives to improve health care. The official journal of the AAN is *Nursing Outlook,* published bimonthly by Elsevier. *Nursing Outlook* provides innovative ideas for leaders in the nursing profession through peer-reviewed articles and timely reports.

American Academy of Nursing (AAN)
555 East Wells Street
Suite 1100
Milwaukee, WI 53202–3823
(414) 287–0289
Fax: (414) 276–3349
E-mail: info@aannet.org

DIANE MANCINO

See Also
American Nurses Association

WEB REFERENCE

American Academy of Nursing (AAN), http://www.aannet.org

American Assembly for Men in Nursing

THE AMERICAN ASSEMBLY FOR MEN IN NURSING (AAMN) provides a national forum for "nurses as a group to meet, discuss, and influence factors which affect men as nurses" (AAMN, 2006). The American Assembly for Men in Nursing had its origins in the National Male Nurses Association (NMNA), founded by Dennis Martin in 1971 with the intention of stimulating interest among men in a nursing career. Although initially quite successful as an organization, NMNA later faltered until being revitalized in 1980, largely through the leadership of Dr. Luther Christman. In 1981, it changed its name to AAMN and adopted objectives to encourage (1) men to become nurses and join with all nurses in humanizing health care; (2) nurses who are men to grow professionally and demonstrate the contributions made by men in nursing; and (3) members to participate fully in the nursing profession and its organizations. Later, an additional objective was added supporting men's health issues (AAMN). Although not stated, fighting discrimination is an implied goal, and the organization is truly nondiscriminatory, with membership "unrestricted by age, color, creed, handicap, sexual orientation, lifestyle, nationality, race, religion or gender" (Pittman, 2005, p. 156). Thus, there are women as well as men among the membership and the current AAMN

Board, chaired over the years by Christman, has female as well as male members (AAMN, 2006). Overall, the association promotes the idea that every professional nursing position and educational opportunity should be equally available to anyone meeting entry requirements, regardless of gender (Bullough, 2006, p. 567). AAMN sponsors annual conferences consistent with its objectives, produces a quarterly newsletter, *Interaction,* and offers annual awards for organizations and individuals who are supportive of men in nursing. The AAMN Web site has a career center, a discussion forum, and links to resources for men in nursing and about men's health (AAMN).

DAVID N. EKSTROM

REFERENCES

American Assembly for Men in Nursing (AAMN). (2006). *Welcome to the American Assembly for Men in Nursing.* Retrieved August 22, 2006, from http://www.aamn.org/index.html

Bullough, V. (2006). Nursing at the crossroads: Men in nursing. In P. S. Cowan & S. Moorhead (Eds.), *Current issues in nursing* (7th ed., pp. 559–568). St. Louis, MO: Mosby.

Pittman, E. (2005). *Luther Christman: A maverick nurse—A nursing legend.* Victoria, BC: Tafford.

American Association of Colleges of Nursing

F OUNDED IN 1969, the American Association of Colleges of Nursing (AACN) is the national voice for baccalaureate and higher degree programs in nursing. Over 500 nursing programs are represented by this organization in its efforts to establish quality standards for nursing baccalaureate and graduate education and influence public policy to improve funding and practices for nursing education, health care, and research. "AACN's educational, research, governmental advocacy, data collection, publications, and other programs work to establish quality standards for bachelor's- and graduate-degree nursing education, assist deans and directors to implement those standards, influence the nursing profession to improve health care, and promote public support of baccalaureate and graduate education, research, and practice in nursing—the nation's largest health care profession" (American Association of Colleges of Nursing, 2007). In 1986, a national panel was established by AACN to develop the *Essentials of Baccalaureate Education for Professional Nursing Practice*. Initially, this document was designed to guide nursing schools in developing standards for undergraduate programs; in 2005, the Commission on Collegiate Nursing Education voted to adopt the *Essentials* document as mandatory for its accreditation practices. In 1994, a task

36

force was appointed to develop a companion document for master's education in advanced practice specialties, the *Essentials of Master's Education for Professional Nursing Practice*. In 2006, a task force was appointed to develop the *Essentials of Doctoral Education for Advanced Practice Nursing*. These were adopted in October 2006 by the AACN membership. Master's and Doctor of Nursing Practice guidelines have also been adopted by the Commission on Collegiate Nursing Education as mandatory for accreditation. In addition, the AACN has developed position papers and white papers to address issues for nursing education and practice, for example, *Faculty Shortages in Baccalaureate and Graduate Nursing Programs, Differentiated Competencies for Nursing Practice, the Role of the Clinical Nurse Leader, the Clinical Practice Doctorate, Position Statement on Nursing Research, Hallmarks of the Professional Nursing Practice Environment,* and *Indicators of Quality in Research-Focused Doctoral Programs in Nursing* (http://www.aacn.nche.edu).

HARRIET R. FELDMAN

REFERENCE

American Association of Colleges of Nursing. (2007). *Homepage.* Retrieved August 12, 2007, from www.aacn.nche.edu

American Association of University Professors

"**T**HE MISSION OF THE American Association of University Professors (AAUP) is to advance academic freedom and shared governance, to define fundamental professional values and standards for higher education, and to ensure higher education's contribution to the common good. Founded in 1915, the AAUP has helped to shape American higher education by developing the standards and procedures that maintain quality in education and academic freedom in this country's colleges and universities" (AAUP, 2007). Membership is represented by individual faculty, librarians, and other academic professionals at public and private universities across the country. The principles and practices of AAUP may be found in its *Statement of Principles on Academic Freedom and Tenure*. The AAUP largely concerns itself with issues of due process and academic freedom. The organization works with legislative leaders to influence higher education legislation. The AAUP publishes statements on such topics as intellectual property, distance education, and the use of part-time and non–tenure track faculty, and an annual faculty salary report that includes detailed salary and benefit information.

HARRIET R. FELDMAN

REFERENCE

American Association of University Professors. (2007). *Mission and description*. Retrieved August 12, 2007, from http://www.aaup.org/AAUP/About/mission/

American Association of University Women

FOUNDED IN 1881, the mission of the American Association of University Women (AAUW) is to promote "equity for all women and girls, lifelong education, and positive societal change" (AAUW, 2007a). Furthermore, the AAUW "contributes to a more promising future and provides a powerful voice for women and girls—a voice that cannot and will not be ignored" (AAUW, 2007c). AAUW sees itself as a "catalyst for change," and in this vein has promoted a number of successful initiatives, for example, *How Schools Shortchange Girls: The AAUW Report* (1992) and implementation of Sister-to-Sister summits for teens. AAUW provides educational and professional support, grants and fellowships, updates on research, conferences that include opportunities for activism, information on up-to-date issues affecting girls and women, a voice in government, and a community network of colleagues around the world. In 2005, AAUW adopted the theme Education as the Gateway to Women's Economic Security, which "represents a shared commitment [of the AAUW Educational Foundation Board and the Association Board] . . . to support and engage members and prospective members . . ."

(AAUW, 2007b). Their comprehensive Web site contains information for members and nonmembers alike.

HARRIET R. FELDMAN

REFERENCES

American Association of University Women. (1992). *How schools shortchange girls: The AAUW report: A study of major findings on girls and education.* Washington, DC: AAUW Educational Foundation and National Education Association.

American Association of University Women. (2007a). *About us.* Retrieved June 14, 2007, from http://www.aauw.org/about/index.cfm

American Association of University Women. (2007b). *Education as the gateway to women's economic security.* Retrieved August 12, 2007, from http://www.aauw.org/newvision/index.cfm

American Association of University Women. (2007c). *The value of belonging to AAUW.* Retrieved June 14, 2007, from http://www.aauw.org/join/value/index.cfm

American Nurses Association

ESTABLISHED IN 1896 as the Nurses' Associated Alumni of the United States and Canada, the American Nurses Association (ANA) is today considered to be the voice of registered nurses in the United States. In 1899, the name was changed to Nurses Associated Alumnae of the United States; in 1911, the name was changed to its current name, American Nurses Association (2007a). The ANA is governed by a federation of 54 Constituent Member Associations, Associate Organizational Members, Organizational Affiliates, Individual Members, and Individual Affiliates. The ANA serves as the parent corporation for the American Nurses Credentialing Center (ANCC), American Nurses Foundation (ANF), and American Academy of Nursing (AAN). The ANA's purposes include: working for the improvement of health standards and the availability of health care services for all people; fostering high standards of nursing; and stimulating and promoting the professional development of nurses and the advancement of their economic and general welfare (ANA, 2006, p. 2). Participation by the majority of registered nurses is through state nurses associations, the Center for American Nurses (CAN), and the United American Nurses (UAN).

As the only national full-service professional organization representing the nation's registered nurse population, ANA's five Core Initiatives are intended to benefit the entire registered nurse population and the populations they serve. The 109th Congress, exemplars of the ongoing work of ANA, had the following Core Initiatives:

1. Nursing Shortage: The ANA has consistently urged Congress to increase funding for nursing workforce development programs administered by the Health Resources and Services Administration under Title VIII of the Public Health Service Act and opposed the use of immigration to solve nursing shortages and efforts to weaken certification requirements for nurses educated in foreign schools of nursing.
2. Appropriate Staffing: The ANA has supported efforts such as mandating valid and reliable nurse staffing systems in acute care and requiring standard, public reporting of nurse staffing levels and mix and patient outcomes; the Safe Nursing and Patient Care Act (S. 357/H.R. 791), which limits the number of overtime hours a nurse may be required to work; the immediate enactment of upwardly adjustable skilled nursing facility nurse staffing ratios that have been shown to reduce harm to residents; and efforts to require nursing homes to collect and report auditable nurse staffing data, and to require the Centers for Medicare and Medicaid Services to post these data on the Nursing Home Compare Web site (ANA, 2007b).
3. Workplace Rights: The ANA has supported such legislation as that protecting the right of nurses to speak out about activities, practices, or conditions that threaten the health and safety of their patients or the environment; removing barriers and discriminatory practices that interfere with full participation by advanced practice registered nurses in the health care delivery system; preserving the right to overtime compensation for registered nurses; enabling advanced practice registered nurses to certify homebound status and develop and sign the plan of care for patients receiving home services; supporting Medicaid coverage for all services that nurse practitioners and clinical nurse specialists are legally authorized to perform under state law; fully including registered nurses in the National Practitioner Data Bank (http://www.npdb-hipdb.com/), which tracks licensing, disciplinary, and medical malpractice actions taken against U.S. physicians; and maintaining that nurses should have the same rights and responsibilities as reported physicians and that reporters should be protected from retribution.
4. Workplace Health and Safety: The ANA has demonstrated its belief that nurses have the right to a safe and secure workplace in which

to provide quality patient care and has worked to protect nurses from workplace violence and urged Congressional action to allow the federal Occupational Safety and Health Administration to promulgate, implement, and enforce an ergonomics standard to control workplace hazards that lead to or worsen musculoskeletal disorders, many of which are found in repetitive handling activities like lifting, transferring, and repositioning patients.

5. Patient Safety/Advocacy: The ANA has long been committed to comprehensive health care reform that will ensure universal access to health care (preferably through a single-payer system); progressive, incremental steps to cover the millions of Americans who lack health care coverage; efforts to exempt new insurance pools, such as association health plans, from state insurance laws and regulations; a Medicaid program that provides coverage based on federal standards that ensure access for poor and special needs populations, reinvesting any saving realized from the restructuring of Medicaid to expand coverage and benefits; legislation that would mandate the reporting of medical errors to a National Center for Patient Safety; whistleblower protection to ensure that nurses who report medical errors are not retaliated against; a balanced, multipronged legislative approach to address the current medical malpractice liability problem; creation of a standard, affordable prescription drug benefit within the Medicare program and this benefit must provide all beneficiaries with access to needed medications; and increased funding for the National Institute of Nursing Research and the National Institutes of Health.

The ANA offers several publications, including *The American Nurse, American Nurse Today, The Online Journal of Issues in Nursing,* and others addressing standards and principles of various areas of nursing practice. For more than a century, the ANA has advanced the profession of nursing and worked to protect the rights and responsibilities of registered nurses. Through its many programs and services, ANA continues to make progress to strengthen the position of registered nurses and to advocate for patients.

American Nurses Association
8515 Georgia Avenue
Suite 400
Silver Spring, MD 20910–3492
(301) 628–5000

DIANE MANCINO

See Also
Center for American Nurses
United American Nurses

REFERENCES

American Nurses Association. (2006). *ANA bylaws*. Retrieved August 17, 2007, from http://www.nursingworld.org/HiddenDocumentVault/ MemberCenter/ANABylaws2006PDF.aspx

American Nurses Association. (2007a). *Where we come from*. Retrieved August 17, 2007, from http://www.nursingworld.org/FunctionalMenuCategories/ AboutANA/WhereWeComeFrom_1.aspx

American Nurses Association. (2007b). *Nurse staffing: Resources on staffing issues*. Retrieved August 17, 2007, from http://www.nursingworld.org/ MainMenuCategories/ThePracticeofProfessionalNursing/workplace/ Workforce/ShortageStaffing/Staffing.aspx#below

American Nurses Association Hall of Fame

I N 1976, THE AMERICAN Nurses Association established their Hall of Fame, coinciding with the year of the bicentennial of the United States. Fifteen charter members were selected to represent the leadership of nursing, nominated because they "affected the health and/or social history of the United States through sustained, lifelong contributions in or to nursing practice, education, administration, research, economics, or literature" (American Nurses Association, 2006). The ANA Hall of Fame serves as an enduring tribute to these dedicated and accomplished nurses. Initially, one criterion for selection was that individuals be deceased; however, following the 1996 induction it was decided that members could be deceased or living. New members are added at each of the American Nurses Association biennial conventions.

HARRIET R. FELDMAN

REFERENCE

American Nurses Association. (2006). *Hall of fame.* Retrieved September 9, 2006, from http://nursingworld.org/FunctionalMenuCategories/AboutANA/WhereWeComeFrom_1/HallofFame.aspx

American Nurses Credentialing Center

T HE MISSION OF THE American Nurses Credentialing Center (ANCC) is to promote excellence in nursing and health care globally through credentialing programs and related services. The American Nurses Association (ANA) established the ANA Certification Program in 1973 to provide tangible recognition of professional achievement in a defined functional or clinical area of nursing. The ANCC became its own corporation, a subsidiary of the ANA, in 1991. More than 150,000 nurses throughout the United States and its territories in 40 specialty and advanced practice areas of nursing carry ANCC certification. The ANCC certifies health care providers; accredits educational providers, approvers, and programs; recognizes excellence in nursing and health care services; educates the public; collaborates with organizations to advance the understanding of credentialing services; and supports credentialing through research, education, and consultative services.

An important and growing program offered by the ANCC is the Magnet Recognition Program®. Developed by the ANCC to recognize health care organizations that are successful in recruiting and retaining registered nurses because they provide the very best in nursing care and uphold the tradition within nursing of professional nursing practice.

Magnet Recognition also provides a vehicle for disseminating successful practices and strategies among nursing systems. The Magnet Recognition Program® is based on quality indicators and standards of nursing practice as defined in the American Nurses Association's *Scope and Standards for Nurse Administrators* (2003) and those derived from the original Magnet Hospital study (McClure, Poulin, Sovie & Wandelt, 1983). As a natural outcome of this, the program elevates the reputation and standards of the nursing profession.

American Nurses Credentialing Center
8515 Georgia Ave, Suite 400
Silver Spring, MD 20910–3492
(800) 284–2378
Source of Information: http://www.nursingworld.org/ancc/

DIANE MANCINO

See Also
Magnet Hospitals

REFERENCES

American Nurses Association. (2003). *Scope and standards for nurse administrators* (2nd ed.). Washington, DC: Author.

McClure, M. L., Poulin, M. A., Sovie, M. D., & Wandelt, M. (1983). *Magnet hospitals: Attraction and retention of professional nurses.* Washington, DC: American Nurses Association.

American Nurses Foundation

FOUNDED IN 1955 AS THE research, education, and charitable affiliate of the American Nurses Association (ANA), the American Nurses
Foundation (ANF) supports the mission of ANA. Incorporated as a
charitable foundation, ANF raises funds and develops and manages grants
to support nursing research, education, and clinical practice. ANF's goals
include: promoting public health; advancing the nursing profession; promoting cultural competency and ethnic diversity; and funding nursing
research. The nursing research grant program provides funding for beginning and experienced nurse researchers in clinical and academic settings.
Since 1955, over $3 million in grant awards have supported the work of 900
nurse researchers. The ANF is nationally recognized as a philanthropic
organization that supports the continued growth and development of
nursing. Through its programs and initiatives, ANF advances the work
of the profession and improves the quality of health care and nursing
services.

The research of ANF Scholars impacts health outcomes, improves
the delivery of nursing services, and enhances the quality of work life
for nurses. The ANF also manages grants and contracts funded externally. Some of the grants are awarded to ANA and managed through

ANF, whereas others are awarded directly to ANF. Funding has been received from private foundations such as W. K. Kellogg for a community coalition-building project and Robert Wood Johnson for the development of smoking cessation programs. Federal grants have come from several government agencies, including the Centers for Disease Control and Prevention, the Division of Adolescent School Health, the Maternal and Child Health Bureau, the Substance Abuse and Mental Health Services Administration, the Health Resources and Services Administration, and the Agency for Healthcare Research and Quality. Many of these funded projects address nurse staffing, workplace health and safety, continuing competency, and patient safety, and health.

One example of an important current ANF program is the Nurse Competence in Aging (NCA) initiative funded by The Atlantic Philanthropies (USA) Inc. Awarded to ANA through ANF, this 5-year initiative represents a strategic alliance between ANA, the American Nurses Credentialing Center (ANCC), the John A. Hartford Foundation Institute for Geriatric Nursing, and the New York University College of Nursing. Designed to maximize and sustain geriatric competency within national specialty nursing associations, NCA seeks to improve nursing care for older adults. The anticipated outcome of this initiative is to enhance the geriatric competence, knowledge, skills, and attitudes of thousands of national specialty nursing organization members, thereby improving the care of our elderly citizens.

American Nurses Foundation
8515 Georgia Avenue
Suite 400 West
Silver Spring, MD 20910
301–628–5227
Web site: http://www.nursingworld.org/anf/

DIANE MANCINO

See Also
American Nurses Association

American Organization of Nurse Executives

FOUNDED IN 1967, the American Organization of Nurse Executives[1] (AONE), a subsidiary of the American Hospital Association, is a national organization of over 5,000 nurses who design, facilitate, and manage care. Its mission is to represent nurse leaders who strive to improve health care. American Organization of Nurse Executives members are leaders in collaboration and catalysts for innovation. The AONE's vision is to shape the future of health care through innovative nursing leadership. The organization provides leadership, professional development, advocacy, and research in order to advance nursing practice and patient care, promote nursing leadership excellence, and shape health care public policy.

The AONE serves its members by: (1) providing vision and actions for nursing leadership to meet the health care needs of society; (2) influencing legislation and public policy related to nursing and patient care issues; (3) offering member services that support and enhance the management, leadership, educational, and professional development of

---

[1] The original name for the group was The American Society of Nursing Service Administrators; the current name was adopted in 1985.

51

nursing leaders; and (4) facilitating and supporting research and development efforts that advance nursing administration practice and quality patient care. For staff nurses who aspire to a career in nursing leadership, nurse managers in a first management position, directors who manage one or many departments, the chief nursing officers of large health care systems, or a nurse consultant or educator, AONE offers the tools, insights, and solutions to help these professionals achieve even more success in their career. American Organization of Nurse Executives offers several publications including a bimonthly journal, *Nurse Leader* and a member newsletter, *Voice of Nursing Leadership*. Timely information on critical topics is available through the weekly *AONE eNews Update*.

American Organization of Nurse Executives Headquarters
Liberty Place
325 Seventh Street, NW
Washington, DC 20004
(202) 626–2240
Fax (202) 638–5499
Chicago Office
One North Franklin
32nd Floor
Chicago, IL 60606
(312) 422–2800
Fax: (312) 422–4503
Web site: http://www.aone.org/aone/contactus.html

DIANE MANCINO

Americans With Disabilities Act

THE AMERICANS WITH DISABILITIES ACT (ADA), which was signed into law in 1990, details the legal rights of disabled U.S. citizens. The ADA is comprised of five titles and is located in volume 42 of the U.S. Code, beginning at section 12101. Although the ADA does not list all impairments that are included in the law, a person with a disability is defined as having a physical or mental impairment that significantly restricts one or more primary life activities, along with a person who has a history of this impairment or who is seen by others as having an impairment (U.S. Department of Justice, 2005). Title I covers employment, requiring employers with 15 or more workers to offer equal opportunities to disabled qualified potential employees. Therefore, this forbids discrimination in any aspect of the work environment, from initial recruitment and interviewing to promotion, pay, social events and other benefits of employment (U.S. Department of Justice, 2005). This title also disallows any potential prehire question about a disability before offer of a position occurs. Title I complaints need to be filed with the U.S. Equal Employment Opportunity Commission inside of 180 days of the date of the potential infringement.

Title II covers two sections: State and Local Government Activities, and Public Transportation. Title II mandates that both state and local governmental agencies provide opportunity for equal access to any or all events, services, and offerings that range from educational to sports to voting options to town meetings (U.S. Department of Justice, 2005). Additionally, governments are required to comply with upgraded building codes and standards that take people with disabilities into consideration. Complaints or concerns can be forwarded to the Department of Justice within 180 days of the potential date of concern. The transportation mandates from Title II cover city uses and all public trains and subways. The authorities must assure that public transportation is available and accessible to those with disabilities, especially with new purchases and renovations (U.S. Department of Justice, 2005). Concerns regarding public transportation may be sent to the Office of Civil Rights within the Federal Transit Administration.

Title III addresses the spectrum of public accommodations that covers diverse businesses and nonprofit offerings that cover restaurants, theaters, medical offices, shelters, recreation options, hotels, private education, and so on (U.S. Department of Justice, 2005). Public accommodations must comply with the same nondiscrimination expectations along with adhering to new building codes and regulations. Concerns regarding public accommodations may be sent to the Office of Civil Rights Division within the U.S. Department of Justice.

Title IV states regulations regarding telecommunication including telephone and television access for those with hearing and speech disabilities. This Title requires telephone companies to offer telecommunication relay services 24 hours a day, 7 days a week. The relay services offer specialized services for the deaf, which include devices and teletypewriters (U.S. Department of Justice, 2005). For additional information, the Federal Communications Commission (FCC) would be the contact source. Title V is a miscellaneous section that contains additional provisions specific to the explanation and enforcement of Title I through the U.S. Equal Employment Opportunity Commission. These additional clarifications address threatening and/or retaliation against people with disabilities (Equal Employment Opportunity Commission, 2006).

RONDA MINTZ-BINDER

REFERENCES

Equal Employment Opportunity Commission. (2006). *The Americans with disabilities act of 1990, titles I and V.* Retrieved August 18, 2006, from http://www.eeoc.gov/policyada.html

U.S. Department of Justice. (2005). *A guide to disability rights laws*. Retrieved August 20, 2006, from http://www.ada.gov/cguide.pdf

WEB REFERENCES

Federal Communications Commission, http://www.fcc.gov/cgb/dro

U.S. Department of Justice: Civil Rights Division, http://www.ada.gov

U.S. Equal Employment Opportunity Commission, http://www.eeoc.gov

U.S. Office of Civil Rights, Department of Transportation, http://www.fta.dot.gov/ada

Assessment of Leadership Styles and Skills

ALVIN TOFFLER SAID, "The illiterate of the 21st century will not be those who cannot read and write, but those who cannot learn, unlearn, and relearn" (The Quotations Page, 2007). The essential abilities of effective leaders may not be measurable by any particular instrument but more by how the person does in the setting or context of the work environment. That being said, there are a variety of personality assessment tools used by employers and others to assess the strength of leaders. Some of these tools are: Multifactor Leadership Questionnaire (MLQ); Myers-Briggs Type Indicator (MBTI), 16PF, The Sixteen Personality Factor Questionnaire; Integration-Leadership Competencies Profile (Integration); Ethical Leadership Culture Change Inventory (LCCI), and Emotional Intelligence Questionaire-Self/360 (http://www.transformationalleadershipgroup.com/index.php). Developed by Bass in 1985, and revised in 1990, the Multifactor Leadership Questionnaire (MLQ) is considered the primary quantitative instrument to measure the transformational leadership construct. The concept measures four factors demonstrated by leaders: idealized influence, inspirational motivation, intellectual stimulation, individualized consideration (Bass & Avolio, 1990).

Strengths that are needed by leaders are the capacity to inspire a shared vision, enable others to act, challenge the status quo, and motivate others within an ethical context. Outcomes desired from nurse leaders are improvements in quality of care, compliance with standards, efficient and effective operations, and individual growth and cultural enhancements. Effective leadership is measured by how well the leader manages real world challenges on a day-to-day basis. The successful leader needs technical skills and emotional competence, and the ability to manage one's own emotions and those of others. The literature consistently emphasizes the "need for technical and cognitive competence while having highly developed emotional and relational skills" (Scott, 2005, p. 24). Some of the day-to-day requirements for successful leadership are to be a visionary, protector, evaluator, negotiator, evaluator, selector, problem solver, and healer, all of this while managing budgets, conducting strategic and fiscal planning, ensuring high quality of care and compliance with regulatory standards, and contributing to organizational growth. Increasingly, nurse leaders have broader and larger spans of control, which may include non-nursing areas (Arnold et al., 2006). The capable leader provides an environment for people to experience caring, healing, and learning. This leader treats others with dignity, respect, honesty, and fairness. The leader also recognizes the value of individual differences and the collaboration of people with different strengths and expertise (Malloch & Porter-O'Grady, 2005).

Leaders who evidence self-knowledge, strategic vision, risk-taking, creativity, interpersonal and communication effectiveness, inspiration, and the ability to lead change ought to be successful transformational leaders (Morjikian & Bellack, 2005).

MARILYN JAFFE-RUIZ

REFERENCES

Arnold, L., Drenkard, K., Ela, S., Goedken, J., Hamilton, C., Harris, C., et al. (2006). Strategic positioning for nursing excellence in health systems: Insights from chief nursing executives. *Nursing Administration Quarterly* *30*(1), 11–20. Retrieved July 11, 2006, from http://infotrac.galegroup.com/itw/informark

Barker, A. M., Sullivan, D. T., & Emery, M. J. (2006). *Leadership competencies for clinical managers.* Boston: Jones and Bartlett Publishers.

Bass, B., & Avolio, B. (1990). *Multifactor Leadership Questionnaire: The benchmark measure of transformational leadership.* Retrieved August 3, 2007, from http://www.mindgarden.com/products/mlq.htm

Drenkard, K. N. (2001). Creating a future worth experiencing. *Journal of Nursing Administration, 31*(7/8), 364–376.

Dunham-Taylor, J. (2000). Nurse executive transformational leadership found in participative organizations. *Journal of Nursing Administration, 30*(5), 241–250.

Goleman, D. (1998). *Working with emotional intelligence.* New York: Bantam Books.

Malloch, K., & Porter-O'Grady, T. (2005). *The quantum leader: Applications for the new world of work.* Sudbury, MA: Bartlett and Jones.

Morjikian, R., & Bellack, J. (2005). The RWJ executive nurse fellows program, Part I: Leading change. *Journal of Nursing Administration, 35*(10), 431–438.

Porter-O'Grady, T., & Malloch, K. (2003). *Quantum leadership.* Sudbury, MA: Jones and Bartlett.

Scott, K. A. (2005, August). The new nurse executive: Thriving in the first 6 months. *Nurse Leader, 3*(4), 24–27.

Swearingen, S., & Liberman, A. (2004). Nursing leadership: Serving those who serve others. *Health Care Manager, 23*(2), 100–109.

The Quotations Page. (2007). *Alvin Toffler.* Retrieved August 13, 2007, from http://www.quotationspage.com/quotes/Alvin_Toffler

Tracey, C., & Nicholl, H. (2006). Mentoring and networking. *Nursing Management, 12*(10), 28–32.

Transformational Leadership Group. (2004). *Homepage.* Retrieved August 13, 2006, from http://www.transformationalleadershipgroup.com/index.php

Vestal, K. (2005, August). Lessons learned: Ensuring organizational sustainability. *Nurse Leader, 3*(3), 10–11.

Associate Degree Nursing Education

ASSOCIATE DEGREE NURSING **(ADN)** education began in 1952 based on the results of a research project initiated by Mildred Montag (National Organization for Associate Degree Nursing, 2006). The focus of this study was to determine whether placing a program within the community colleges to prepare technical nurses was feasible (Haase, 1990). The results proved the viability of this approach and the number of ADN nursing programs now number over 940 with more than 600 within community colleges across the United States (National Organization for Associate Degree Nursing, 2006). Associate degree registered nursing programs average four semesters of theory and clinical content across medical-surgical, maternity, pediatrics, and psychiatric/mental health nursing. Other program content includes pharmacology, communication, nursing process, and leadership. The units, content, theoretical framework, philosophy, and student learning outcomes are state board of nursing approved; programs also are accredited on a voluntary basis by groups such as the National League of Nursing Accrediting Commission (NLNAC). As indicated in the position statement of the National Organization for Associate Degree Nursing (N-OADN) (2006), associate degree education is focused on evidence-based practice while instilling critical thinking, clinical practice competency, and technical expertise. Students completing an ADN program are eligible to take the National Council Licensure Examination for Registered Nurses (NCLEX-RN). In 2004, 42.2% of RNs entering the workforce did so with associate degrees compared to 30.5% with baccalaureate degrees (BSN), 25.2% with diplomas, and 0.5% with graduate degrees (Health Resources and Services Administration, 2006). Registered Nurses in practice nationally include 33.7% prepared at the ADN level, compared to 34.2% with BSN degrees (Health Resources and Services Administration, 2006). Leadership at the ADN level is primarily spearheaded by organizations such as N-OADN and the National League for Nursing (NLN). N-OADN is the national leader and advocate for associate degree nursing and registered professional nursing practice. NLN represents all accredited academic programs of nursing with many members and board of governor members from associate degree programs. American Association of Community Colleges (AACN) also has been a strong proponent for associate degree nursing education.

Issues regarding associate degree nursing education are generally the same across the United States; however, the timing of such issues coming forward often is legislatively driven. The primary issue confronting associate degree education has been the debate over what academic degree should be the basis for entry into nursing practice. Associate degree nursing proponents believe that this degree is the minimum for entry and should remain as such. Proponents for Baccalaureate education as the minimum degree for entry into practice believe that a 4-year education enriched with research, community health, and a stronger theoretical knowledge base is essential for entry into practice. Examples of this debate include several attempts in various states and nationally to change entry into practice to the BSN level, starting in 1965. Furthermore, in 2006 legislation was introduced in New York State to mandate that associate degree nurses educated after a specific date would be required to obtain the BSN within 10 years after graduation. In mid-2006, New Jersey legislature followed suit with similar legislation. In 2005, legislation in California was passed to align all ADN prerequisites across all 76 programs for ease of entry into the California state university system by spring 2006. Another major issue in California has been the continued debate over meeting Title 5 Open Access Community College legislative mandates and allowing for selection criteria for ADN students. At present, there are no screening criteria other than a basic 2.5 grade point average in both core and overall college courses; however, a 29.4% attrition rate within the ADN program (Board of Registered Nursing, 2006) resulted in a loss of 1,753 students in 2004–2005.

Many issues have faced the leaders of associate degree education, such as unfilled faculty vacancies, titling for administrative heads of ADN programs, faculty retention, and fiscal restraints in college education. For example, in the early to mid-2000s, associate degree nursing leaders were faced with limited nursing faculty, overwhelming numbers of applying students, and budgetary constraints (Milone-Nuzzo & Lancaster, 2004), accompanied by an aging faculty and administrative workforce and few anticipated future replacements (Health Resources and Services Administration, 2006). Associate degree nursing leaders attempted to counter these issues through stronger mentorship programs for new faculty as well as operating programs with smaller budgets and seeking outside funding to provide resources to accommodate increases in the number of students.

RONDA MINTZ-BINDER
JOYCE J. FITZPATRICK

See Also
Entry Into Practice
Licensure

REFERENCES

Board of Registered Nursing. (2006). *California board of registered nursing 2004 annual school report*. Retrieved June 12, 2006, from http://www.rn.ca.gov/forms/pdf/schoolrpt04–05.pdf

Haase, P. T. (1990). *The origins and rise of associate degree nursing education*. Durham, NC: Duke University Press.

Health Resources and Services Administration. (2006). *Preliminary finding: 2004 national sample survey of registered nurses*. Retrieved June 17, 2006, from http://bhpr.hrsa.gov/healthworkforce/reports/rnpopulation/preliminaryfindings.htm

Milone-Nuzzo, P., & Lancaster, J. (2004). Looking through the right end of the telescope: Creating a focused vision for a school of nursing. *Journal of Nursing Education, 43*(11), 506–511.

National Council of State Boards of Nursing. (2006). *NCLEX fact sheet*. Retrieved June 17, 2006, from https://www.ncsbn.org/2006_NCLEX_Fact_sheet.pdf

National Organization for Associate Degree Nursing. (2006). *Position statement of associate degree nursing*. Retrieved June 12, 2006, from http://www.noadn.org/all. Php?1 =home&w=800

WEB REFERENCES

American Association of Community Colleges, http://www.aacc.nche.edu

All Nursing Schools: A Complete Directory of U.S. Nursing Schools, http://www.allnursingschools.com

Discover Nursing: Johnson & Johnson Campaign for Nursing's Future, http://www.discovernursing.com

National League for Nursing, http://www.nln.org

National Organization for Associate Degree Nursing, http://www.noadn.org

National Institutes of Health, Office of Science Education, http://www.science.education.nih.gov

B

Background Screening for Foreign Educated Nurses

U.S. **LAW REQUIRES** that foreign-born health care professionals pass an independent credentials review to qualify for certain occupational visas. Among these professions are: registered nurses, licensed practical nurses, occupational therapists, physical therapists, speech language pathologists and audiologists, medical technologists, medical technicians, and physician assistants. A certificate indicating applicants have passed such credentials evaluation is required before the U.S. Citizenship and Immigration Service can issue an occupational visa for them to live and work as a health care professional in the United States. In short, as a foreign-educated nurse, if one is interested in obtaining an occupational visa to work in the United States, one is required by Section 343 of the Illegal Immigration Reform and Immigrant Responsibility Act (IIRIRA) of 1996 to obtain a *VisaScreen*™ certificate.

VISASCREEN™

VISA **CREDENTIALS** Assessment is a program offered by the International Commission on Healthcare Professions (ICHP), a division of the Commission on Graduates of Foreign Nursing Schools (CGFNS). The *VisaScreen*™ Certificate is issued after a complete evaluation of a professional's credentials to verify that he or she meets the minimum federal requirements. The certificate must be received before the U.S. Citizenship and Immigration Services (USCIS) will issue an occupational visa to the applicant to live and work as a professional in their field in the United States. The *VisaScreen*™ program is comprised of three parts: a credentials review of the candidate's entire professional education and all registration/licensure that he or she has held and currently holds, successful completion of either the CGFNS Certification Program or the NCLEX-RN® (for registered nurses), and successful completion of a group of English language proficiency examinations. Minimum passing scores for these examinations are set by the U.S. Department of Health and Human Services (HHS) and the U.S. Department of Education. Criminal background checks and finger printing of foreign health professionals are done at U.S. embassies, where visas are granted. State licensing boards have state-specific requirements regarding criminal background checks and licensing.

BARBARA L. NICHOLS

REFERENCES

Department of Homeland Security. (2003). Rules and regulations. Certificates for certain health care workers. *U.S. Federal Register, 68*(143) 43901–43921.

Department of Homeland Security. (2004). Rules and regulations. Extension of the deadline for certain health care workers required to obtain certificates. *U.S. Federal Register, 69*(140) 43729–43732.

Commission on Graduates of Foreign Nursing Schools. (n.d.). *ICHP visa credentials fact sheet*. Philadelphia: Author.

Commission on Graduates of Foreign Nursing Schools. (2005). *VisaScreen*™: *A crucial step toward working in the United States*. Philadelphia: Author.

Commission on Graduates of Foreign Nursing Schools. (2006). *2005 Annual report: A world of experience*. Retrieved September 13, 2007, from http://www.cgfns.org/files/pdf/annualreport/2005_annual_report.pdf

Commission on Graduates of Foreign Nursing Schools. (2007). *Frequently asked questions: VisaScreen*™ *Visa Credentials Assessment*. Retrieved July 2007, from http://www.cgfns.org/files/pdf/req/vs-requirements.pdf

Trilateral Initiative for North American Nursing. (1996). *An assessment of North American nursing*. Philadelphia: Commission on Graduates of Foreign Nursing Schools.

Barton, Clarissa Harlowe

CLARISSA [CLARA] HARLOWE BARTON was born on December 25, 1821, in North Oxford, Massachusetts. Barton was 90 years old when she died on April 12, 1912, in Glen Echo, Maryland (Faust, 1986). Although Clara Barton received most of her schooling from her brothers and sisters, she taught for 10 years in Massachusetts before pursuing writing and language instruction at the Liberal Institute in Clinton, New York (Pryor, 1987). Barton was extremely influential in global politics and health care abroad as well as domestically. She is remembered as the founder of the American Red Cross (1881) and was president of that organization for 22 years. Miss Barton fueled the movement of public health nurses both in this country and internationally. Her efforts in Europe assisted the United States to sign the Geneva Agreement in 1882. Clara Barton was a recipient of the Iron Cross, the Cross of Imperial Russia, and the International Red Cross Medal. She wrote the American amendment to the Red Cross constitution and founded the National First Aid Society in 1904. Barton was also instrumental in locating missing soldiers after World War I (1918). She assisted the entire field of nursing through her work as a global health care advocate and philanthropist. Clara Barton is regarded as a truly dedicated American patriot for her devotion in

67

bringing quality health care practices to the United States (Halamandaris, n.d.). She was inducted into the National Women's Hall of Fame at Seneca Falls, New York, in recognition of her commitment to the well-being of society.

M. JANICE NELSON

REFERENCES

Faust, P. I. (Ed.). (1986). *Historical times illustrated encyclopedia of the Civil War.* [Online]. Retrieved November 20, 2005, from http://www.civilwarhome.com/bartonbio.htm

Halamandaris, V. J. (n.d.). *Profiles in caring* (Column 101). [Online]. Retrieved November 20, 2005, from http://www.nahc.org/NAHC/Val/Columns/SC10.html

Pryor, E. B. (1987). *Clara Barton: Professional angel.* Philadelphia: University of Pennsylvania Press.

Benchmarking

BENCHMARKING is a method to compare certain aspects of business or clinical performance in order to drive improvement in productivity and quality. The process of benchmarking entails collating an organization's performance data on a wide variety of practices and then comparing that performance to other similar organizations in order to set goals that will improve processes, operations, and quality. The American Productivity and Quality Center (http://www.apqc.org) describes benchmarking as the process of identifying, understanding, and adapting outstanding practices and processes from organizations anywhere in the world to help organizations improve.

Benchmarking can lead organizations to new methods, ideas, and tools to improve effectiveness. Although benchmarks are not necessarily industry standards, regulatory guidelines, or rules, they are a mark against which an organization compares itself in the continuous search for better practices that will lead to superior performance. Investigating the practices of other organizations helps an organization to focus on how to do things better (improve efficiency) and to do things right (improve effectiveness).

For example, a hospital may look at its average length of stay for a particular diagnosis-related group (DRG), compare it to length of stay results in a set of similar competitor facilities, and set a goal of decreasing the average length of stay by a certain percentage. Using benchmarking to help guide improvement targets helps health care facilities, for example, to examine the average length of stay in other hospitals, and then set an improvement goal based on the data from the other hospitals. In the academic setting, benchmarking data might relate to student enrollment and retention or to outcomes such a licensure and certification.

A benchmarking methodology includes the following activities:

* Set objectives to define the scope of the effort
* Select a benchmarking approach
* Identify benchmarking partners or benchmark sources
* Gather information (research, surveys, quantitative analyses)
* Determine what constitutes the benchmark calculation; that is, what is included/excluded in the numerator and denominator of the benchmark
* Compare actual data to the benchmark
* Identify variances; some variances will be favorable (current performance is better than the benchmark) and some will indicate an opportunity improve by achieving an outcome that other organizations are able to achieve (current performance is not as good as the benchmark)
* Calculate the gap in performance
* Select ideas for improvement tactics for areas that are not favorable compared to the benchmark
* Develop an action plan
* Plan and implement the change
* Measure the result and compare to benchmark

The end goal is not to mimic the practices and goals of other institutions. Instead, it is to understand why their productivity, quality, or processes are performing more effectively or producing better outcomes. Additionally, it is not necessarily the case that a higher expenditure compared to a benchmark for a particular service should automatically be labeled as inappropriate. Rather, it would be an area meriting further examination. For example, only by understanding the reasons and processes behind a competing hospital's effectiveness can a benchmarking hospital develop a plan to improve. Likewise, educational institutions have begun to value benchmarking as an increasingly competitive environment.

Benchmarking has become a meaningful practice at many hospitals. Many organizations that have received continually high national rankings have established profitable benchmarking centers, which other hospitals visit in order to see firsthand the operations and processes that help the leading hospital to succeed. Additionally, other sources for comparative clinical, financial, and operational benchmarks are available, including Premier, Inc. and *The DRG Handbook* (Solucient, 2007). These sources allow comparison groups to be composed based on a wide range of possible groupings, such as bed size, teaching status, system affiliation, urban or rural location, profitability, payer mix, or case mix complexity.

Benchmarking, however, is not an easy exercise. Perhaps the most challenging aspect of benchmarking is that it needs to be an ongoing assessment tool, rather than a one-time initiative. Continuous collection of data surrounding competing hospitals can be difficult, because most hospitals do not report their statistics publicly; however, the trend toward greater transparency in the health care industry is slowly making benchmarking data more readily available. Several public and private organizations now track various metrics for individual hospitals. Because changes and innovations occur constantly within the health care industry, if benchmarking is not conducted continuously, the institutions risks becoming a "reactor" to industry changes, rather than a leader.

NANCY HOLLINGSWORTH

REFERENCES

Bhavnani, S. M. (2000). Benchmarking in health-system pharmacy: Current research and practical applications. *American Journal of Health-System Pharmacy, 57*(20s) 13–20.

Baptist Health Care Corp. (2003). *Health care organization shares the wealth with "benchmarking days"; site visits from other institutions yield two-way learning process.* Retrieved October 9, 2006, from http://www.findarticles.com/p/articles/mi_m0NUZ/is_3_10/ai_98469406

Solucient. (2007). *The DRG handbook: Comparative clinical and financial benchmarks.* Evanston, IL: Thomson Healthcare.

Trimble, D. (2004). *Benchmarking—Uncovering best practices and learning from others.* Retrieved September 13, 2007, from http://www.prosci.com/benchmarking.htm

Breckinridge, Mary

MARY BRECKINRIDGE was born of Southern aristocratic parents on February 17, 1881, in Memphis, Tennessee. She died in 1965 at the age of 84. Breckinridge is undoubtedly best known for her commitment to the practice of nurse midwifery in the United States, which resulted in a remarkable improvement in the health care of women and children in rural Kentucky. Her politically prominent family included Thomas Jefferson's attorney; a vice president under Buchanan; and her father, a congressman, a U.S. ambassador to Russia, and Commissioner of Indian Affairs. Breckinridge was not only a world traveler; she also was educated by the best of tutors and in the best of private schools (American Association of the History of Nursing [AAHN], 2000). Breckinridge was twice married. Influenced by the illness of a friend's child, she completed requirements for a diploma in nursing at St. Luke's Hospital School of Nursing in New York City. She subsequently remarried and had two children, neither of whom survived childhood. Following additional studies in community health and then midwifery in Great Britain, Breckinridge turned to nursing, and she involved herself with supervising nurses during the influenza epidemic of 1918. After World War I, she went to France with the "American Committee for Devastated France." She was awarded

72

the *Medaille Reconnaisance Française* for establishing a Visiting Nurse Service there (AAHN, 2000). Breckinridge eventually settled in impoverished rural Kentucky, where she established the "Kentucky Committee for Mothers and Babies," later to become the Frontier Nursing Service (1925). The service was initially underwritten by Breckinridge's personal funds, but she soon became adept at publicity and fund-raising essential to keeping the service growing. That service remains operational to this day (Bullough, 1998). Breckinridge was inducted into the American Nurses Association Hall of Fame in 1982; she was admitted into the National Women's Hall of Fame in Seneca Falls, New York, in 1995.

M. JANICE NELSON

See Also
ANA Hall of Fame

REFERENCES

American Association of the History of Nursing. (2000). *Mary Breckinridge. 1881–1965.* [Online]. Retrieved March 29, 2006, from http://www.aahn.org/gravesites/breckinridge.html

American Nurses Association. (1995). *Mary Breckinridge (1881–1965) 1982 inductee.* [Online]. Retrieved September 13, 2007, from http://www.nursingworld.org/FunctionalMenuCategories/AboutANA/WhereWeComeFrom_1/HallofFame/19761982/brecmx5517.aspx

Bullough, V. L. (1998). Mary Breckinridge. In V. L. Bullough, O. M. Church, & A. P. Stein (Eds.), *American nursing: A biographical dictionary.* New York: Garland.

Wilkie, K. E., & Moseley, E. R. (1996). *Frontier nurse: Mary Breckinridge.* New York: Julian Messner.

Budget Management

THE NURSING leadership role in financial management of an organization or unit affects control of nursing practice, nursing service delivery, and program management. Budgeting concepts are focused on money as a resource and for many years were often deemphasized in nursing practice and education. Allocation of resources is an important consideration for the nurse executive and frontline leader-manager because decisions regarding the cost of supplies or personnel have a direct influence on the financial health of an organization, as well as the quality of the services that the consumers receive.

A budget is a plan with a timetable that guides an organization's activities. It is a continuous process of predicting monies needed to provide a service, implement the service, and evaluate outcomes of the service. A budget is based on *revenue* (income generated or owed for services) and *expenses* (expenditures and costs of activities needed for the organization's operations). The difference between the projected cost and actual cost of services is called a *variance*. The major types of budgets include the *operating* budget (the daily income and costs in one year for workload, personnel and labor requirements, supplies, and overhead), the *capital* budget (buildings, land, long-term investments, or durable expensive equipment), the *cash* budget (actual/expected monthly income and cash disbursements), and the *long range* budget (a strategic plan of goals over a 3- to 10-year period). A *program* budget looks at a certain existing or future program that needs evaluation, a *product-line* budget analyzes income and costs with a specific patient group, for example, patients with myocardial infarction, and a *special-purpose* budget is used for an ad hoc service or program that was previously unaccounted for. An organization generally will have a *master budget* that includes all of the major budgets (Finkler & Kovner, 2000). The master budget will have many sub-budgets, depending on the size of the organization. For example, the operating budget may have a sub-budget for personnel only that would include the actual worked time (*productive time*) and the time paid to an employed for not working (*nonproductive time*).

Two typical approaches to budgeting that are most often utilized are the traditional or incremental format, in which the budget is simply increased a certain percentage based on historical operations and projected revenue; and the *zero-based* format, in which the budget starts anew each cycle with all expenses requiring specific justification.

The budgeting process is concerned with cost control. *Direct* costs in nursing service relate to a specific activity (unit) such as provision of nursing care, and include the costs of personnel and other resources used in patient care. *Indirect* costs relate to secondary costs within the organization such as overhead (electricity), administrative and insurance costs, and other support services (housekeeping). Variables of volume and cost measures also drive the budget. *Volume* measure is a unit of service adopted by an institution, for example, bed occupancy per day, average daily census, or nursing care hours per patient. A *cost* measure is usually nursing salaries.

MARTHA J. GREENBERG

REFERENCES

Finkler, S. A., & Kovner, C. T. (2000). *Financial management for nurse managers and executives* (2nd ed.). Philadelphia: Saunders.

Huber, D. L. (2006). *Leadership and nursing care management* (3rd ed.). Philadelphia: Saunders.

Marquis, B. L., & Huston, C. J. (2006). *Leadership roles and management functions in nursing: Theory and application* (5th ed.). Philadelphia: Lippincott Williams & Wilkins.

Yoder-Wise, P. S. (2007). *Leading and managing in nursing* (4th ed.). St. Louis, MO: Mosby/Elsevier.

Bullough, Vern L.

VERN L. BULLOUGH was born in Salt Lake, Nevada, on July 24, 1928; he died on June 21, 2006. Bullough earned a BA from the University of Utah, and Master's and doctoral degrees in history at the University of Chicago. Together with his wife, Bonnie, a graduate of the Salt Lake City General Hospital School of Nursing with advanced degrees in nursing and sociology, the Bulloughs generated numerous academic publications and coauthored the first history of nursing text, which was generated by a trained historian and a nurse (Brodie, 2006). Following the loss of their 13-year-old son while they were on Fulbright Scholarships in Egypt, the Bulloughs returned to the United States, where Vern Bullough spent three decades authoring a nursing history bibliography, editing a three-volume set of biographies of nurses that contributed to the shaping of American nursing from the 1850s to the 1990s, and publishing numerous articles and books that "illuminated the development of the profession and the issues it faced" (Brodie, 2006). Responding to criticism from the nursing community regarding his lack of a nursing background that would authorize him to speak to nursing issues, Bullough pursued a BS in nursing at California State University, which he completed in 1981 (Brodie, 2006). In addition to his expertise in the history of medicine and nursing, Bullough was a compassionate humanitarian who was not only a prolific writer but also an ardent activist involved in securing equal rights for all people regardless of their sexual orientation, race, creed, lifestyle, or physical limitations. Both Bulloughs received the Kinsey Award for research on human sexuality in 1993. Vern Bullough was a Fellow of the American Academy of Nursing.

M. JANICE NELSON

See Also
American Academy of Nursing

REFERENCES

Brodie, B. (2006). Vern L. Bullough, PhD, RN, FAAN. *The American Association of the History of Nursing Bulletin, 91,* 6–7.

Bullough, Vern L. (n.d.). *Distinguished professor. A history in the natural and social sciences.* Retrieved August 31, 2006, from http://www.vernbullough.com/bullough/publications/books.html

Lewis, B. (2006). *Newsroom. Bonnie Bullough dies.* Retrieved August 31, 2006, from http://www.usc.edu/uscnews/stories/1848.html

Nalick, J. (2006). *Vern Bullough PhD, F.A.A.N., RN.* Retrieved September 4, 2006, from http://uscnurse.usc.edu/faculty/vern.htm

C

Case Management

C ASE MANAGEMENT is a type of nursing care delivery or work design to organize patient care and meet patient needs. The Case Management Society of America (CMSA) defines case management as "a collaborative process of assessment, planning, facilitation and advocacy for options and services to meet an individual's health needs through communication and available resources to promote quality cost-effective outcomes."

In the United States, case management originated from managed care and prospective payment reimbursement and is used by many health care providers and systems. Although the nursing profession has a long history of using case management in community and other settings, contemporaneous nursing case management focuses on individual patients rather than populations of patients, and manages patient care by major medical diagnoses or diagnosis-related groups (DRGs). DRGs are predetermined payment schedules reflecting anticipated costs for treatment of specific patient conditions.

In nursing case management, patient care is planned using predetermined patient outcomes with specific time frames and the use of specific resources through the use of critical pathways (also called clinical

81

pathways or care pathways) and multidisciplinary action plans (MAPs). Critical pathways are tools or guidelines, developed by interdisciplinary teams, which provide direction for managing the care of a specific patient concern with specific and expected care outcomes and strategies at certain points in time. A MAP is a combination of a nursing care plan and critical pathway. Regardless of the nomenclature, critical pathways identify crucial and predictable occurrences that (1) must take place at established times; (2) organize time-dependent multidisciplinary provider interventions; (3) utilize best practices; (4) aid the standardization of care; and (5) reduce health care costs. A variance on a critical pathway is any deviation from the standard or expected time frame that alters the patient's progress through the pathway. Case managers track variances, documenting when and why a patient's care varies from the pathway, and may recommend changes to the plan.

There are many case management frameworks, perspectives, and meanings, because case management exists in many settings. Case management is a *service* for insured patients aimed at identifying the most financially effective health care service providers, treatments, and settings for the individual. The *role* of the case manager is one of coordination of a patient's care. Case management is a *system* that focuses on the continuum of care across settings with a patient's specific episode of illness. The system uses and evaluates time dependent patient outcomes, strategies, and resources. Case management occurs in acute care settings and outpatient settings such as hospice, home health, psychiatry, and insurance companies. CMSA reiterates that "case management serves as a means for achieving client wellness and autonomy through advocacy, communication, education, identification of service resources and service facilitation."

Further, CMSA states, "the case manager helps identify appropriate providers and facilities throughout the continuum of services while ensuring that available resources are being used in a timely and cost-effective manner in order to obtain optimum value for both the client and the reimbursement source. Case management services are best offered in a climate that allows direct communication between the case manager, the client, and appropriate service personnel, in order to optimize the outcome for all concerned." Huber (2006) asserts that nursing case management embodies leadership and management behaviors. To be effective the nurse case manager must coordinate and evaluate multidisciplinary care, integrate clinical nursing practice, communicate care concepts, direct others, and influence policy and organizational systems.

MARTHA J. GREENBERG

REFERENCES

Huber, D. L. (2006). *Leadership and nursing care management.* (3rd ed.). Philadelphia: Saunders.

Marquis, B. L., & Huston, C. J. (2006). *Leadership roles and management functions in nursing: Theory and application.* (5th ed.). Philadelphia: Lippincott, Williams & Wilkins.

Sullivan, E. J., & Decker, P. J. (2005). *Effective leadership and management in nursing.* (6th ed.). Upper Saddle River, NJ: Pearson Prentice Hall.

WEB REFERENCE

Case Management Society of America, http://www.cmsa.org/

Case Statements

CASE STATEMENTS are formal printed documents that are used in fund-raising campaigns to communicate the institution's vision to the public, primarily those who are prospective donors. The Council for Advancement and Support of Education (CASE; 2006), which is an organization serving many institutions of higher education as well as non-profit organizations throughout the United States, recommends that the case statement include attention to the following questions: What about your institution would make a prospect want to donate? How does a donor go about giving to your institution? What makes your institution a good financial investment?

The campaign case statement typically begins with the mission statement of your institution, and includes your vision for the future. Many case statements include a brief history of accomplishments so that the prospective donor understands the institution's past success and can be comfortable that there will be future successes. Basic facts about the institution are included. For example, for schools of nursing it would be important to include types of academic programs offered, overall enrollment within each academic program, percentage of students who receive financial aid, and graduation and pass rates on the required licensing and certification examinations. The case statement often includes information about past successes with fund-raising, even if it is minimal. Donors like to know that there is a beginning infrastructure for accomplishing the institution's goals. The specific fund-raising goals are often detailed in the case statement, although at times these are included as inserts so that the case statement can be used for a number of requests. Most important, the case statement must include a compelling message for why the institution needs additional support. Donors invest where there is both vision and need so it is important to tie these components together in the case statement and let the donor know what difference their investment will make. In the case statement, it is most important for the institution or organization to distinguish itself from other like institutions or organizations as fund-raising is extremely competitive and there are many places for possible investment by donors. Prospective donors often choose to invest based on the distinguishing factors that they perceive.

The case statement is used externally with prospective donors. It may be accompanied by an internal case statement that includes more details and is made available to the volunteers who will help with the fund raising initiative. The internal case statement should be consistent with the external case statement; it serves as a resource document for the Board, the volunteers, and the staff.

CASE is a membership organization that provides many useful tools for fund-raising campaigns. This organization also makes available sample case statements for campaigns and sponsors an awards program for excellent case statements (CASE, 2006).

JOYCE J. FITZPATRICK

REFERENCE

Council for Advancement and Support of Education. (2006). *Write-minded: Is anyone reading your case statement?* Retrieved July 16, 2006, from http://www.case.org

Center for American Nurses

THE CENTER FOR AMERICAN NURSES is a professional association that was established in 2003 to create a community of nursing organizations that serve individual, nonunion nurses by providing programs, tools, and policies that address their workforce concerns. Based in Silver Spring, Maryland, the Center currently serves 39 nursing organizations and more than 45,000 nurses seeking workforce solutions through its organizational and individual memberships. The Center accomplishes its goals by offering workforce solutions designed to make nurses their own best advocates in their practice environments. Through research, continuing education, and knowledge sharing among today's nursing community, the Center offers powerful resources to nurses seeking to overcome workforce challenges and realize opportunities. The Center's tools, services, and strategies support nurses at all levels of experience who are striving to improve their practice environments, meet their personal and professional goals, and promote excellence in patient care.

Membership is represented by organizational and individual nurse members throughout the country. Addressing both the professional and personal needs of nurses, the Center works to identify working conditions that affect nurses and, in turn, equips nurses with positive power strategies such as effective communication, collaboration, cooperation, and appreciative inquiry, to advocate for themselves within their practice environment. Together, these working conditions are termed the *Workforce Ecosystem*© and include staffing, workflow design, physical environment, organizational culture, and personal/social factors that can enhance or hinder a nurse's effectiveness and well-being. Major initiatives include a focus on the mature nursing workforce, worker's rights and responsibilities, and conflict resolution. Publications, audio-conferencing, and online continuing education offerings are available through the Center. To learn more, visit http://www.centerforamericannurses.org

Center for American Nurses
8515 Georgia Avenue
Suite 400
Silver Spring, MD 20910-3492
(301) 628-5243
Fax: (301) 628-5297

CARRIE HOUSER JAMES
WYLECIA WIGGS HARRIS

Center for
Nursing Advocacy

ESTABLISHED in 2001, the Center for Nursing Advocacy was established by seven graduate nursing students at Johns Hopkins University School of Nursing who came together to help address the nursing shortage. The founders hoped that using informal, alternative, or hybrid approaches to media analysis would help to dispel myths and commonly held beliefs about the nursing profession that made it less attractive to pursue for employment. This mission of the Center, to increase public understanding of the central, front-line role that nurses play is health care, is accomplished by attempting to promote positive portrayals of nurses in the media and encouraging the media to consult with expert nurses. Using comic or irreverent elements to critique the media, the Center seeks to capture the attention and interest of those who create media. Center activities include ranking best and worst media portrayals of nursing (annual Golden Lamp Award); the use of letter-writing campaigns to make nurses' voices heard; reviewing and analyzing media; discussion forums for exchange of ideas; encouraging nurses to create nurse-friendly media, and monitoring the media. In addition, the Web site has links for frequently asked questions (FAQs), general information on nurses and nursing, an archive of news about nurses and nursing in the media, individual media reviews, literature supporting the work of the Center, a press room for information available to the media, and an opportunity to contact the Center and use their search function. A press kit is also available through the Center, as is information about success stories about a number of large and small corporations that have modified their advertising to be more sensitive to how nurses are portrayed and their image exploited for financial gain. Donations are welcome because the Center is nonprofit and needs donations to sustain its mission of advocacy. Ultimately, the Center seeks to improve the image of nursing, which, in turn, will attract people to the nursing profession, thereby providing a long-term solution to the fluctuating global nursing shortage.

The Center for Nursing Advocacy
203 Churchwardens Road
Baltimore, MD 21212-2937
410-323-1100
www.nursingadvocacy.org

HARRIET R. FELDMAN

Centers for Disease Control and Prevention

T HE **CENTERS FOR DISEASE CONTROL AND PREVENTION (CDC)** is an agency of the U.S. Department of Health and Human Services (HHS) located in Atlanta, Georgia. Recognized as the leading U.S. government agency for protecting the health and safety of its people, the CDC does this by providing credible information that "enhances health decisions and promotes health through strong partnerships with state health departments and other organizations" (CDC, 2007). In addition, the CDC also directs quarantine activities, conducts epidemiological research, and provides consultation on an international basis for the control of preventable diseases.

The CDC was established in 1946 as the Communicable Disease Center. It quickly acquired an Epidemiology Division when it took over the Public Health Service Plaque Laboratory in San Francisco. Within a year, the CDC gained worldwide recognition for quality and quantity of its contributions to the taxonomy of the *Enterobacteriaceae*. In the next 25 years, the CDC investigated several epidemics, including polio, cholera, and smallpox. During this time, the CDC was also successful in eradicating smallpox and measles. It also traveled overseas in response to health care needs, made advances in research, and continued to grow. In 1970, the Communicable Disease Center became the Center for Disease Control. This agency continued to advance, working globally, eradicating diseases, and diagnosing new diseases, such as AIDS. In the past six decades since its founding, the CDC has grown dramatically in size and stature, scope and science, and reputation and reach. In addition, the CDC addresses issues related to chronic diseases, disabilities, workplace hazards, injury control, threats to environmental health, and terrorism preparedness. Today the CDC is considered the nation's premier health promotion, prevention, and preparedness agency and a global leader in public health.

The CDC's mission states "healthy people in a healthy world" (CDC, 2007). They seek to accomplish this mission by working with partners throughout the nation and the world. One of these partners is *Healthy People 2010*. *Healthy People 2010* consists of a set of national objectives to achieve over the first decade of the new century. Its goals are to "increase the quality and years of healthy life, and to eliminate health disparities" (HHS, 2000).

Healthy People 2010 provides health objectives in a way that enables different groups to combine their effects and work as a team. The objectives are integrated into current programs, special events, publications, and meetings involving health care or health promotion. Schools can carry out activities to further the health of the community. Health care providers can encourage patients to pursue healthier lifestyles and to participate in community programs. Nurses specifically play an important role in health promotion by educating and encouraging their patients toward a healthier lifestyle.

The goal for the CDC is for people around the world to live safer, healthier, and longer lives through health promotion, health protection, and health diplomacy. Health promotion consists of improving global health by sharing knowledge, tools, and other resources with people and partners around the world. Implementing protection strategies involves a transnational prevention, detection, and response network that protects Americans from health threats at home or abroad (CDC, 2005). Also, the CDC and U.S. government want to be seen as a trusted and effective resource for health promotion and health protection globally.

There are 12 centers, institutes, and offices that make up the CDC. These include the National Center for Environmental Health, the National Center for Injury Prevention and Control, and the Epidemiology Program Office. Individually, they each respond to their area of expertise but they pool all of their resources and expertise on cross-cutting issues and specific health threats (CDC, 2007). In the last 2 years, the CDC has reorganized its centers, institutes, and offices to meet 21st-century health and safety threats. By doing so, the CDC is becoming a more integrated, adaptable, and faster agency. One way that the CDC is meeting the needs of the 21st century is by preparing for emerging health threats so that people in all communities are protected from infectious, occupation, environmental, and terrorist threats. The goal is to address scenarios that include natural and intentional threats. The CDC has sub-goals for pre-threat, during the threat, and post-threat activities. These goals give the CDC something to work toward; accomplishing these goals may give people a way to feel prepared and ready.

As the largest group of health care professionals, nurses may be viewed as important leaders for implementing the stated objectives of the CDC. Nurses are uniquely positioned to assist in prevention and promotion efforts in a multitude of health care settings and in various levels of the community. They play a pivotal role in carrying out the CDC's mission. The CDC works with nurses in "state and local health departments to implement disease prevention and health promotion on a variety of issues on an ongoing basis" (CDC, 2004). Because of their high level of public trust, nurses have shown to be effective communicators, counselors, educators, advocates, and mentors to individuals and groups striving to maintain healthier lifestyles. Nurses demonstrate an important leadership role by their involvement in the prevention of diseases and promotion of health as well as being equipped to respond to disaster situations. Nurses who are leaders of their professional organizations and who are often leaders through their practice of key public health efforts are important consumers of research and technical assistance available through the CDC.

The CDC remains committed to its vision of healthy people in a healthy world. They consistently apply research findings to improve people's daily lives. Although the CDC has grown in tremendous ways since 1946, the heart of the CDC is still its people. They are still determined to make a difference in the lives around the world.

STEPHANIE J. OFFORD
DINA GREENFIELD

REFERENCES

Centers for Disease Control and Prevention, Office of Women's Health. (2004). *Lillian Wald: (1867–1940)*. Retrieved September 22, 2006, from http://www.cdc.gov/Women/owh/wominspire/wald.htm

Centers for Disease Control and Prevention. (2005). *CDC health protection goals: Factsheet*. Retrieved September 22, 2006, from http://www.cdc.gov/about/goals/pdf/hpg-list.pdf

Centers for Disease Control and Prevention. (2007). *CDC organization.* Retrieved August 9, 2007, from http://www.cdc.gov/about/organization/cio.htm

U.S. Department of Health and Human Services. (2000). *Healthy People 2010: What are its goals?* Retrieved September 24, 2006, from http://www.healthypeople.gov/about/goals.htm

Certificate of Need

A CERTIFICATE OF NEED (CON) standard is established by state law. It prohibits identified health facilities/services/equipment from being initiated, upgraded or modernized, expanded, relocated, or acquired without a certificate from that state determining that the need exists in the specified area. Criteria for the approval or denial of a certificate of need are established by law or regulation as review standards, and include cost, quality, and access considerations. The types of facilities, services, and equipment that are covered as well as the review standards vary from state to state. More than half of U.S. states use this concept with regard to the health care services that they provide (Citizens Research Council of Michigan, 2005). Certificate of need applications are reviewed against the following criteria: public need, financial feasibility, character, and competence (New York State Department of Health, 2005).

> **Public Need:** Determination of public need is based on a variety of factors, including population, demographics, and service utilization patterns, epidemiology of selected diseases and conditions, and access to services.

Financial Feasibility: Financial feasibility is based on expenses, projected revenues, current financial status, and capacity to retire debt.

Character and Competence: Assessment of the character and competence of an applicant is based on experience and past performance in operating a health care service, including records of violations, if any, and whether a substantially consistent high level of care was maintained. Applicants without experience in health care services are evaluated based on compliance with laws and practices pertinent to their professional experience.

By using a Certificate of Need evaluation system, the government can evaluate the need for specific health care services in a specific region, determining whether there is a lack or surplus of services provided. Although attention is given to the construction and related costs of capital expansion and improvements, the focus of participating states is on the increase in health care costs that can arise from the availability of unneeded service capacity and total operating expenses that are more costly than necessary. Applicants are required to demonstrate that the service is needed, that it is not duplicative, and that the service will be provided at the lowest cost possible (Citizens Research Council of Michigan, 2005).

Health care service providers are also required to demonstrate the need for the initiation, upgrading, expansion, relocation, and acquisition of services and beds, which are all subject to Certificate of Need review. Each state's certificate of need program has individual features that differentiate it from other states with similar programs. Categories regulated by certificate of need programs include: acute care, air ambulance, burn care, cardiac catheterization, CT scanners, gamma knives, long-term care, mobile hi-tech, MRI scans, neonatal care, obstetric services, open heart services, organ transplant services, PET scans, psychiatric services, rehabilitation, renal dialysis, rescue care facilities, subacute care, substance abuse, swing beds, and ultrasound diagnostic tests (Certificate of Need Application, State of Alaska, 2006; Citizens Research Council of Michigan, 2005). Some states evaluate projects according to general criteria, whereas others make distinctions as to what entity provides the service, usually including hospitals while excluding other providers.

DINA GREENFIELD

REFERENCES

Certificate of Need Application, State of Alaska. (2006). *Health and Social Services, Office of the Commissioner, Health Planning and Systems*

Development. Retrieved March 11, 2007, from http://www.hss.state.ak.us/commissioner/Healthplanning/cert_of_need/forms/default.htm

Citizens Research Council of Michigan. (2005). *The Michigan Certificate of Need Program.* Retrieved September 28, 2006, from http://www.crcmich.org/PUBLICAT/2000s/2005/rpt338.pdf#search=%22who%20needs%20a%20certificate%20of%20need%22

New York State Department of Health. (2005). *Introduction to the CON process.* Retrieved September 28, 2006, from http://www.health.state.ny.us/nysdoh/cons/cons_application/page_00_intro_to_con_process.htm

Certification

THE AMERICAN NURSES ASSOCIATION'S scope and standards of practice handbook state that nursing is a dynamic profession blending evidenced-based practice with intuition, caring, and compassion to provide quality care. The nursing profession contracts with society to promote health, to do no harm, and to respond with skill and caring when change, birth, illness, disease, or death is experienced (American Nurses Association [ANA], 2004). The health care industry has been challenged to improve patient safety, patient and practitioner satisfaction, patient outcomes, and the profitability of the health care organization (Kennedy, 2006). These challenges, along with the rapid advancements in technology, have brought about so many changes in the delivery of care. Registered nurses must proactively deal with constant change and must be prepared for an evolving healthcare environment that includes advanced technology (ANA, 2004).

The practice of nursing involves skills in assessment, diagnosis, outcome identification, planning, implementation, and evaluation. It is the nurse's responsibility to provide the utmost patient care using these skills. How can nurses enhance and improve their practice? Quality of practice is enhanced through education. The eighth standard of nursing practice states that "the registered nurse attains knowledge and competency that reflects current nursing practice" (ANA, 2004, p. 35). The measurement criteria of this standard are that the nurse participates in ongoing educational activities and demonstrates a commitment to lifelong learning. Another measurement criterion is that nurses acquire knowledge and skills appropriate to the specialty area, practice setting, role, or situation.

Nurses are ethically and professionally responsible for obtaining specialized knowledge or skills as their careers progress (American Association of Colleges of Nursing, 2006). This is the rationale for certification in certain specialty areas of nursing practice. "Certification is the process by which a non-governmental agency validates based upon predetermined standards, an individual registered nurse's qualifications and knowledge of practice in a defined functional or clinical area of nursing. The purpose is to assure the public that the nurse has completed all eligibility criteria and earned a specific credential. Another is to promote the development of specialty areas of nursing by establishing minimum competency standards and recognizing those who have met the standards" (Oncology Nursing Certification Corporation, 2006). Specialty areas of nursing certification are in the fields of anesthesia, critical care, midwifery, and oncology.

Why is certification important in the field of nursing practice? The process of certification ensures that the nurse has attained a standard of practice that is beyond the minimum required for practice. This process involves meeting a rigorous predetermined standard requirement of the agency that involves test taking, obtaining classes that fulfill accreditation requirements, and being current in practice. Although licensure measures entry-level competence, certification validates specialty knowledge, experience and clinical judgment (Redd & Alexander, 2003). On December 11, 2002, American Association of Colleges of Nursing (AACN) took a bold step when it released to the media a definitive report on the benefits that specialty certification for nurses bring to the public, employers, and nurses themselves. Titled *Safeguarding the Patient and the Profession: The Value of Critical Care Nurse Certification*, this paper stated that nurses whose clinical judgment has been validated through certification make decisions with greater confidence. The paper further stated that the more knowledgeable the nurses, the better they can recognize problems and intervene appropriately, resulting in few medical errors (Redd & Alexander, 2003). As health care becomes more competitive and complex as well as more legally defined, nurses are challenged to advance their education and obtain certification in their areas of practice.

JUDY L. VALLARELLI

REFERENCES

American Association of Colleges of Nursing. (2006). *Advancing higher education in nursing: 2006 Annual report: Annual state of the schools.* Retrieved June 8, 2006, from http://www.aacn.nche.edu/2006AnnualReport.pdf

American Nurses Association. (2002). *Scope and standards of practice for nursing professional development.* Washington, DC: Author.

American Nurses Association. (2004). *Scope and standards of nursing practice.* Washington, DC: Author.

Kennedy, M. (2006). In the courts: Class action lawsuits target nurse staffing and pay. *American Journal of Nursing, 106*(8), 22.

Oncology Nursing Certification Corporation. (2006). *Certification makes a difference.* Retrieved March 2006 from http://www.oncc.org/publications/pdf/certification.pdf

Redd, M. L., & Alexander, J. W. (2003). Safeguarding the patient and the profession: The value of critical care nurse certification. *American Journal of Critical Care, 12,* 154–164.

Change

A **SIMPLE DEFINITION** of change comes from Roget's II Thesaurus (1995) "the process or result of changing from one appearance, state, or phase to another" (http://www.bartleby.com/62/74/C0237400.html). In fact, there are many ways that change manifests itself. Most leaders need to understand that a distinction exists between a first-order change and second-order change (Watzlawick & Weakland, 1974). First-order changes are differences that occur in a system that itself remains unchanged. An example of first-order change is water boiling in a pot on a stove. As the water boils, first-order change is taking place. The water is becoming different as the molecules jostle together because of the heat of the stove. In this instance, even though there is difference-taking place, the water remains water.

First-order change generally involves the application of a problem-solving model. First-order change is rule- or principle-based, and is circular in nature. First-order change is often incremental and more frequently than not maintains the status quo – hence the adage – "the more things change the more they stay the same." First-order change often involves a search for a singular antecedent cause or problem to solve. Characteristics of first-order change identified by the National Academy for Academic Leadership (http://www.thenationalacademy.org/ready/change.html #defining) include adjustments within existing structures, doing more or less of something. First-order change is reversible, nontransformational and does not involve new learning or understanding of the systems thinking required in a second-order change effort.

Large system changes involve attention to multiple players, roles, rules, levels, values, beliefs, issues, and questions of politics and resources. So second-order change requires a shift in thinking to other logical levels. Second-order change exists when there is a change in the state, structure, rules, or principles by which a system operates. Second-order change may seem illogical, however, because it focuses on a *system of causes* with *multiple effects and consequences*. Second-order change answers questions of *what, how, and why* with attention to *systems thinking and patterns of relationships in mind* (Richmond, 1994). Second-order change requires an understanding of the web of reciprocal causality among the variables involved. Causes and effects are linked together in loops and become dynamic rather than static. Consider what happens when the water in the pot reaches a certain temperature. The water changes state, and operates with a different set of rules as the water is transformed into steam. Water turning to steam is an example of second-order change.

As the National Academy for Academic Leadership notes, other characteristics of second-order change involve new ways of seeing things, and shifting gears. Second-order change involves new learning and transformational change. In organizational development change circles, there is a growing awareness that focusing on problems and first-order change efforts may not be that useful. A problem-oriented approach to change mostly poses these questions: What is wrong? Why is it wrong? How does the problem limit us? This is in contrast to an appreciative approach to change that focuses on what is working and specifying desirable outcomes instead of focusing on the problems. An outcome approach to change poses these questions: What is the change that is wanted? How will the change be defined and made explicit? Where, when, and with whom is the change desired? If the change is achieved, what else will be affected or changed? What stops a group from realizing the changes desired? What are the resources that exist to make the change possible? Appreciative Inquiry (AI) (http://appreciativeinquiry.case.edu/) is an approach to change that focuses more on what is working rather than on what is broken or not working. Such positive, outcome-oriented thinking often requires attention to a second-order change rather than first-order change frame of mind.

DANIEL J. PESUT

REFERENCES

The National Academy for Academic Leadership. (n.d.). *Leadership and institutional change resource page.* Retrieved August 13, 2007, from http://www.thenationalacademy.org/ready/change.html#defining

Richmond, B. (1994). *Systems dynamics, systems thinking: Let us just get on with it.* Retrieved August 13, 2007, from http://iseesystems.com/resources/Articles/SDSTletsjustgetonwithit.pdf

Roget's II: The new thesaurus (3rd ed.). (1995). Boston: Houghton Mifflin. Retrieved August 13, 2007, from http://www.bartleby.com/62/74/C0237400.html

Watzlawick, P., & Weakland, J. (1974). *Change: Principles of problem formation and problem resolution.* New York: Norton.

WEB REFERENCE

Appreciative Inquiry, http://appreciativeinquiry.case.edu/

Change Agents and Change Agent Strategies

C HANGE AGENTS are people who lead change projects or business-wide initiatives by defining, researching, planning, and building coalitions as part of a business or organizational change effort. According to the National Aeronautics Space Administration (NASA) (2001) change agents value and create climates that support change and know how to use power and influence. They deal with both logical and psychological aspects of change. They start the change process with themselves rather than with others. They facilitate rather than force change. They are able to let go of old ideas and experiment with alternatives that support their own enthusiasm. They seek out and accept criticism of their ideas. They are able to get others to "buy into" their ideas for change. Given this set of characteristics change agents need the following skill set. Change agents need to be trustworthy, reliable, honest, competent, and credible within respective organizations. They must possess persuasion, negotiation, and effective listening skills. Successful change agents embody leadership through demonstration of a strong work ethic supported by enthusiasm and respect for individual differences. They have the ability to think conceptually and organize thoughts logically as well as the skill to plan and execute activities and plans. They have good judgment and strong communication skills and are able to coach and facilitate others. "Change Agents must have the conviction to state the facts based on data, even if the consequences are associated with unpleasantness" (Bhardwaj, 2003). Irrespective of the change model or theory that change agents use, successful change depends on purposeful networking (Desantis, 2006). Purposeful networking is a three-phase process of creating, managing, and deploying networks. Change agents are "bridgers" in networks. That is, change agents connect and weave together people and information or "nodes" in a network of relationships in a way that links the social and intellectual capital of the network in service of well-defined outcomes and the desired change. Such "bridgers" are also known as network weavers who build smart communities through actively managing their networks. Network weavers (Krebs & Holley, 2006) know their networks and weave the network together in an iterative connecting and bridging process of communication and interaction in service of an identified vision, goal, or change.

Change agents are masters of change management, defined as "the process, tools and techniques to manage the people-side of change processes, to achieve the required outcomes, and to realize the change effectively within the individual change agent, the inner team, and the wider system" (Nauheimer, 2006). Change management consists of a four-phase process of visioning, planning, implementing, and reviewing and learning. In each phase, both strategies and competencies are needed to influence and achieve effective change. In the visioning phase, the strategies of information-gathering, conceptualizing, and pattern recognition are integrated into coalition building, diagnosis, and outcome specification. In the planning phase's recruitment, team development and delegating parallel and dovetail with the change agent competencies of team building, coalition building, influencing, communicating, and project implementation. In the implementation phase, the change strategies of influencing, negotiating, communicating, listening, monitoring, controlling, and delegating support project management and performance standard setting and resistance and anxiety management, along with training and management of the technical, functional, or operational systems involved with the organization. Finally, reviewing and learning requires expertise in analyzing, reflecting, learning, development of staff, and disengaging. There are many business and process improvement models change agents use in change management efforts depending on the nature of the change. For a complete description of the development needs and change strategies associated with change agent competencies, see Angehrn and Atherton (2006).

DANIEL J. PESUT

REFERENCES

Angehrn, A., & Atherton, J. (2006). *A conceptual framework for assessing development programs for change agents*. Fountain Bleau, Cedrex, France: Center for Advanced Learning Technologies INSEAD. Retrieved September 1, 2006, from http://www.calt.insead.edu/eis/documents/Conceptualframework.pdf#search=%22change%20agents%22

Bhardwaj, M. (2003). *Six sigma dictionary of terms*. Retrieved September 1, 2006, from http://www.isixsigma.com/dictionary/Change_Agent-393.htm

Desantis, M. (2006). *Leading change: Creating, managing and deploying networks for change*. Retrieved September 1, 2006, from http://www.managementfirst.com/change_management/articles/leading_change.php

Krebs, V., & Holley, J. (2006). *Building smart communities through network weaving*. Retrieved September 1, 2006, from http://www.orgnet.com/BuildingNetworks.pdf

National Aeronautics Space Administration. (2001). *Core financial project change agent selection criteria. Huntsville, AL: Marshall Space Flight Center*. Retrieved September 1, 2006, from http://corefinancial.ifmp.nasa.gov/pilot_centerv2/toolkit/documents/ChangeAgentSelectionCriteria.doc

Nauheimer, H. (2006). *The change management toolbook*. Retrieved September 1, 2006, from http://www.change-management-toolbook.com/home/introduction.html

Chi Eta Phi Sorority, Incorporated

CHI ETA PHI SORORITY, INCORPORATED is a professional nursing organization guided by the motto, *Service for Humanity*. This motto is embedded in the mission of promoting higher education, collaborating with other professional groups, developing leaders, and stimulating friendly relationships. Established in 1932 by Ailene Carrington Ewell and 11 other courageous nurses at Freedman's Hospital in Washington, DC, Chi Eta Phi is shaped by the attributes of character, education, and friendship.

From the inception of the organization, members have implemented national programs in their communities that support the mission of service. The national programs are the vehicles by which members engage in service activities that encourage wellness through disease prevention and health promotion. Members engage in health screenings in targeted populations to identify potential and actual health problems and sponsor health education programs in order to address health issues. Programs for the elderly embrace various services for seniors through Chi Care Calls. In addition, there are various programs for boys and girls including health education sessions, mentoring, and support to youth of all ages.

In light of increasing health disparities in underrepresented populations, the increasing aging population, the tremendous shortage of professional nurses in health care, and nursing faculty in academia, Chi Eta Phi Sorority, Inc., is continuing to engage in recruitment activities, and partner with national organizations to maximize current health promotion and disease prevention programs that cut across the life span. In addition to the service that is rendered to the community, Chi Eta Phi also provides opportunities within the nursing field. The organization provides educational scholarships to undergraduate and graduate nursing students as part of supporting retention in nursing programs. Moreover, through financial, tutoring and mentoring activities, issues relating to recruitment, and retention of student nurses are addressed. Three leadership development programs are designed to assist members in fostering effective leadership skills.

The organization sponsors biennial conferences, produces biannual newsletters (*Chi Line*), annual journals, one focused on scholarship and the other, on reporting programs and projects of chapters. The sorority published biographies of Mary Eliza Mahoney, America's first Black Professional Nurse, and Lillian Harvey, a nurse educator and leader. Organization headquarters are located in Washington, DC. Actively seeking to promote diversity in the field of nursing, Chi Eta Phi's membership includes both men and women. Membership is by invitation and extended to registered nurses and student nurses enrolled in professional schools of nursing that are committed to service. In 2007, there were more than 8,000 members located throughout the United States, St. Thomas, U.S. Virgin Islands, and Liberia, West Africa.

LILLIAN GATLIN STOKES

REFERENCES

Miller, H. S. (2007). *The history of Chi Eta Phi Sorority, Inc. Vol. II, 1968–1997*. Washington, DC: Chi Eta Phi Sorority, Inc.
Chi Eta Phi Sorority, Inc. (2007). *Fact sheet, Chi Eta Phi Sorority, Inc.* Washington, DC: Author.

WEB REFERENCE

Chi Eta Phi Sorority, Incorporated, http://www.chietaphi.com

Clinical Evaluation

NURSING EDUCATORS, like those in other fields, are concerned with outcomes. Clinical evaluation is one way to measure the outcomes of a nursing program. The work of the educator is not complete until there is an appraisal of how well students have met course objectives and eventually the overall outcomes of the program. Evaluation is the capstone activity of nursing faculty. Faculty need to learn early in their careers about the art of talking to students about their performance. Clinical days, mid-semester, and end-of-semester activities include the responsibility of student evaluations. Teachers must determine if students have or have not met the course objectives. In addition, faculty has to determine a grade, distinguishing among below average, average, above average, and excellent. The use of a rubric that distinguishes excellent to failing performances is a superb tool that enables faculty to be objective and fair when grading students. Use of a rubric by faculty for grading leads to less confusion about grades, as it is easier to explain and/or defend grade variations that may otherwise be perceived by others as too subjective.

A major portion of faculty time is spent evaluating student performance and providing feedback to students. In nursing education, this assessment is very detailed and is ongoing throughout the semester. Most clinical nursing faculty begin evaluating students on the first day of the clinical practicum. The regular use of anecdotal notes that carefully describe the assignment and how well the student met the objectives is necessary, as it is difficult to remember all of the specifics for each student in a clinical group. It is important to write positive comments as well as negative comments. These notes need to be written as soon after clinical as possible and shared on a weekly basis with the student. It is important to include students in this process, asking them for self-evaluation of their performance throughout the semester. Mid-semester for most students is a major turning point. This is when students talk in depth with faculty about how well they are meeting the objectives and what they have left to accomplish. At that time, any student who is failing didactic or clinical coursework should be notified both in writing and in person. Department chairs, deans, and lead teachers also may be notified of an impending failure, depending on the organizational structure and individual school policies and procedures. There also may be systems of remediation in place to assist the students and these may be included in the notice.

At the end of the semester, a final student evaluation is filed in the student's record. This evaluation should identify whether or not the student met the objectives, if there are any strengths and/or weaknesses in the student's performance, and any recommendations for improvement going forward. These evaluations must be signed by the student. This does not mean that the student agrees with the findings; rather, it signifies that the student has talked to the faculty member about his/her performance. Course evaluations must be filed in a timely fashion, as it is imperative that all students have complete records; incomplete records may affect financial aid opportunities, future enrollment, and employer requirements. These records become part of the permanent file and are used throughout the student's career, including the preparation of after graduation references. Faculty also examines records as the student progresses throughout the curriculum. The record may demonstrate consistent growth or indicate a behavioral trend that is problematic. Deans also may return to the records years after students graduate if they are asked to write recommendations or answer questions about past clinical and classroom experiences.

DAYLE JOSEPH

REFERENCES

ILTE Workshop: *Creating grading rubrics*. Retrieved March 24, 2006, from http://ilte.ius.edu/pdf/creating_a_grading_rubric.pdf

Kearns, L. E., Shoaf, J. R., & Summey, M. B. (2004). Performance and satisfaction of second-degree BSN students in Web-based and traditional course delivery environments. *Journal of Nursing Education, 43*(6), 280–284.

Liberto, T., Roncher, M., & Shellenbarger, T. (1999). Anecdotal notes: Effective clinical evaluation and record keeping. *Nurse Education, 24*(6), 15–18.

Neary, M. (2000). Supporting students' learning and professional development through the process of continuous assessment and mentorship. *Nursing Education Today, 20*(6), 463–474.

Reising, D. L., & Devich, L. E. (2004). Comprehensive practicum evaluation across nursing program. *Nursing Education Perspective, 25*(3), 114–119.

Ruthman, J., Jackson, J., Cluskey, M., Flannigan, P., Folse, V. N., & Bunten, J. (2004). Using clinical journaling to capture critical thinking across the curriculum. *Nursing Education Perspective, 25*(3), 120–123.

Schaffer, M. A., Nelson, P., & Litt, E. (2005). Using portfolios to evaluate achievement of population-based public health nursing competencies in baccalaureate nursing students. *Nursing Education Perspective, 26*(2), 104–112.

Winters, J., Hauck, B., Riggs, C. J., Clawson, J., & Collins, J. (2003). Use of videotaping to assess competencies and course outcomes. *Journal of Nursing Education, 42*(10), 472–476.

Clinical Ladder

BECAUSE one of the greatest threats to nursing staff satisfaction is lack of recognition for excellent work, it became clear in the 1980s that some new creative ways to acknowledge staff nurses needed to be developed. Until this time, most nurses were recognized for quality work by being channeled into administrative positions. Even in the 1980s, job satisfaction translated into nurse retention. With the advent of Patricia Benner's work (1984), *From Novice to Expert*, however, it seemed possible to develop additional pathways to recognize outstanding clinical nurses. One of these methods became known as the Clinical Ladder. In the clinical ladder concept, nurses advanced in the organization by demonstrating their growth in knowledge and experience. Each additional level of recognized skills advanced the financial remuneration of the nurse. Often skills were divided into descriptions of practice, such as beginner, advanced beginner, competent, proficient, and expert. Skill sets describe the various levels of accomplishment. For example, in the area of recognizing and responding to clinical emergencies:

Beginner: learns by observing and asking questions and understands that critical thinking is involved.

111

Advanced beginner: Has practice skills required in emergent situations but may lack experiential knowledge to fully appreciate the situation.

Competent level: Has developed necessary skills to function in the emergent situation but may become overwhelmed by multiple tasks or the pressures of leading in the situation.

Proficient nurse: Organization for patient care is automatic and dynamic; picking up on changes in condition and taking appropriate action.

Expert Nurse: Is able to take immediate action in the situation, access both nursing and interdisciplinary team resources quickly, function seamlessly and automatically in the situation, and calm others in the midst of a crisis (Schoessler et al., 2005).

Each level builds on knowledge and skills from the previous level as well as adding continuously increasing critical thinking and reasoning, holistic intuition, and experience-guided behaviors. These levels of functioning are on a continuum.

Numerous clinical ladder models exist today. Some have outcome-based criteria and staff selects a specific number of behaviors from among various categories. For example, categories could include competency, customer service, teamwork, quality, and continuous learning. Within the quality category, the nurse might choose one of the following behaviors:

* Assume an active role in the quality or practice outcome project
* Complete special projects with leadership approval and communicate outcomes to the staff
* Participate in an approved research study
* Attend research or quality educational workshop and share learning with other staff members
* Review a nursing research article and present to staff
* Initiate a cost-saving initiative on the unit with documentation of outcomes (Goodrich & Ward, 2004)

In many institutions, formal education is a significant part of the program. Regardless of how the program is structured, the clinical ladder concept encourages and rewards nurses who develop in depth expertise while choosing direct patient care involvement.

KARREN KOWALSKI

REFERENCES

Benner, P. (1984). *From novice to expert*. Menlo Park, CA: Addison Wesley.

Goodrich, C., & Ward, C. (2004). Evaluation and revision of a clinical advancement program. *MEDSURG Nursing, 13*(6), 391–398.

Schoessler, M., Akin, R., Body, R., Falconer, K., Kaiel, C., Moore-Stout, D., et al. (2005). Remodeling a clinical ladder: An action research design. *Journal for Nurses in Staff Development, 21*(5), 196–201.

Coaching Nurses

COACHING for job performance is a key role of the nurse leader. Similar to an athletic coach, the nurse leader uses continuous reinforcement and feedback loops to guide staff to a desired outcome or performance level. Coaching includes observing and obtaining feedback on employee performance and using that information to reinforce positive behaviors and suggest ways to improve weaknesses. Effective coaching evolves over the course of employment and should not be viewed as a one time intervention. When the leader establishes rapport with an employee and begins the coaching process, the employee is more likely to be engaged in supporting a positive work culture and less likely to be surprised with developmental feedback at the annual review.

According to Frankel and Ofuzo (1992), the following are some actions of an effective coach:

* Listens
* Views the employee as a person
* Cares about the employee and helps with personal problems
* Sets a good example
* Encourages the employee

114

* Helps get the work done
* Keeps the employee informed
* Praises the employee for a job well done, and provides criticism in a straightforward manner

When coaching ceases to be effective in enhancing employee performance, the nurse leader changes roles from coach to counselor and generally moves the employee into a formal disciplinary process. It is important to note that coaching for effective performance is not always a precursor to disciplinary action, but may be the first step in formal action should the employee choose not to respond to coaching methods. For this reason, a written coaching plan can be a helpful tool. A written plan outlining expectations of both the coach and the employee as well as the objectives of the coaching relationship can be very helpful in holding each party accountable for the outcome of the coaching process. In addition, should coaching move to formal disciplinary action, the written coaching plan can provide additional support to the nurse leader by demonstrating a sincere effort to improve performance outside of the disciplinary action process.

Coaching employees can be one of the most rewarding aspects of the nurse leader's role. The ability to engage employees in the process and observe positive changes and growth creates an environment of mutual trust and respect for both the coach and the employee. The most important facet of being a good coach is being a great role model by consistently demonstrating the behaviors and attitude that you as a coach expect of your team.

JEFFREY N. DOUCETTE

REFERENCE

Frankel, L. P., & Ofuzo, K. L. (1992). Employee coaching: The way to gain compliance. *Employment Relations Today, 5,* 311–320.

Collective Bargaining and Unions

STAFF NURSES in many hospitals have been organizing themselves into unions since World War II. In the 1940s, nurses in New York, California, Pennsylvania, and Ohio formed nursing unions. In 1946, with urging from state nurses associations representing nurses for collective bargaining, the American Nurses Association (ANA) started its national economic security program (Foley, 2002). In 1999, the ANA formed an independent affiliate known as the United American Nurses (UAN) that is also a member of the AFL-CIO. In 2003, the most recent year with available data, 19.5% (472,000) of all RNs (2.4 million) in the United States were represented by unions. Some nurses belong to the UAN, some to independent unions, and some to traditional labor organizations. Totally, unions represent 14.3% of all workers in the United States (UAN, 2005). The National Labor Relations Act governs proprietary and not-for-profit health care facilities. Some states have additional laws that govern employee relations in public health care facilities. The Fair Labor Standards Act sets minimum wages, overtime rules, and workweek hours. The Equal Pay Act of 1963 addresses wage disparities based on sex while the Equal Employment Opportunity Act (1972) prohibits discrimination on the basis of age, race, color, religion, sex, or national origin. The

American with Disabilities Act (1990) prohibits discrimination against an otherwise qualified individual by reason of a physical or mental disability and requires that the employer bring the physical environment into compliance with ADA requirements.

Employee rights include the right to organize and bargain collectively; solicit and distribute union information during nonworking hours; picket and strike; grieve and arbitrate issues; be free from termination unless there is "just cause"; and negotiate benefits and conditions of employment. Management rights include the right to: a 10-day advance notice of a bargaining unit's intention to strike, picket, or engage in other concerted work activity; hire replacement workers in the event of a strike; prohibit employees from engaging in union activity during working hours; reasonably restrict union organizers to certain locations and time periods to avoid interference with facility operations; and prohibit supervisors from participating in union activity.

KAREN A. BALLARD

See Also
Americans With Disabilities Act

REFERENCES

Foley, M. F. (2002). Collective action in the workplace. In D. Mason, J. Leavitt, & W. Chaffee (Eds.), *Policy and politics in nursing and health care* (4th ed.) (pp. 387–397). Philadelphia: W. B. Saunders.

United American Nurses. (2005). *RN union difference*. Retrieved September 5, 2006, from http://www.uannurse.org/organize/organize.html

Commission on Collegiate Nursing Education

THE COMMISSION ON COLLEGIATE NURSING EDUCATION (CCNE) is a nationally recognized accrediting organization for baccalaureate and graduate degree programs in nursing education. Established in 1996, CCNE is the autonomous accrediting arm of the American Association of Colleges of Nursing—the national voice for baccalaureate and graduate degree nursing education programs since 1969. CCNE is formally recognized by the U.S. Secretary of Education and the Council for Higher Education Accreditation and serves the public interest by assessing and identifying programs that engage in effective educational practices. With a national scope, CCNE accredits nursing programs in 49 states, the District of Columbia, and the Commonwealth of Puerto Rico. For a complete listing of CCNE-accredited programs, go to the CCNE Web site: http://www.aacn.nche.edu/CCNE/reports/accprog.asp. To be eligible for CCNE accreditation, nursing programs must be at the baccalaureate or master's degree levels, and in 2008, the professional nursing doctorates level and post-baccalaureate nurse residency. In addition, programs must be offered by an institution of higher education that is accredited by an organization recognized by the U.S. Secretary of Education.

CCNE is governed by a 13-member Board of Commissioners that includes nursing deans, nursing faculty, practicing nurses, professional consumers, and public consumers. The work of CCNE is supported by a professional and administrative staff, more than 700 volunteer evaluators who are trained by the organization to serve as peer reviewers in the accreditation process, and several committees. In general, CCNE accreditation is conferred for up to 5 years for new programs and for up to 10 years for programs pursuing continuing accreditation. Programs are evaluated against a set of established standards during a comprehensive on-site evaluation. A four-pronged monitoring process ensures that a program's compliance with the standards continues between evaluations. This process includes submission of annual reports, continuous improvement progress reports, substantive change notifications when warranted, and special reports on areas of noncompliance. CCNE accreditation activities are designed to reflect good accreditation practices and are premised on a statement of principles or values that are published by the organization.

JENNIFER PAUP BUTLIN

WEB REFERENCE

American Association of Colleges of Nursing, http://www.aacn.nche.edu/Accreditation/index.htm.

Commission on Graduates of Foreign Nursing Schools

THE COMMISSION ON GRADUATES OF FOREIGN NURSING SCHOOLS INTERNATIONAL (CGFNS) is a not-for-profit, immigration-neutral, internationally recognized leading authority on the education, registration, and licensure of nurses and other health care professionals, worldwide. CGFNS protects the public by assuring the integrity of professional credentials in the context of global migration. CGFNS offers four credentials evaluation and verification services that meet U.S. immigration and state licensure requirements. These programs are:

* Certification Program (CP)
* Credentials Evaluation Service (CES)
* *VisaScreen*™ (VS)
* Credentials Verification for New York State (CVS)

CERTIFICATION PROGRAM (CP)

THE CGFNS CERTIFICATE is used by over 80% of U.S. Boards of Nursing as a prerequisite for licensure in the United States and may be required to obtain certain occupational visas to practice nursing in the United States. The CGFNS Certification Program (CP) is a three-part program designed for first-level, general nurses (RNs) educated outside the United States. The program includes a credentials review, qualifying exam of nursing knowledge, and test of English language proficiency. On successful completion of all three parts of the program, the applicant is awarded the CGFNS Certificate.

CREDENTIALS EVALUATION SERVICES (CES)

A S WITH THE CGFNS CERTIFICATION PROGRAM, the CGFNS Credentials Evaluation Service is a prerequisite for state licensure in certain U.S. states and territories. CES is also used by U.S. schools to determine academic placement of international students; however, there is no examination component in the Credentials Evaluation Service. The program is based on an evaluation of a health care professional's educational and professional licensure/registration credentials. The resulting report compares the health care professional's education and licensure credentials in terms of U.S. comparability.

VisaScreen™ **(VS)**

S ECTION 343 of the Illegal Immigration Reform and Immigrant Responsibility Act of 1996 requires that foreign-born health care professionals who wish to practice in the United States successfully complete a screening program before receiving an occupational visa. This includes registered and licensed vocational nurses, physical therapists, speech-language pathologists and audiologists, medical technologists, medical technicians, occupational therapists, and physician assistants. *VisaScreen*™: Visa Credentials Assessment is a program offered by the International Commission on Healthcare Professions (ICHP)—a division of CGFNS—enabling health care professionals to meet this requirement by verifying and evaluating their credentials to ensure that they meet the U.S. government's minimum requirements. The *VisaScreen*™ program is comprised of an education analysis, licensure validation, English language proficiency assessment, and in the case of registered nurses, an exam of nursing knowledge.

CREDENTIALS VERIFICATION FOR NEW YORK STATE (CVS)

F OR HEALTH care professionals wishing to practice in the state of New York, the CGFNS Credentials Verification Services collects and verifies

122

COMMISSION
ON GRADUATES
OF FOREIGN
NURSING
SCHOOLS

the authenticity of an applicant's educational and licensure/registration credentials so they can be evaluated by the New York State Education Department. These services and programs validate credentials and enhance international regulatory and educational standards for health care professionals around the globe.

BARBARA L. NICHOLS

REFERENCE

Nichols, B. (Ed.). (2005, October). *Annual report*. Philadelphia: Commission on Graduates of Foreign Nursing Schools.

Complex Adaptive Systems (Chaos Theory)

I N 2001 THE INSTITUTE OF MEDICINE (IOM) published the second in a series of reports on the quality of health care in America. The committee's first report, *To Err is Human: Building a Safer Health System*, focused on patient safety as a systems issue that needs attention. Patient safety, however, is embedded in a context of complexity. *Crossing the Quality Chasm*, the second IOM report, focused on the need to redesign health care systems in order to foster innovation and improve care. Quality was defined as a system property and the IOM established an agenda for change that intends to recast and recraft the American health care system for the 21st century. Zimmerman, Lindberg, and Plsek (2001), in an appendix to the *Crossing the Quality Chasm* report, suggest that redesign of the health care system for the 21st century may well be strategically accomplished through the use of complex adaptive systems thinking. Redesign of health care through complexity science inspired innovations is an interesting and useful theoretical framework. Complex adaptive systems consist of context sensitive adaptable elements, which respond to simple rules. The emergent evolutions of complex systems reveal they are nonlinear and support emergence through novel behavior, which is nonpredictable, yet inherently

124

COMPLEX
ADAPTIVE
SYSTEMS
(CHAOS
THEORY)

orderly. Complexity science provides a new paradigm to guide systems design and suggests a series of questions to consider when confronted with wicked and sticky problems. To learn more about complexity science, visit the Plexus Institute (http://www.plexusinstitute.com/). The mission of this not-for-profit organization is to foster the health of individuals, families, communities, organizations and our natural environment by helping people through the new science of complexity. Plexus offers a complexity science primer for those new to the concepts and science (http://www.plexusinstitute.com/services/E-Library/show.cfm?id=150).

DANIEL J. PESUT

REFERENCES

Institute of Medicine. (2001). *Crossing the quality chasm: A new health system for the 21st century*. Washington, DC: National Academies Press.

Zimmerman, B., Lindberg, C., & Plsek, P. (2001). *Edgeware insights from complexity science for health care leaders*. Irving, TX: Voluntary Hospital Association.

Conflict Management for Nurse Leaders

CREATING A HEALTHY WORK environment has been demonstrated to be one of the most significant factors in reducing medical errors, improving patient safety, reducing work-related stress, and enhancing patient care delivery systems. Creating a positive and healthy work environment is a challenge for all nurse leaders. Inherent in this work is a need to understand the organization's culture in handling conflict, the costs of conflict, the impact of organizational complexities, barriers to managing conflict, and strategies for effective conflict resolution (Filley, 1980).

Changes in the health care delivery system over the past two decades and the trend to move decision making to the bedside have resulted in the dismantling of traditional hierarchal models and left many to wonder who is really making decisions in health care organizations. This uncertainty coupled with the increasing complexity in the patient care environment creates many opportunities for conflict. Although intuitive to health leaders, Forte (1997) showed that conflict among health care workers is counterproductive to patient care. According to a study of the American Management Association, nursing managers spend an average of 20% of their time dealing with conflict management. Furthermore, the study identified that conflict management skills are rated equally important or slightly more important than planning, communication, and decision making (McElhaney, 1996).

CAUSES OF CONFLICT

U NDERSTANDING how conflict arises can be very helpful to the nurse leader in anticipating situations and dealing with escalating issues in the workplace. Although sources of conflict in health care may seem endless, they are generally limited to several root causes. A common source of conflict in health care is incompatible goals between individuals or groups of individuals at work. For example, an employee does not agree with a new management policy regarding time and attendance. The employee wants flexibility in his schedule and the manager expects employees to be ready to work on time. One can easily see how this level of differing goals could lead to conflict. A second source of conflict is the inherent in the different personal values we bring to work. There are employees who, for example, enjoying going out for a drink after work, whereas others prefer to leave work and go home to spend time with family. It is only a matter of time before a divide exists in the two groups and this distancing can frequently lead to conflict. A third factor contributing to conflict in the workplace is the extent to which we rely on others to complete our work. A fair amount of conflict can arise between nurses and ancillary support staff around the interdependence on one another to achieve outcomes for patient care.

In addition to interpersonal sources, conflict can arise between individuals and the organization. The availability and distribution of resources in the workplace can be a significant source. Resources can be anything from budgetary dollars to office space or even time spent with your boss. Employees consistently report in numerous published surveys that "having the equipment I need to do my job" is a top ten job satisfier. Another source of organizational conflict is inherent in the distribution of power. Many times, people are working in the best interest of the organization and inadvertently create conflict by "stepping on someone else's toes" because they do not understand the organizational hierarchy or politics that are part of any group. Finally, employees in health care organizations generally feel that polices are unpredictable and constantly changing. Working in a highly regulated environment, there is a tendency to have a policy in place for every action an employee is expected to perform. When these policies are not congruent with accepted practice standards or are not consistently enforced, they can be a major source of conflict between the organization and its employees.

EFFECTIVELY MANAGING CONFLICT

T HERE are some basic principles that apply to any counseling session with employees that will always help leaders prepare for the discussion. First, write out your thoughts about the situation and how you might handle it with the employee. Ask yourself if your thoughts are rational and if they are painting a view of the situation that is as objective and free from emotion as possible. Second, write down some key phrases or outline the conversation that you will have with the employee when you meet. Third, always schedule a time to meet with an employee. This gives credibility to the fact that the meeting is serious and important enough to you as a leader for dedicated time on your schedule. When you are meeting with the employee, deal with only one topic at a time and be specific. Use concrete examples and always keep the conversation focused on the issue at hand. Finally, focus your expectations on the specific behavior that you want from the employee. For example, "I need you to clock in and out every time you are working" is more direct than "I need you to pay more attention to detail when you come to work and go home."

One of the most effective methods for dealing with conflict is active listening. It is imperative that the nurse leader has a clear understanding of the perceptions of the parties involved in the conflict. It is also helpful to paraphrase the issue to the employee to ensure that everyone is on the same page. Powell (1986) suggests the following techniques for effective active listening:

* Do not share anger. Remain calm and matter-of-fact.
* Respond constructively in both verbal and nonverbal language.
* Ask questions and listen to the answers.
* Separate fact from opinion, including your own.
* Do not respond hastily. Plan your response.
* Consider the employee's perspective first.
* Help the employee find the solution. Ask questions and listen to responses. Do not be paternalistic.

Many times, employees simply want to be heard and, this in and of itself can be an effective way to deal with conflict.

Valentine (2001) identified five potential conflict management strategies and related these strategies to nurse leaders. Avoiding, compromising, collaborating, accommodating, and competing are widely accepted strategies for dealing with conflict. The study further identified that staff nurses most frequently chose avoidance as their dominant conflict management style, whereas nurse leaders were split between avoiding and compromising. Avoidance is a strategy that allows both parties to cool down. Giving the parties time to think about the situation and scheduling a time to meet at a later date is effective when the issue is not critical. The nurse leader must follow through on scheduling the follow-up meeting as soon as possible. Compromise is closely related to avoidance in that taking middle ground may lead to a resolution of the conflict. Compromise is also a temporary solution used to allow the parties to work out a more permanent solution. Accommodation is effective when the issue is more important to the other person. This technique maintains a spirit of cooperation and develops employees by allowing them to make decisions about the situation. Collaboration is generally viewed as a win-win approach to conflict management. When a collaborative approach is used, both parties make concessions to improve the overall outcome of the issue that resulted in conflict. This method is widely practiced and accepted in health care organizations. Finally, competition is used when the nurse leader exerts his position power over subordinates. This approach is viewed as disciplinary in nature and does not allow the subordinate to participate in the conflict resolution process.

As a nurse leader, choosing the most effective method to resolve conflict is a critical step in the coaching process with employees. The challenge of managing multiple levels of providers with varying levels of autonomy requires skills beyond basic management theory. The ultimate goal in conflict management is to minimize the long-term effects of conflict on the group's performance and to keep the parties "whole" in the process.

JEFFREY N. DOUCETTE

REFERENCES

Filley, A. C. (1980). Types of sources of conflict. In M. S. Berger, D. Elhart, S. C. Firsich, S. B. Jordan, & S. Stone (Eds.), *Management for nurses: A multidisciplinary approach* (pp. 154–165). St. Louis, MO: C. V. Mosby.

Forte, P. S. (1997). The high costs of conflict. *Nursing Economics, 15,* 119–123.

McElhaney, R. (1996). Conflict management in nursing administration. *Nursing Management, 24,* 65–66.

Powell, J. T. (1986). Stress listening: Coping with angry confrontations. *Personnel Journal, 65*(5), 27–30.

Valentine, P. (2001). A gender perspective on conflict management strategies of nurses. *Journal of Nursing Scholarship, 33*(1), 69–74.

Conflict of Interest

THE DICTIONARY OF LAW (*Merriam-Webster's Dictionary of Law*, 2006) defines conflict of interest as: "a conflict between the private interests and the official or professional responsibilities of a person in a position of trust, or a conflict between competing duties." Examples of this concept may include city workers who are prohibited from accepting gifts from vendors, because this might cause them to favor these vendors (Conflicts of Interest Board of the City of New York, 2006); health care practitioners' personal interests or preferences may alter the type of care they provide to clients from the same or different backgrounds. Many research institutions have policies and procedures to manage conflicts of interest. Additionally, authors of scientific journals have established policies to protect the integrity of the conflict of interest among scientists. Furthermore, many government officials will not even take gifts from vendors, because that might sway their feelings, which would be unethical. Also, many institutions have conflict of interest policies to which employees must adhere.

The 1993 Code of Ethics of the American College of Healthcare Executives defines conflict of interest as something that potentially exists when a health care administrator holds a managerial position that allows them to use authority or classified information. This includes allowing significant others to benefit from the information as well. This may go

129

as far as to allow the administrator to make decisions that are potentially detrimental to the organization, as long as they benefit the administrator's needs (Bross, 2005). In other words, people in power use their influence to help others gain advantage in exchange for a favor, product, or remuneration.

Potential conflicts of interest can occur when insiders benefit from an organizational decision (Duronio, 2004). Nurses may be involved in conflict situations as a result of competing loyalties in the work setting, including those related to patients, families, physicians, colleagues, health care organizations, and health plans (American Nurses Association [ANA], 2001). A nurse may be the scheduler of an OR or procedure room and use the personal relationship with a friend to move a given patient ahead of others on the schedule in exchange for a gift of some sort. In many cases, the interactions that have potential conflicts of interest are those that offer some financial benefits to the parties involved.

A conflict of interest occurs when a nurse's personal or private interests interfere with a client's best interests or the nurse's own professional responsibilities. This is the utmost dilemma because it is hard to determine who is benefiting most from the arrangement; the patient or the caregiver. The interest at hand may be personal, commercial, political, academic, or financial. The conflict can be actual, perceived, or potential. When a conflict of interest influences or appears to influence a nurse's judgment, this may adversely affect the client's trust in the nurse (College of Registered Nurses of British Columbia, 2006). Nurses may encounter conflict of interest in situations involving clinical practice, education, or management of research, which all have the potential to cause unfavorable effects. The nurse may not even recognize or confess that the conflict in actuality exists. Even small gifts from patients or pharmaceutical companies can manipulate a nurse's judgment. If such a conflict is unavoidable, nurses are encouraged to offer full disclosure and to speak with the appropriate people in order to be able to manage the conflict properly and ethically. When resolving such a conflict, the nurse must remember to guarantee patient safety, while protecting the patient's best interests and upholding the professional integrity of the nurse.

Additional conflicts of interest that the nurse may encounter are related to a differing of opinions of the nurse and the client with regard to the client's care. In such a case, the nurse would have to consider whether his or her own actions are ethically justifiable. This can be done by balancing the interests of everyone involved, which may include the client, his or her immediate family, and the nursing staff, followed by analysis of all possible modes of action. The nurse must gain the client's confidence to ensure that the client will not become noncooperative, aggressive, or depressed. The nurse should listen to the client's needs and wishes to determine why a client might be refusing care (Bolmsjo & Hermeren, 2003).

Another form of conflict may be the use of incentive programs that reward nurses for patients that they refer to a specific facility. "These types of rewards raise questions about the need or quality of the services provided or, in some cases, not provided" (Monet, 1999). The patient may have been referred to this clinic for a legitimate reason, or it may be a result of an incentive that entices the nurse. Nurses in leadership positions with budgetary responsibilities and those who are in advanced practice positions and bill directly for services must be especially cognizant of the potential for conflicts of interest (ANA, 2001).

DINA GREENFIELD

REFERENCES

American Nurses Association. (2001). *Code of ethics for nurses with interpretive statements*. Washington, DC: Author.

Bolmsjo, I., & Hermeren, G. (2003). *Nursing ethics: Conflicts of interest: Experiences of close relatives of patients suffering from amyotrophic lateral sclerosis.* Retrieved October 4, 2006, from http://web.ebscohost.com/ehost/pdf?vid=97&hid=102&sid=5c5dbfef-21ec-44fd-a553-e8329aa2d532%40sessionmgr102

Bross, W. (2005). *Ethical issues—clinical research.* Retrieved September 28, 2006, from http://www.findarticles.com/p/articles/mi_qa4090/is_200412/ai_n9477083

College of Registered Nurses of British Columbia. (2006). *Conflict of interest.* Retrieved on September 28, 2006, from http://www.crnbc.ca/downloads/439.pdf#search=%22conflict%20of%20interest%20%2B%20nurses%22

Conflicts of Interest Board of the City of New York. (2006). *Introduction to the conflicts of interest board.* Retrieved September 28, 2006, from http://www.nyc.gov/html/conflicts/html/about/intro.shtml

Duronio, C. D. (2004). Dealing with conflicts of interest. *Clinical Journal of Oncology Nursing, 8*(2), 115–116. Retrieved October 4, 2006, from http://web.ebscohost.com/ehost/pdf?vid=44&hid=102&sid=5c5dbfef-21ec-44fd-a553-e8329aa2d532%40sessionmgr102

Merriam-Webster's Dictionary of Law. (2006). Conflict of interest. Retrieved September 29, 2006, from http://dictionary.reference.com/browse/conflict of interest

Monet, S. (1999). *Hawaii nurse: Cost containment & healing from the heart.* Retrieved October 4, 2006, from http://web.ebscohost.com/ehost/pdf?vid=97&hid=102&sid=5c5dbfef-21ec-44fd-a553-e8329aa2d532%40sessionmgr102

Salladay, S. A. (2003). *Nursing 2003: Conflict of interest; Prescription for trouble.* Retrieved October 4, 2006, from http://web.ebscohost.com/ehost/pdf?vid=81&hid=102&sid=5c5dbfef-21ec-44fd-a553-e8329aa2d532%40sessionmgr102

Conflict of Interest in Research

CONFLICT OF INTEREST FOR INDIVIDUAL SCIENTISTS

ONE OF THE critical underlying assumptions of science is that researchers conceptualize, implement, and disseminate their research free from bias. Scientists building on and extending others' research must trust that the findings from previous studies are as reflective of actual reality as possible and that neither the data reported nor the interpretations of the data were influenced by outside forces. A conflict of interest (COI) in research exists "when the individual has interests in the outcome of the research that may lead to personal advantage and that might, therefore, in actuality or appearance, compromise the integrity of the research" (Rubenstein, 2002, p. 38). COI has the potential to bias a researchers' conduct of research in a variety of ways.

There are several types of situations that can create a conflict of interest for an individual scientist. The most common are financially related conflicts in which an investigator has a financial interest in a source that funds the research itself. This conflict might be present for someone who is a member of a governing board of a company funding the research, an investigator who holds stock in the company that supports the research, or an investigator who is a paid speaker for a company that funds his/her research. If successful recruitment of an adequate number of participants is crucial and an investigator has a financial investment that relies on the outcomes of a particular study, many different aspects of a study can be affected. Throughout the research process, from conceptualization of the problem, through dissemination of findings, a conflict of interest on the part of any investigator has the potential to influence:

* how potential participants are recruited (e.g., application of inclusion/exclusion criteria),
* how the informed consent process is implemented (e.g., subtle coercive techniques applied),
* how requests by participants to withdraw from a study are handled,
* how decisions are made about what data represents a true outlier,
* which findings are chosen for inclusion in a report, and
* timeliness of a published report.

Strategies for managing conflicts of interest at the individual level include: (1) institutional reviews for potential conflicts of interests for investigators and research staff (Federman, Hanna, & Rodriguez, 2003); (2) disallowing individuals who hold significant financial interest in research involving human subjects from conducting the research; and (3) promoting disclosure and transparency of financial interests (National Institutes of Health, 2002).

CONFLICTS OF INTEREST AT THE INSTITUTIONAL LEVEL

THERE is a clear expectation that institutions in which research is conducted will provide oversight of scientific activities and researchers by creating an ethical environment that promotes research integrity and discourages scientific misconduct (Rubenstein, 2002). Institutional conflicts of interest include relationships with agencies or industries that promote a real or perceived impression that could compromise the trust the public places in them as credible sources of information and protection of human subjects. These relationships can be engaged in by individuals at any administrative level and include deans, vice presidents, presidents, trustees, and others who are thought to "represent the institution."

Every institution should have a written policy and procedures that address conflict of interest on both the part of the individual investigator and the institution. This policy should include:

* offering educational opportunities to all employees engaged in research about research integrity;

* providing for external review of arrangements or relationships that could represent a potential compromise or conflict of interest;
* having procedures to oversee the commitments of those involved in the conduct, design, and review of research, including all levels of personnel such as research assistants, principal investigators, students, and administrators;
* listing acceptable activities and financial relationships and those that require review;
* having a plan to evaluate the ethical climate of the institutional environment and monitor compliance of individuals equitably; and
* implementing procedures that guide investigations of allegations of scientific misconduct or potential conflict of interest (Rubenstein, 2002).

The ethical climate of an institution is thought to be one predictor of the strength of research integrity held by the investigators who conduct science and the administrators and trustees of the organization itself (Gaddis, Healon-Fauth, & Scott, 2003). Development of educational venues and policies and procedures about conflict of interest are primary responsibilities of an institution. Monitoring conflict of interest is the responsibility of all individuals involved in research. An ethical climate that promotes research integrity will help assure that the public's trust is maintained in the credibility of research findings and those who conduct research.

MARION E. BROOME

REFERENCES

National Institutes of Health. (2002). *Conflict of interest workshop summary*. Retrieved October 10, 2006, from http://www.grants.nih.gov/grants/policy/coi/COIworkshopsum.doc

Federman, D. D., Hanna, K., & Rodriguez, L. (2003). *Responsible research: A systems approach to protecting research participants*. Washington, DC: National Academies Press.

Gaddis, B., Helton-Fauth, W., & Scott, G. (2003). Development of two measures of climate for scientific organizations. *Accountability in Research, 10*, 253–288.

Rubenstein, A. (on behalf of the Committee on Assessing Integrity in Research Environments). (2002). *Integrity in scientific research*. Washington, DC: National Academies Press.

Consultation

NURSES ARE ALL CONSULTANTS. There are many different types of consultants, both internal and external, but nurses are consulting every time they try to make a change or make something better, but without real control over the implementation of the changes. If you are advising or teaching, but have little control over the process of implementation, you are consulting. If you *do* have control over the implementation, you are managing. So, in the broadest sense of consultation, nurses are routinely involved in advising and consulting. Consultants are in a position of having little direct control or authority to implement recommendations and this can be a very frustrating position in which to be. The challenges of consulting are to have leverage and impact that will enable the consultant's advice and expertise to be utilized and to enable recommendations to be implemented and make a difference. I believe that nurses make good consultants and the profession is improved by their expertise.

The *Merriam-Webster Desk Dictionary* (McKechnie, 1995, p. 118) defines consultation as "the process of utilizing an expert for professional or technical advice or opinions." An expert is further defined as someone who is very "skilled; having much training and knowledge in a special field." Although it can be debated what makes an expert and what knowledge is needed, in general, nurses who function as consultants have an area of expertise that is valued and needed by others. The role of the consultant is to transfer knowledge, be a trainer or problem solver, or enable others to better accomplish their role or ensure the needed results. Broadly, consulting can cover many functions. Nurses who teach patients, advise other employees, or have staff roles in the organization are internal consultants. They offer expertise and advice to others but usually do not have the positional power to make sure something is done. That is the role of the manager. Organizations today have many staff roles that support specific areas, and the nurses in these roles are in effect consulting to bring a level of expertise and advice that is needed. Outside consultants are experts who are not employed by the organization and are invited in to provide expertise and advice in areas where the organization does not have internal expertise. It is increasingly common that health care organizations cannot afford to employ someone with niche knowledge on a full-time basis. So it is appropriate to be able to contract with those experts on an "as needed" basis.

INTERNAL CONSULTATION

INTERNAL consultation takes place everyday in organizations. As an internal consultant, you have a job in the organization and need to juggle respect for and challenge of the status quo. You must work through the line manager to get things done so all of the organization's managerial, clinical, and political issues may come into play. You are, in effect, expected to "sell your solutions" so that they are implemented and make a difference. And, in some ways, it is more difficult to be "a prophet in your own land," so getting changes adopted may be frustrating and challenging. As health care organizations rapidly add more complex technology and major clinical information systems, the number of internal consultants will undoubtedly increase.

EXTERNAL CONSULTATION

CONSULTATION is considered "external" if the advisors are not employed by the organization and bring expertise into the organization on a contractual basis. External consultants can be solo consultants or employees of a consulting firm. Nurse consultants are employed in a variety of companies that focus on managerial consultation, clinical consultation, financial consultation, or technology consultation. Additionally, there are many niche companies that focus on a narrower spectrum of health care, such as case management or recruitment. As you might imagine the variety of consulting opportunities for nurses is enormous, given the complexity of health care and nursing. For example, consultation associated with such areas as information systems often requires a nurse that has expertise in clinical delivery, technology, and change management in order to support major initiatives involved in implementing a new system.

External consultants are often viewed as a threat. That is because they are unknown to the staff and are by the nature of the consultation often involved in disruption to the status quo. External consultants spend time learning about the organization, understanding the issues surrounding the consultation, and soliciting information and knowledge from staff and managers. With what they learn about the organization and their own expertise and experience, they work to craft a plan to implement changes that will address the issues they were hired to solve. One of the advantages of external consultants is that because they are not a part of the formal organization, they have the freedom to think and act independently of the internal hierarchy. This independence in thinking enables them to honestly craft the best approaches to the situations that are under consultation. Because staff initially may be very wary of the questions that consultants ask, full information may not be conveyed or the nurses may be afraid to engage in the process itself. It is important to understand clearly the nature of the consultative process, the input needed from staff, and the expected outcomes. This clarity will go a long way toward facilitating the process and ensuring good results.

CONSULTATION PROCESSES IN NURSING

B ECAUSE of the complexity of nursing, there will always be a need for consulting expertise in organizations. Consultation in nursing generally focuses on areas of clinical, education, research, and administration/management. Although rarely is a consulting assignment purely in one area, it is usually mainly in one of the four. For instance, consultation may be used to determine the optimal model of care needed for defined patient populations. Or consultation may be used to facilitate research processes that will guide clinical innovation. Increasingly, consultants provide support to the installation of clinical technology and information systems. Whatever the need, it is possible to find experts in the field who are engaged in consulting. Internally, expert nurses such as educators, clinical nurse specialists, and advanced practice nurses are employed by the organization to support learning and practice on an ongoing basis. These experts typically have a reporting relationship to a manager of education and practice, but deliver consultation to nurses who are practicing in the delivery system. In this case, the expert nurses advise, teach, and support nurses but have no direct control or authority to implement. In seeing the value of their advice, the manager hopefully will follow through to be sure that changes are made and evaluated.

THE CONSULTATION PROCESS

THE consultation process is similar to the nursing process, beginning with discussions to clarify issues to be resolved. Who will be involved in defining the problems and framing the consultation? What methods of consultation will be utilized? And what kind of information and data will be necessary to support the decision making? Next, the data collection and problem diagnosis phase will typically involve a lot of people who will be interviewed, questioned, and observed to gather as much information as possible. The ability to efficiently gather data is a big determinant of how rapidly the project can be done. Collected data will need to be organized and reported in some fashion. The consultant will synthesize data into a manageable number of issues. The client will then be able to give feedback, think through potential resistance, and determine the most acceptable way to proceed with the project. Goals can be clearly set and action plans developed. Only after this important groundwork is laid can the project proceed. The last phase involves implementation and measurement of results. The consultant may or may not be involved in the implementation phase, which will be accomplished by the line organization under the direction of a director or manager. Because the actual changes are taking place, the plan and the process are continuously reviewed to ensure that desired outcomes are being met. This is also the time when there is a degree of anxiety in the organization and there may be resistance to change. Therefore, it is an imperative that measurement systems are in place to monitor progress and document results.

The process of consultation is clearly a commitment to find the best ways to build and start new plans, and may be conducted to improve existing processes or define and implement innovation. Whatever the impetus, it is the role of the consultant to support and facilitate the process in a way that brings expertise to the organization and streamlines the work to be accomplished. It is more than just another pair of hands. Rather, consultation involves melding expert knowledge with the strengths of the organization.

PREPARATION TO BECOME A CONSULTANT

A NURSE who is interested in becoming a consultant will need to develop an inventory of skills necessary to be successful. Although the skills may vary widely depending on the area of expertise, there are some basic skills that should be a part of every consultant's tool kit. First, there are skills and knowledge specific to one's discipline and in some cases clinical area of expertise, which should be well grounded in fact and current for the practice area. Second, skills specific to the processes and phases of the consultation must be developed, including negotiation skills, dealing with conflict, extensive analytical ability, presentation skills, and the ability to see things from many vantage points. In all situations, consultants must be able to act assertively, express support, listen and learn, confront issues, and manage group process. Most of these characteristics can be learned and mastered with experience. For the person who is introverted, developing a public persona and confidence may require experience and practice. By contrast, for the extrovert, learning to step back and listen may be the biggest challenge. Above all, a consultant must be authentic, genuine, and honest. Learning when to walk away from opportunities that may not fit one's skill set is an important lesson. No one can be an expert in everything so an honest assessment of skills and attributes is essential to build a portfolio of successful consultation.

Successful consultation is a complex blend of gaining an understanding of the client's need, outlining a process for the consultation, developing a budget, and designing a contract to guide the project. It is important to get the agreement of all parties to the consultation in writing so that it is clear what the deliverables will be so that all expectations are met. It is common during consultations to have the scope of the project expand. This will require an addendum to the original contract. Consultation is a serious endeavor and should be guided by clear and achievable goals and contractual agreements. The business skills of developing work plans and contracts can be learned from a variety of sources including written guidance, other experienced consultants, or lawyers.

In summary, consultation is a fascinating career path for nurses, which expands with expertise in one's field. As an early career pathway, it is possible to receive extensive training in tools and methodologies as a member of a consulting firm. Regardless of the route, the trip is always fascinating and challenging. Whether consulting internally or externally arriving at recommendations is much the same and includes a carefully crafted set of activities that define needs, determine approaches, provide data support, and develop implementation plans. The discipline of project management will help any initiative to come in on time, on budget, and with good results.

KATHERINE VESTAL

REFERENCES

Block, P. (1981). *Flawless consulting*. San Diego, CA: Pfeiffer & Company.

McKechnie, J. (Ed.). (1995). *Merrian-Webster desk dictionary*. New York: Simon and Schuster.

Norwood, S. (1998). Making consultation work. *Journal of Nursing Administration, 28*(3), 44–47.

Smeltzer, C., & Hope, C. (2002). Can I be a healthcare consultant? *Journal of Nursing Administration, 32*(1), 12–14.

Wong, L. (2000). *The Harvard Business School guide to careers in management consulting*. Boston: HBR Press.

Consumer Satisfaction

CONSUMER SATISFACTION is key to the financial success of any marketing enterprise, regardless of profit or nonprofit status, religious or secular affiliation, and regardless of the product, whether it is automobiles, computers, cosmetics or hair products, toiletries, or health care. Given the competitive nature of health care facilities over the last 30 years or so, it is imperative that these organizations concentrate on quality improvement strategies that will "capture" a certain population needing health care services, and will concomitantly lead to a high level of consumer satisfaction. Administrators or administrative teams (including the Chief Nursing Officer) have a dual responsibility: employee satisfaction and consumer satisfaction. Consumers are more likely to respond favorably to employees who enjoy what they are doing, and they are more likely to return for additional services. Dissatisfied employees will more than likely cause dissatisfaction among consumers (Neff, 2002).

Consumer satisfaction can be determined in a number of ways:

* *Face-to-face interviews*: this is particularly effective when the consumer has registered a complaint

* *Questionnaires*: to be completed either while the consumer is still on the premises, or by mail, to be returned at the consumer's convenience
* *Critical Incident*: "What did you like best about your service?" "What did you like least about your service?"
* *Telephone interviews* to ascertain service satisfaction
* *Consumer surveys*: surveying the community at large, whether or not they have sought or received services at a given institution.

Stopper (2004) asserts that trusting the people you work for, having pride in what you do, and enjoying the people you work with has a positive effect on employee morale and results in a high level of client satisfaction.

M. JANICE NELSON

See Also
Employee Satisfaction

REFERENCES

Neff, T. M. (2002). What successful companies know that law firms need to know: The importance of employee motivation and job satisfaction to increased productivity and stronger client relationships. *Journal of Law & Health, 17*(2), 385ff.

Stopper, W. G. (2004). Creating a great place to work [R]—Lessons from the "100 Best." *Human Resources Planning, 27*(2), 20ff.

Continuing Professional Education

CONTINUING PROFESSIONAL EDUCATION (CPE) in its most general definition is education intended for adult learners, especially for those beyond traditional undergraduate college or university age. Typically in the United States, CPE can involve enrollment in college/university credit-granting courses, often by students enrolled part-time, and is offered through a division or school of continuing education of a college/university. It also means "courses, programs, or organized learning experiences usually taken after a degree is obtained to enhance personal or professional goals" (http://www.oln. org/student_services/definitions.php).

Continuing Professional Education is a category that indicates a collection of courses for completion of a specialized program of study. The continuing education category includes for-credit programs of study (awarding a specific number of college/university credits), Continuing Education Units (CEU), and the broader noncredit program of study commonly known as Continuing Professional Education (http://www.iseek.org/static/awards.htm). Rapid changes and increasing complexity in health care have increased the challenges in nursing education. According to Williams (2004), the rapid changes in health care, diminished life span of useful information, and increasing complexity of practice make it essential that nurses maintain competence by continuing to learn throughout their careers (Williams, 2004, p. 277). Nurses are constantly challenged to update old knowledge as well as gain new knowledge.

The adult learning model is based on assumptions such as the following: adult "need to know," learner self-concept, the role of learner's experiences, readiness to learn, orientation to learning, and motivation (Knowles, Holton, & Swanson, 1998). Before undertaking something new, adults need to know why it has to be done. This is one source of motivation: to learn aside from other internal motivators, such as self-esteem, job satisfaction, quality of life, and external motivators that include job-mandated education and financial incentives. This makes CPE very important, not only in nursing but in other disciplines as well.

JUDY L. VALLARELLI

REFERENCES

Knowles, M. S., Holton, E. F., & Swanson, R. A. (1998). *The adult learner: The definitive classic in adult education and human resource development*. Woburn, MA: Butterworth-Heinemann.

Williams, B. (2004). Self direction in a problem based learning program. *Nurse Education Today, 24*(4), 277–285.

WEB REFERENCES

Ohio Learning Network, www.oln.org/student_services/definitions.php
ISEEK, www.iseek.org/static/awards.htm

Continuous Quality Improvement

QUALITY AND SAFETY are major foci in health care today and are important not only professionally for nursing, but strategically important for institutions (Reinertsen, 2006). Quality has taken on a renewed and intense focus following reports such as "To Err is Human," "Crossing the Quality Chasm," and, most recently, "Preventing Medication Errors" (Institute of Medicine, 2001, 2006; Kohn, Corrigan, & Donaldson, 1999). Today, terms such as continuous quality improvement (CQI), total quality management (TQM), and performance improvement (PI) are used to describe a process and common thread, regardless of the name, which is to improve the care and outcomes of patients. Parenthetically, it should be noted that higher education in nursing has taken a similar path with CQI (see Yearwood, Singleton, Feldman, & Colombraro, 2001). The movement from quality assurance (QA) to CQI in the clinical setting represents a complete paradigmatic shift and significant cultural change for healthcare organizations. Traditional QA focused on individuals, using a reactive process that evaluated issues retrospectively to prevent their reoccurrence. Quality assurance decisions often were based on assumptions of causes; therefore, solutions potentially would not completely resolve problems and issues recurred. Often, substandard

QA data resulted in disciplinary means and blamed human error for noncompliance (Al-Assaf, 2005). In contrast, CQI mandates a top-down promulgation of quality and a cultural change for the organization. Continuous quality improvement focuses on processes and systems of care, not individuals, requiring a multidisciplinary approach and focusing on all aspects of patient care related to both process and outcome. Continuous quality improvement requires the health care organization to constantly evaluate and revise processes to better meet the needs of patients and stakeholders.

CONTINUOUS QUALITY IMPROVEMENT IN NURSING

NURSING has long been involved in CQI initiatives, reporting not only to evaluate specific nursing practice, but also to evaluate patient care in the broader context. Nursing has specific indicators which are monitored; examples include the National Database for Nursing Quality Indicators (NDNQI), Veterans Administration Nursing Outcomes Database, National Voluntary Consensus Standards for Nursing-Sensitive Care (JCAHO), and Transforming Care at the Bedside (Institute for Healthcare Improvement and Robert Wood Johnson Foundation). In 2006, the National Quality Forum (NQF) released the NQF-endorsed™ National Voluntary Consensus Standards for Nursing–Sensitive Care (National Quality Forum, 2006). These include 15 "nursing sensitive" measures of processes and outcomes that are affected, provided, or influenced by nursing personnel—but for which nursing is not exclusively responsible.

FUTURE TRENDS

CQI combines quality improvement initiatives involving multiple disciplines with evidence-based practice to provide the best possible care for patients (Baker, 2006). Nursing will play an important role in four key trends that will shape quality and safety: (1) transparency; (2) 100K Lives Campaign and standards of care; (3) pay for performance/pay for reporting; and (4) patient centeredness and coordination of care (Reinertsen, 2006). Transparency in health care quality is just beginning and will become more common as hospitals strive to distinguish themselves in this era of health care business coalitions, health care savings accounts, and consumer-directed plans. In addition, an institution's quality performance is now visible not only internally and to specific accrediting or regulating agencies but widely available to the public. One example of transparency is quality data on the Centers for Medicare and Medicaid Services' core measures. These data are available on the Hospital Compare Web site and include not only process and outcome measures for specific conditions but include patient satisfaction data as well (U.S. Department of Health and Human Services, 2005). Also, as institutions begin to publish or share their quality information through various media (e.g., Web sites), it is essential that information and data are clearly described, simple to understand, and truly useful to patients and the public in decision making.

A second trend is the development of extensive quality initiatives nationally and internationally. In 2005, more than 2,600 health care organizations and associations joined together to reduce 100,000 hospital deaths (100K Lives Campaign) by mid-June 2006. The 100K Lives Campaign was successful in meeting this goal and is ongoing (Institute for Healthcare Improvement, 2006). This unique program is committed to implementing six evidence-based practices in the hospital setting and other initiatives will be added. This program has been widely publicized and is successful. It requires hospitals to join together and accelerate the pace at which evidence-based practices in quality and safety are implemented (Reinertsen, 2006). Pay for performance or pay for reporting in quality has received much attention. The number of quality indicators which institutions are required to monitor either voluntarily or via requirements is increasing at a frenetic pace and these external pressures continue to grow. Examples of organizations with quality indicators include: The Centers for Medicare and Medicaid Services (CMS), Agency for Healthcare Research and Quality (AHRQ), accrediting agencies (Joint Commission of Accreditation of Hospital Organizations-JCAHO; National Committee on Quality Assurance-NCQA), purchasers of care, coalitions (The Leapfrog Group), and private organizations (National Quality Forum). The fourth trend is a focus on patient-centered systems of care versus patient-centered individual care. Institutions will focus on the entire episode of care across all settings, especially with chronic diseases. No longer will the accountability for quality processes and outcomes be focused in one setting (e.g., hospital), but will focus on the coordination of care across the continuum of care.

Nursing leadership plays a key role in the successful development and implementation of programs related to quality and safety. Nursing has an in-depth understanding of systems and the ability to lead teams and bring together multiple stakeholders toward a common goal. Essentials of nursing leadership in quality include knowledge of CQI techniques, current knowledge of external organizations driving the quality reporting agenda nationally, benchmarking techniques, and knowledge of health information technology. Nursing education must also be involved in this process. It is crucial that undergraduate and especially graduate programs in nursing incorporate information on CQI and a working knowledge of the national agenda related to health care quality.

JO ANN BROOKS

See Also
Agency for Healthcare Research and Quality
National Quality Forum
The Leapfrog Group

REFERENCES

Al-Assaf, A. (2005). Organizational quality infrastructure: How does an organization staff quality? In S. B. Ransom, M. S. Joshi, & D. B. Nash (Eds.), *The healthcare quality book*. Chicago: Health Administration Press and Washington, DC: AUPHA Press.

Baker, G. R. (2006). Strengthening the contribution of quality improvement research to evidence based health care. *Quality and Safety in Health Care, 15*, 150–151.

Institute for Healthcare Improvement. (2006). *100K lives campaign*. Retrieved August 18, 2006, from http://www.ihi.org

Institute of Medicine. (2001). *Crossing the quality chasm: A new health system for the 21st century*. Washington, DC: National Academies Press.

Institute of Medicine. (2006). *Preventing medication errors*. Washington, DC: National Academies Press.

Kohn, L. T., Corrigan, J. M., & Donaldson, M. S. (Eds.). (1999). *To err is human: Building a safer health system*. Washington, DC: National Academies Press.

National Quality Forum. (2006). *National quality forum: Nursing care quality at NQF*. Retrieved August 18, 2006, from http://www.qualityforum.org/nursing/default.htm

Reinertsen, J. L. (2006). Quality and safety: Quality is now strategic. *Futurescan: Healthcare trends and implications 2006–2011* (pp. 20–24). Chicago: Health Administration Press.

U.S. Department of Health and Human Services. (2005). *Hospital compare*. Retrieved August 13, 2007, from www.hospitalcompare.hhs.gov

Yearwood, E., Singleton, J., Feldman, H. R., & Colombraro, G. (2001). A case study in implementing CQI in a nursing education program. *Journal of Professional Nursing, 17*, 297–304.

WEB REFERENCES

Institute for Healthcare Improvement, http://www.ihi.org
Hospital Quality Alliance, http://www.hospitalcompare.hhs.sgov

National Quality Forum, http://www.qualityforum.org
National Database of Nursing Quality Indicators, http://www.nursingworld.org/
    quality/database.htm
The Leapfrog Group, http://www.leapfroggroup.org

Council of the Advancement of Nursing Science

THE COUNCIL OF THE ADVANCEMENT OF NURSING SCIENCE (CANS) was officially launched in 2000 as an open membership group of the American Academy of Nursing. The mission of the Council is *Better Health Through Nursing Science*. The aims of the Council are to: (1) be a strong voice of nurse scientists at the national, and international levels that supports the development, conduct, and utilization of nursing science; (2) share research findings with individuals, communities, institutions, and industry; and (3) facilitate lifelong learning opportunities for nurse scientists (http://www.nursingscience.org/). The need to establish a national body of nurse scientists was recognized by the American Academy of Nursing's (AAN) Board of Directors in 1997 since the American Nurses Association had disbanded its Council of Nurse Researchers several years earlier. It took several task forces and meetings of Academy members to formulate a proposal to establish CANS that met the concerns of Academy members. Academy members were also leaders in other national or regional nursing research societies and there was concern for the duplication and potential competition among these groups. Significant energy was expended to be as inclusive as possible in the conceptualization, implementation, and structure of CANS.

150

The Nursing Research Roundtable that meets informally, cohosted by the National Institute of Nursing Research and other nursing organizations with interest in the development and support of nursing research, discussed the development of CANS as well. CANS' initial steering committee was comprised of the presidents of the four regional nursing research associations (Eastern Nursing Research Society, Midwest Nursing Research Society, Southern Nursing Research Society, and the Western Institute of Nursing), a representative from Sigma Theta Tau International, representatives of the American Nurses Foundation and several specialty organizations, along with AAN. The leadership at the National Institute of Nursing Research (NINR) strongly supported the concept of establishing a national representative group that could support nursing science independent of NIH.

After several years of collaborative planning, CANS took on responsibility for the biennial *State of the Science in Nursing Research* meeting, usually held in Washington, DC. In addition, CANS sponsors one national program during the off year from the State of the Science meeting focusing on topics relevant to building capacity in nursing science. CANS has active individual membership that is open to all scientists who support its mission. Additional information about the history of CANS, current members of the Steering Committee, and ongoing programs can be found at the CANS Web site (http://nursingscience.org).

WILLIAM L. HOLZEMER

See Also
American Academy of Nursing

Credentialing

CREDENTIALING is a process through which registered nurses who have developed expertise in a particular specialty have this specialized knowledge base acknowledged. One such mechanism is certification, "the formal recognition of specialized knowledge, skills, and experience demonstrated by the achievement of standards identified by a nursing specialty to promote optimal health outcomes" (American Board of Nursing Specialties, 2000). In order to become certified by the American Nurses Credentialing Center (ANCC) (http://nursingworld.org/ancc/) or one of the specialty nursing organizations (SNOs) offering such a process, the nurse usually has to submit a professional portfolio demonstrating applicable education, years of work experience, a nursing license, references, and evidence of successful completion of the organization's certification examination. Certifications are usually renewed every 5 years by completion of continuing education requirements or submission of professional accomplishments and/or additional examination. According to ANCC, certification does not confer a protected, legal scope of practice but does aid the public by identifying competent nurses within a nursing specialty (ANCC, 2003). Additionally, certification recognizes professional achievement within the profession, in the workplace, and among one's peers and enhances professionalism; in some federal and state statutes such as the federal Balanced Budget Act of 1996 credentialing serves as a criterion for third-party reimbursement of the nurse specialist's practice.

KAREN A. BALLARD

See Also
Certification

REFERENCES

American Board of Nursing Specialties. (2000). *Fact sheet*. Retrieved September 16, 2006, from www.nursingcertification.org/

American Nurses Credentialing Center. (2003). *ANCC certification: Opening a world of opportunities*. Retrieved September 16, 2006, from www.nursingworld.org/ancc/cert/

Cultural Diversity

THERE IS ABUNDANT evidence that both the public and private sectors of this country are struggling with issues of diversity, which brings the challenge of balancing anxiety and opportunity. Abraham Maslow's work is being confirmed once again. We are a country obsessed with safety whether it's about protecting our borders or patient safety. In health care, diversity is a complex issue because it has so many facets. It is a social issue. The societal trends and a rapidly changing demographic picture make it virtually impossible to ignore. In 1900, one in eight Americans were nonwhite; today, this nation is one in four. By 2050, one in three Americans will be African American, Hispanic, Native American or Asian/Pacific Islander (Institute of Medicine, 2004). In California, Hawaii, New Mexico, and the District of Columbia, minority groups already make up more than half the population. And Hispanics now surpass African Americans as the largest minority group in the United States. According to the National Institutes on Health, "the diversity of the American population is one of the nation's greatest assets; one of its greatest challenges is reducing the profound disparity in health status of American's racial and ethnic minorities" (Smedley & Stith, 2002).

It is a legislative issue. The Civil Rights Act of 1964 was signed into law on July 2, 1964. This legislation was intended to ensure that the financial resources of the federal government would no longer subsidize racial discrimination (Smith, 1999). Every recipient of federal funds is required to provide written assurances that nondiscrimination is practiced throughout the entire institution and protections for individuals that speak English as a second language are also provided. Nearly one in five people over 5 years of age speak a language other than English at home.

It is a care delivery issue, a care provider issue, and a health care system issue. Nursing is still predominantly comprised of white females and so are faculty that prepare future nursing care providers. In the examination room, four cultures intersect: the cultures of the patient, clinician, organization, and the United States. As defined by Office of Minority Health (OMH), "Cultural and linguistic competence is the ability of health care providers and health care organizations to understand and respond effectively to the cultural and linguistic need brought by patients to the health care encounter" (http://www.omhrc.gov/clas/finalpo.htm). In pursuit of this aim, in December 2000 OMH published the National Standards for Culturally and Linguistically Appropriate Services (CLAS). Currently large inconsistencies exist, for those in the majority and those who comprise the minority members of the population, in the ability of the United States to provide access to high-quality health care, to communicate to its citizens the risks and mitigation strategies concerning bioterrorism, and to provide the same degree of education for all.

It is a patient-driven issue and, although not acknowledged in the literature, a patient safety issue. Every patient encounter is a cultural encounter and therefore a significant encounter. The presence and absence of nurses impacts the care patients received and the ability to be the surveillance system that health care systems rely upon to know and sense the need to rescue. It stands to reason that being culturally appropriate and relevant is necessary for that surveillance system to function properly for all. Diversity, holding multiple perspectives without judgment, is not the crux of the issue. It is the judgment based on the value systems and norms of those who by number are in the majority and, because of numbers, have the power to define what is considered to be different. So what difference does difference make? In terms of cultural diversity and patient care, a great deal. Nurses have an obligation to fulfill their social contracts with society and, above all, do no harm to those in their care.

G. RUMAY ALEXANDER

REFERENCES

Institute of Medicine. (2004). *In the nation's compelling interest: Ensuring diversity in the health care workforce.* Washington, DC: National Academies Press.

Office of Minority Health. (2000). *Assuring cultural competence in health care: Recommendations for national standards and an outcomes-focused research agenda.* Retrieved November 10, 2006, from http://www.omhrc.gov/clas/finalpo.htm

Smedley, B. D., & Stith, A. Y. (2002). *Unequal treatment, confronting racial and ethnic disparities in health care.* Washington, DC: National Academies Press.

Smith, D. B. (1999). *Health care divided: Race and healing a nation.* Ann Arbor: University of Michigan Press.

D

Delegation

DELEGATION IS AN essential skill, process, and art, learned by nurses, managers, and leaders. In today's world of nursing practice, management, and leadership, delegation is a necessity. Although definitions of delegation may differ, the purpose of delegation remains constant, to get the work done efficiently. The nurse, manager, and leader do this through others by directing the work or performance of others to accomplish patient or organizational goals. The American Nurses Association (ANA) defines delegation as transferring responsibility of performing a task from one person to another. The National Council of State Boards of Nursing (NCSBN) specifies that delegation is transferring authority to a competent person to perform a select nursing task in a select situation. The NCSBN further describes steps in the process of delegation, which include: (1) identifying the task to be done; (2) selecting the most capable/competent person; (3) using clear communication of the goals and purpose of the task; (4) establishing a time frame for task completion; (5) monitoring the progress of the job; (6) providing guidance; and (7) assessing the performance and accomplishment of the goal or task.

Key components of delegation are *legal liability or accountability, responsibility, and authority*. In direct patient care a registered nurse (RN) is liable for his/her actions and must be cognizant of the state nurse practice act, standards of practice, organizational policies, and legal-ethical behaviors. Generally, acceptable delegated tasks fall within the implementation phase of the nursing process. The RN may not delegate the other phases of the nursing process involved in direct patient care, for example, assessing, analyzing, diagnosing, teaching, and evaluating. Nurses may delegate tasks that do not involve direct patient care which may carry fewer legal risks. Delegation involves responsibility and the duty for the person accepting the task to follow through and accomplish the task at an appropriate level. The person who the nurse has delegated the task to must have an appropriate level of education and skill or training to assume the task.

Several factors and contexts influence the delegation of authority. In patient care, the state nurse practice act gives the RN the authority to delegate. In organizations, managers and leaders have legitimate authority to direct personnel and anticipate compliance. Nurses in direct patient care, management, and leadership positions may transfer responsibility and authority for the delegated task; however, each retains accountability for the process. Because many organizations utilize unlicensed assistive personnel (UAP) such as nurses' aides, orderlies, and technicians, it behooves the nurse-leader to be cognizant of the state nurse practice act, job description, knowledge and training, and skill level of each UAP before delegating.

Errors and pitfalls in delegation can occur particularly when the manager or leader is in a new position. The most common errors include overdelegation, underdelegation, and improper delegation. Overdelegating often occurs when time management skills are poorly developed in an individual or when one is insecure in his/her own ability to perform a task. Underdelegation can occur when a leader-manager lacks trust in subordinates' ability, may assume their subordinates will resent or feel overburdened with delegated work, or thinks that delegation connotes weakness and inability to get the work done. Improper delegation is delegating to the wrong person, or at the wrong time, or for the wrong reason, or delegating beyond the capability of a person.

Last, delegation is highly impacted by cultural diversity. Poole, Davidhizar, and Giger (1995) identify six cultural phenomena to consider when delegating: *communication, space, social organization, time, environmental control, and biological variations*. These can potentially affect the process and outcome of delegation because a select culture may have differing expectations concerning these behaviors or values. *Communication* refers to dialect, volume, eye contact, and touch. Interpersonal *space* differs between cultures. *Social organization*, particularly the family unit, is of greatest importance in some cultures. Cultures tend to be past-, present-, or future-oriented to *time*. Cultural groups have internal or external locus of control or *environmental control*. *Biological variations* such as susceptibility to disease and physical stamina or physical differences, for example, size, should be considered when delegating.

MARTHA J. GREENBERG

See Also
American Nurses Association
Cultural Diversity
The National Council of State Boards of Nursing, Inc. (NCSBN)

REFERENCE

Poole, V. L., Davidhizar, R. E., & Giger, J. N. (1995). Delegating to a transcultural team. *Nursing Management, 26*(8), 33–34.

WEB REFERENCES

American Nurses Association (ANA), http://www.nursingworld.org
National Council of State Boards of Nursing (NCSBN), http://www.ncsbn.org

Differentiated Nursing Practice

THE TERM "differentiated practice" is one that entered the nursing lexicon during the time that associate degree preparation for the registered nurse (RN) license came into being. At that time, the thinking was that professional practice would be within the realm of the nurse prepared at the baccalaureate degree level and the new associate degree graduates along with their colleagues prepared in hospital diploma programs would practice as "technical" nurses. Since the middle of the 20th century, then, there has been interest in developing models of care delivery that differentiate care and responsibilities based on the educational differences of the practitioners involved. It should be noted that the terms "professional" and "technical" are no longer the labels used in the 21st century for such differentiation discussions.

There has never been a successful and lasting model of differentiation implemented in spite of many discussions. There are several likely causes for this failure. First and probably foremost, there has always been an uneven distribution of graduates from the several programs. Although hospital diploma schools have all but disappeared, associate degree programs have been established in most geographical areas and provide a consistent supply of nurses to their respective communities;

162

by contrast, baccalaureate programs are less available, particularly in certain areas of the country, and, therefore, cannot produce the number of graduates necessary for health care organizations to adequately fill the differentiated roles that they might wish to create. Second and equally important is the fact that patients/clients do not tend to emit their needs in neat bundles that are labeled as requiring the presence of either the Bachelor of Science in Nursing (BSN) or the Associate Degree in Nursing (ADN) prepared nurse at any given time. Rather, they generally have needs that are emitted in "... muddled, unsorted and quite unpredictable bundles ..." (McClure, 1976), making suitable staffing plans for differentiated models all but impossible. Third, and perhaps least important, the profession made the decision to license the graduates of the differentiated educational programs with identical credentials. Although to some this may seem like a technicality, it has contributed to the view that there is, in fact, a registered nurse practice that is similar enough for all of these populations in most respects to make any differentiation almost an academic exercise.

Because of this, there has been very little movement toward the creation of differentiated practice models. South Dakota during the 1980s, attempted one effort worth noting. They created a large demonstration project over several years and involved intense work between a major health care provider and several nursing education programs (Koerner & Karpiuk, 1994). Other smaller efforts also have proven unsuccessful and this record of accomplishment, coupled with predicted nursing shortages, will undoubtedly make the pursuit of differentiated models less attractive in the years to come.

MARGARET L. MCCLURE

REFERENCES

American Association of Colleges of Nursing, American Organization of Nurse Executives & National Organization for Associate Degree Nursing. (1995). *A model for differentiated nursing practice.* Washington, DC: American Association of Colleges of Nursing.

Koerner, J., & Karpiuk, K. L. (1994). *Implementing differentiated practice: Transformation by design.* Gaithersburg, MD: Aspen.

McClure, M. L. (1976). Entry into professional practice: The New York proposal. *Journal of Nursing Administration, 6*(5), 12–17.

Disaster Nursing and Emergency Preparedness

T HE UBIQUITOUS THREAT of terrorism combined with the dramatic increase in the frequency and intensity of natural disasters in recent years has reinforced disaster response and emergency preparedness as critical components of our health care system, with significant implications for the profession of nursing. Hurricane Katrina in 2005 was a catastrophic disaster whose scope and destruction overwhelmed state and local first responders, and ultimately the federal disaster response system as well. A heroic effort on the part of many saved hundreds of lives, but the event was a decisive condemnation of our national lack of preparedness.

In the event of a major disaster or public health emergency, America's nurses will comprise a significant percentage of the responding workforce. Yet nurses remain underprepared and grossly underrepresented in positions of power with respect to disaster planning at the major federal agencies, and often at the state planning level as well. Nursing workforce preparedness, current state and national disaster response plans, as well as public confidence in these plans are based on several erroneous assumptions. First, these plans assume that we will have a sufficient number of nurses available to respond. Given the severity of the nursing shortage and the current state of emergency department overcrowding, this seems highly unlikely. The second assumption, that all of our nation's nurses have been exposed to, through education and training, and currently possess the knowledge base and skill set required to respond to these unique types of events, particularly those involving the use of weapons of mass destruction or catastrophic natural disasters is erroneous. Finally, these plans assume that nurses will be both available and willing to respond to any type of public health emergency.

Although there were multiple initiatives established between 2000 and 2006 to increase overall national preparedness (e.g., surge capacity plans and increased electronic surveillance), limited attention has been paid to addressing the issue of workforce readiness. There have not been systematic efforts to address *preparing nurses to respond appropriately to a major terrorist or public health event*. In the event of a disaster or any major public health emergency, will nurses be adequately prepared to recognize that an event has occurred and to respond to it? Will we be able to triage and mobilize nurses to areas of need? Do we have the policies in place to ensure nurses' safety in responding to chemical and radiological emergencies? Nurse executives and other health care administrators openly acknowledge the deficits in nursing education and training programs with regard to this content and the absence of national standards for disaster nursing care. Most important, how will we address the issues related to emergently expanding practice parameters and accommodate altered standards for nursing care during disaster events? There is an urgent need to take ownership as a profession of these issues and their possible solutions.

Federal U.S. agencies such as the Department of Homeland Security, Office of Public Health Emergency Preparedness, and the Federal Emergency Management Agency (FEMA), along with the leading national nursing organizations, have called for the development of *a national nursing workforce that is adequately prepared to respond to any disaster or public health emergency*. Much work remains to be done to achieve this goal. Nurses must continue to define their roles across the disaster continuum and across many diverse types of organizations. There must be safe and supportive work environments created. Disaster nursing requires new strategies and interventions in order for nurses to render care in non-traditional care settings to potentially large numbers of patients while under great stress and with limited resources.

Nursing as a profession has a long history of being creative and visionary in its continuous efforts to meet the needs of patients and their families. Nursing leadership in tumultuous times, such as during the disaster continuum or at a mass casualty incident, also will require significant amounts of the same creativity and vision. When the opportunities and challenges of disaster management in the future are considered, the following arenas will require effective nursing leadership:

* Clearly articulated organizational roles and functions
* Crisis communications and control of the media
* Emergently expanded clinical practice parameters
* Allocation of scarce resources
* Protections surrounding altered standards for care
* Provision of competency-based education and training
* Disaster and public health policy development

Nurses need to seek leadership positions in *all types of health care and public health organizations* to assist with the design of disaster response plans and the development of future change in these organizations. In this capacity, nurses can serve as advocates for communities, and in particular for vulnerable populations such as infants and children, the elderly, the disabled, the mentally ill, and for the safety of other nurses in disaster response. Nurses also need to move into leadership positions in politics, public policy, civic administration, education administration, and emergency management systems. Nurses will have the executive competencies to be in these positions *if they prepare themselves to do so*. Preparation in all phases of disaster planning and management, health promotion, risk reduction, disease prevention, and illness and disease management, information and health care technologies, and human resource management will prepare nurses for such positions of leadership. Effective leadership in Disaster Management requires personal integrity, strength, flexibility, creativity, and the use of collaborative approaches.

TENER GOODWIN VEENEMA

WEB REFERENCES

American Nurses Association: Bioterrorism and Disaster Response
http://nursingworld.org/news/disaster/
American Red Cross: Disaster Nursing
http://www.redcross.org/services/nursing/0,1082,0_327_,00.html
Centers for Disease Control and Prevention: Emergency Preparedness
http://www.bt.cdc.gov/
Centers for Disease Control and Prevention: Crisis Communications Course
http://www.bt.cdc.gov/erc/cerc.asp
Department of Homeland Security: Preparedness & Response
http://www.dhs.gov/xprepresp/

Federal Emergency Management Agency (FEMA)
http://www.fema.gov/
Disaster Nursing and Emergency Preparedness for Chemical, Biological Radio-
    logical Terrorism and Other Hazards
http://www.springerpub.com/prod.aspx?prod_id=21438
National Response Plan
http://www.dhs.gov/xprepresp/committees/editorial_0566.shtm
National Strategy for Pandemic Influenza
http://www.dhs.gov/xprevprot/programs/editorial_0760.shtm

Dock, Lavinia Lloyd

AVINIA LLOYD DOCK, the ardent suffragette and political activist, was born in Harrisburg, Pennyslvania, in 1858; she died in April 1956. Dock graduated from the Bellevue Training School for Nurses in 1886 at 28 years of age. A contemporary of Robb, Nutting, Stewart, and Wald, Dock kept life interesting for this group of early American nursing leaders by insisting that nursing would never be accepted as a respectable profession until women "get the vote" (Christy, 1969)! Dock held a number of positions, including Assistant Superintendent of Nurses under the leadership of Robb at the Johns Hopkins Training School for Nurses in Baltimore. For a short time, she was Superintendent of Nurses at the Illinois Training School, and she worked with Wald at the Henry Street Settlement for some 20 years (American Association of the History of Nursing, 2006). Dock authored one of the first nursing textbooks, *Materia Medica for Nurses;* she served as the foreign editor for the *American Journal of Nursing*, and she authored the four volume *History of Nursing*, the first two volumes of which were coauthored with Nutting. Along with other nursing notables, Dock was one of the founders of the Society for Superintendents of Nursing (later to become the National League for Nursing Education). There is evidence to suggest her involvement with the founding and early days of the Nurses Associated Alumnae of United States and Canada (later known as the American Nurses Association); however, more evident is the 20 years she served as secretary to the International Council of Nurses. Although Dock maintained her ties with nursing, after the age of 50 she devoted most of her time to women's suffrage and political action. In an autobiographical sketch, Dock wrote that she was most satisfied with two events in her life, "... doing the history with Miss Nutting and going to jail with the Women's Party" (Dock, c. 1930). Dock was inducted into the American Nurses Association Hall of Fame in 1976.

M. JANICE NELSON

REFERENCES

American Association of the History of Nursing. (n.d.). *Gravesites of prominent nurses.* Retrieved March 22, 2006, from http://www.aahn.org/gravesites/dock.html

American Nurses Association. (2006). *1976 inductee: Lavinia Lloyd Dock, 1858–1956.* Retrieved March 22, 2006, from http://www.nursingworld.org/hof/dockll.htm

Christy, T. E. (1969). *Cornerstone for nursing education: A history of the division of nursing education of Teachers College, Columbia University, 1899–1947.* New York: Teachers College Press.

Dock, L. L. (c. 1930). Autobiographical sketch. *Lavinia L. Dock by Lavinia Lloyd Dock.* Typewritten manuscript. Archives of the Alumnae Association of the Bellevue School of Nursing, Inc. Veronica M. Driscoll Center for Nursing, Albany, NY.

Downs, Florence S.

A PROMINENT NATIONAL and international figure in nursing research, Florence Stimpson Downs was born in 1925 and died at the age of 80 in 2005. She graduated with a diploma in nursing from St. Luke's Hospital School of Nursing in New York City, and earned her baccalaureate in nursing from St. John's University in Brooklyn. She earned both the master's degree in Psychiatric Nursing and a doctorate in education at New York University—finishing in 1964. Throughout a 40-year academic career, Downs was responsible for formalization of the doctoral program in nursing at New York University. She subsequently moved to the School of Nursing of the University of Pennsylvania as Associate Dean of Graduate Studies where she developed both the Master's and doctoral programs. Downs assumed the editorship of the financially troubled *Journal for Nursing Research* in 1979 and maintained that position for 17 years, during which time she was successful in doubling the subscription rate (Meleis, 2005). Downs served as a curriculum consultant and a consultant in nursing research, both nationally and internationally. She authored some 50 articles, 9 books, and 81 editorials across the span of her career (University of Pennsylvania, 2005). She was designated a Living Legend in Nursing by the American Academy of Nursing in 2004.

M. JANICE NELSON

REFERENCES

Meleis, A. (2005). *Penn Nursing tribute to Dr. Florence Downs*. Retrieved March 29, 2006, from http://www.nursing.upenn.edu:8080blojsom/blog/meleis/2005/10/12/Penn_Nursing

New York University College of Nursing. (2005). *Obituary for Florence Downs*. Retrieved March 5, 2006, from http://www.nyu.edu/nursing/news/florencedowns.html

University of Pennsylvania. (2006). *Almanac: Deaths: Dr. Downs, Nursing*. Retrieved March 5, 2006, from http://www.upenn.edu/almanac/v52/n03/obit.html

E

Electronic Health Record

A**N ELECTRONIC HEALTH RECORD (EHR)** is not a universally defined term. In 2002, Englebardt and Nelson referred to an EHR as a computerized database used in health care to capture data about an individual or patient. In 2004, the Stark regulations (71 FR 45140) defined an EHR as a "repository of consumer health status information in computer processing form used for clinical diagnosis and treatment for a broad array of clinical conditions." Electronic health records can also refer to a system that pulls data together from multiple sources at a point of care. The Office of the National Coordinator for Health Information Technology (http://www.hhs.gov/healthit/) is in the process of supporting work to establish criteria for the function, interoperability, security, and privacy features essential to a certifiable EHR. Additional information about EHR certification can be found at http://www.CCHIT.org. It is also noted that there are no universal definitions for related terms such as electronic medical record computerized patient record (CPR) or computer health record (CHR). These terms can refer to systems with distinctive purpose, content, and functional differences. In many cases, present-day EHRs contain only patient demographics, and financial data and clinical documentation. Secure exchange of information between various providers, including radiologists, laboratories, and other clinicians, would allow for comprehensive information to be available at the point of care. Interest in a comprehensive EHR was generated in 1991 when the Institute of Medicine (IOM) released results of a study that reiterated the problems with a paper-based medical records system and advocated for the development and adoption of computer-based patient records throughout the United States.

BENEFITS

M ANY ORGANIZATIONS are introducing key components and functionality toward meeting the goal of a fully implemented EHR system. As implementations of EHRs become more widespread, evidence will develop as to the expected benefits of such systems as they relate to improved quality of care. The obvious benefits are a legible, organized, more complete patient record. Integrating and coordinating functions of the technology will decrease redundancy. Because the volume of clinical data required for clinical practice is far beyond what can be retained and used without support, computers can provide the powerful storage and information processing assistance that is needed for quality care. Computer-based systems improve access to patient data by multiple users at the same time and can be accessible from remote sites. Decision support tools such as reminders and alerts are safety measures that may ultimately benefit patients. EHRs also may support the development of innovative care models and processes. Despite these benefits, adoption and diffusion of EHRs has been slow. Efficiencies have been noted as a result of successful implementations of EHRs; however, systems that are improperly installed, inadequate, or underutilized generally do not produce the expected efficiencies or benefits.

KEY ISSUES

H UMAN-FACTORS RESEARCH has begun to uncover unintended consequences of computerization. The complexities of the technology that make up an EHR add to the concern that new types of errors are emerging. An extensive qualitative study conducted by Ash, Berg, and Coiera (2004) reported two categories of errors that occur with the use of electronic health care systems. They were identified as errors in data entry and retrieval and errors in communication and coordination. Data entry and retrieval errors occurred with outdated or complex human-computer interfaces that intensified the workload of an already busy clinician. Cognitive workload was increased by imposing clerical tasks, overly structured data entry requirements, and fragmented patient data retrieval formats. They also reported a mismatch between the linear processing of a computer and the interruptive nature of providing health care. This had a significant impact on communication and coordination of patient care. Decision support tools designed to prevent errors can have the opposite effect when misused or poorly designed. Too many alert messages can lead to overload and clinicians may ignore important warning messages. An inappropriate overreliance on these tools also may result. A poorly designed computer system may not reflect the reality of the care tasks or workflow causing the clinician to seek alternative approaches.

Issues of protection of privacy and maintaining the confidentiality of individually identified patient information are also a continuing concern. The Health Insurance Portability and Accountability Act (HIPAA) is the federal law that has established a foundation to address some aspects of the protection of privacy in electronic health records (Tang, 2000); however, there is still variability in the privacy laws across states. Another key issue with EHRs is related to the training required to use such systems; user instruction may not always be adequate to optimize patient privacy protections. In addition, many clinicians have not been exposed to the use of EHRs in their educational programs, which increases the learning curve for mastering use of such systems in the clinical practice environment.

STATE OF THE EVIDENCE

T HE MANAGEMENT OF MEDICAL ORDERS is considered the connective tissue in any EHR. Orders are necessarily complex and integrate patient-specific interventions across departments. Orders management in an EHR crosses customary boundaries and is just as likely to integrate applications and functions as it is to disintegrate traditions when new work processes are crafted. A synthesis of the research on electronic medical orders, referred to as computerized provider order entry (CPOE), notes that the term CPOE is used imprecisely in the literature, which limits our ability to translate the findings of research. CPOE can refer to electronic systems that do or do not include: the electronic transmission of orders to ancillary departments, the use of order sets, capabilities for complex intravenous, total parental nutrition (TPN) or oncology protocol orders, integrated alerts and reminders, pharmacy interfaces, or connections with clinical documentation (Hughes, 2006).

Implementation of an electronic health record as a means of reducing medical errors has received a lot of attention (Ash et al., 2004; Bates et al., 1999; Kohn, Corrigan, & Donaldson, 2000). Koppel and others (2005)

researched CPOE related factors that may increase the risk of medication errors and found that clinicians reported new errors with CPOE
because of fragmented data and processes, lack of integration among
systems, and human-computer interaction issues. Recommendations to
address these issues focus on providing communication and education to
providers and consumers, system designs that support communication
and clinical work processes, user participation in the implementation
and on-going monitoring of safety, and the use of qualitative multidisciplinary research methods to provide deeper insight into the benefits
and issues surrounding EHR (Ash & Bates, 2005; Ash et al., 2004). The
evidence from 23 studies that focused on efficiency, medication errors,
or quality suggests that transcription errors can be eliminated with electronic communication and interfaces and structured order entry. CPOE
can substantially reduce overall and many serious medication errors *if:* (a)
electronic communication and automatic order interfaces are in place, (b)
basic order checks for completeness are present, and (c) decision support
at its most basic level is available—interaction checking for drug/drug,
drug/allergy, and dosing ranges (Hughes, 2006).

NATIONAL INITIATIVES

T HE MAJOR CHALLENGES in health care including high costs, medical errors, variable quality, administrative inefficiencies, and lack
of coordination are all often connected to inadequate use of health information technology (HIT) as an integral part of health care (Thompson
& Brailer, 2004). In April 2004, President Bush issued an Executive Order calling for widespread adoption of interoperable electronic health
records within 10 years. The adoption of interoperable electronic health
records and a nationwide network for appropriate sharing of health information is envisioned as the means for realizing the vision of medical
information that follows the consumer across settings, of clinicians that
have complete, computerized patient information, of quality initiatives
that measure and drive performance, and of public health and bioterrorism surveillance that are seamlessly integrated into care. Within the context of a strategic framework, four goals were asserted for the HIT Decade,
each with specified strategies intended to contribute to the vision for improved health care. The goal of informing clinical practice is to improve
patient care, for example, reducing medical errors, and making health
care more efficient, including reducing duplicative work. Strategies here
include creating incentives for health care providers to adopt and implement electronic health records, decreasing the risk of investment, and
diffusing health information technology to rural and underserved areas. The goal of connecting clinicians focuses on creating interoperable

electronic health records so that data are more easily portable and can follow patients as they move through care settings. Strategies here include fostering regional collaborations, developing a nationwide health information network (NHIN), and coordinating federal health information systems. The goal of personalizing care focuses on assuring that individuals have tools and information to manage their own wellness. The strategies for this goal are to encourage the use of personal health records, enhance informed consumer choice, and promote the use of telehealth systems. Finally, the goal of improving population health includes the collection of timely, accurate clinical information that allows for evaluation of care, public health surveillance, clinical research, and feedback to clinicians. Strategies for this goal are to unify public health architectures, to streamline quality health status monitoring and to accelerate research and the dissemination of evidence (Thompson & Brailer, 2004).

NURSING IMPLICATIONS

T HE USE OF EHRs has the potential to improve quality, safety, and efficiency of care delivery. Further research is needed in the areas of nursing impacts in CPOE and EHR, human-computer interaction, and the science of implementation of such systems (Hughes, 2006). Nurses need to be aware of the specific functionality of EHRs that they use and provide diligent clinical and administrative monitoring if decision support and interfaces are not available in such systems. Because EHRs create professional interdependence, work design, roles, and communication changes need to be carefully analyzed. In addition, the design of such systems must be tailored for patient safety, and nurses need to play an important role in the development and implementation of the EHR to ensure success in health care settings. And, finally, it is critical for nurses to be informed and involved in national initiatives directed to improve the health and safety of the nation through the safe and appropriate application of the tools of our time.

CAROL A. ROMANO
CHARLOTTE SECKMAN

REFERENCES

Ash, J. S., & Bates, D. W. (2005). Factors and forces affecting EHR system adoption: Report of a 2004 ACMI discussion. *Journal of the American Medical Informatics Association, 12*(1), 8–12.

Ash, J. S., Berg, M., & Coiera, E. (2004). Patient care information system-related errors. *Journal of the American Medical Informatics Association, 11*(2), 104–112.

Bates, W. D., Teich, J. M., Lee, J., Seger, D., Kuperman, G. J., Ma'Luf, N., et al. (1999). The impact of computerized physician order entry on medication error prevention. *Journal of the American Medical Informatics Association, 6*(4), 313–321.

Dick, R. S., Steen, E. B., & Detmer, D. E. (Eds.). (1997). *The computer-based patient record: An essential technology for health care.* Washington, DC: National Academies Press.

Englebardt, S., & Nelson, R. (2002). *Health care informatics: An interdisciplinary approach.* St. Louis, MO: Mosby.

Hughes, R. G. (2006). *Patient safety and quality: An evidence-based handbook for nurses.* Rockville, MD: Agency for Healthcare Research and Quality.

Kohn, L. T., Corrigan, J. M., & Donaldson, M. S. (Eds.). (2000). *To err is human: Building a safer health system.* Washington, DC: Institute of Medicine.

Koppel, R., Metlay, J. P., Cohen, A., Abaluck, B., Localio, A., Kimmel, S. E., et al. (2005). Role of computerized physician order entry systems in facilitating medication errors. *Journal of the American Medical Association, 293*(10), 1197–1203.

Tang, P. C. (2000). The HIPAAcratic oath: Do no harm to patient data. *Physician Executive, 26*(3), 50–56. Retrieved July 31, 2006, from http://www.findarticles.com/p/articles/mi_m0843/is_3_26/ai_102450894

Thompson, T. G., & Brailer, D. J. (2004). *The decade of health information technology: Delivering consumer-centric and information-rich health care.* Washington, DC: U.S. Department of Health and Human Services.

Emotional Intelligence

EMOTIONAL INTELLIGENCE (EI) developed as a topic of scientific interest when Salovey and Mayer (1990) used the term to refer to people's ability to monitor emotions in themselves and others and then to use this information to guide actions. Rooted in the work of Edward Thorndike on social intelligence, the recent popularity of EI stems from writings of supporters who believe EI is important for personal and professional success, represents a component of effective leadership, and can be enhanced through training.

Although there is a growing consensus that EI contributes to success beyond what might be predicted by other established constructs, such as cognitive intelligence (e.g., IQ) and personality (e.g., extroversion), there is still debate about the extent to which EI contributes to success and the degree to which it can be enhanced.

There is considerable interest in three models of EI, that is, Salovey and Mayer (1990), Goleman (1995), and Bar-On (2000), and the measures of EI derived from these models (Cherniss, 2004). In 1996, the Consortium for Research on Emotional Intelligence in Organizations (CREIO) (http://www.eiconsortium.org/) was founded to advance research and practice related to EI in organizations. Their Web site provides information about recent EI research and offers a generic framework that identifies personal, for example, self-regulation, and social, for example, social skills, competencies. CREIO and others (Vitello-Cicciu, 2003) have proposed various strategies for enhancing EI, and a 2004 issue of *Psychological Inquiry* (Vol. 15[3]) is devoted to debating and clarifying what research-based information is known about this topic.

CECILIA R. BARRON

REFERENCES

Bar-On, R. (2000). Emotional and social intelligence: Insights from the Emotional Quotient Inventory. In R. Bar-On & J. D. A. Parker (Eds.), *The handbook of emotional intelligence* (pp. 363–388). San Francisco: Jossey-Bass.

Cherniss, C. (2004). Intelligence, emotional. In C. Spielberger (Ed.), *Encyclopedia of applied psychology* (Vol. 2, pp. 315–319). Oxford: Elsevier Academic Press.

Goleman, D. (1995). *Emotional intelligence*. New York: Bantam Books.

Salovey, P., & Mayer, J. D. (1990). Emotional intelligence. *Imagination, Cognition, & Personality, 9*(3), 185–211.

Vitello-Cicciu, J. M. (2003). Innovative leadership through emotional intelligence. *Nursing Management, 34*(10), 28–33.

Employee Performance Appraisal Process

O NE OF THE MOST IMPORTANT responsibilities of a manager is evaluating the work performance of employees. The employee appraisal provides the opportunity to review expectations and the employee's attainment of these expectations. It is a formal time when the review of past work and future goals is discussed. The appraisal should address opportunities for growth and professional development regardless of the position the employee holds. Ideally, it is a two-way communication that will motivate and encourage the employee and stimulate professional growth. Furthermore, it is a time to clarify the mission and goals of the institution and let the employee know if she/he is contributing to achieving the goals. Not only is the appraisal a time to look at past performance, but also it is a valuable time to look toward the future and align with organization priorities.

APPRAISER ANXIETY

T HE annual employee appraisal is a responsibility often fraught with anxiety for the manager and dread for the employee. What gets in the appraiser's way emotionally? The appraiser's own anxiety about anticipated results based on past history with this employer or other employees has an impact. The manager has personal feelings/biases that get in the way of looking at performance. The appraiser has the responsibility of evaluating feelings and preconceived ideas about the employee and focusing on clear, measurable outcomes with concrete examples.

Most health care managers have risen to their position because they are clinically competent. Many have not had formal training and have had little experience in giving employee evaluations. In the role of appraiser, the manager often has anxiety about anticipated results. What should be done if there is an emotional reaction such as crying, denial, or defensiveness? The evaluation process requires specific people and counseling skills (Chandra, 2006). If the manager has been attentive all year and addressed concerns when they occurred as well as offered praise when appropriate, there are no surprises for the employee. This allows for a more productive meeting; however, the formal review carries more weight with the employee and is likely to cause more apprehension if the review is tied to compensation. Therefore, it is wise to give some thought to handling employee tension and possible emotional reactions. Performance reviews are not the time to give negative criticism for things that have gone wrong all year long. The review is not an opportunity to place blame. If an individual has failed to reach targets, this is addressed when the failure is discovered, not at the time of the annual review (Armstrong, 2006).

EMPLOYEE ANXIETY

A NXIETY for the employee is caused by a fear of the unknown. Even if they have open communication with their manager, the anticipation of an evaluation causes tension. To eliminate some of this fear and tension, a standard approach is used for evaluating employees. The position description specifies preemployment competencies and what competencies the employee needs to attain. This becomes the basis for the annual evaluation. Agency human resource policies guide the manager and provide standardized forms for each position description. A standardized measurement-based performance evaluation process creates objectivity and makes the process predictable. When the manager has solid measures, employees are more focused (de Koning, 2005). Outcome measures instill clarity of role expectations.

Evaluating employees is an ongoing process. It takes the form of the required annual appraisal mandated by the organization and regulatory agencies and the ongoing evaluation of work and performance addressed whenever the employee is not fulfilling the expectations of the role. In addition, incorporated into a manager's routine is the praise and recognition of a job well done. Frequently, feedback focuses on the negative. The Gallup Organization researchers and others have reported that people remember criticism but respond to praise. Criticism makes them defensive, whereas praise produces confidence and a desire to be more productive (Morgan, 2005).

EMPLOYEE SELF-ASSESSMENT

A PROACTIVE approach for the employee has been recommended by Jackman and Strober (2003). They recommend a manageable four-step approach, consisting of self-assessment, external feedback, absorbing the feedback, and absorbing the change. This approach is not to be confused with the 360-degree method (Peiperl, 2001). In the Jackman and Strober method, the feedback is from trusted colleagues. When employees are open and deal with feedback constructively, the organization benefits. Their work better aligns with the mission and goals of the institution. Employees can improve communication throughout their department by openly seeking feedback from management and coworkers.

Another popular approach is the 360-degree feedback. The focus of this approach is feedback from peers, supervisors, and subordinates. Although it is time-consuming, it has value in that it is comprehensive. It is always a work in progress because all employees need coaching to understand the method and the potential hidden conflicts (Peiperl, 2001). Ideas from this method should be incorporated into employee evaluation in health care. Consumer satisfaction is a valuable outcome measure. Every employee is responsible for this measure. Peer review is also a useful measure in evaluating teamwork. When the health care team works well together, everyone benefits.

The classic work regarding employee self-assessment by Drucker (1999) still has validity today. McGregor (1957) described this process that ultimately creates an objective review that ensures employee participation in the process. The employee starts the process by doing a self-analysis, identifying strengths and weaknesses, and then defining short-term goals or targets for himself/herself. The manager then enters the process to help the employee relate the self-appraisal to targets that are in alignment with organization goals. With coaching from the manager, the employee identifies specific steps to take to achieve these targets. This is to be accomplished within a specific time frame. The approach described by McGregor shifts the emphasis from appraisal to analysis, which is a more positive approach. Performance is tied to goals or targets, not employee personality. This allows the manager to focus on coaching the employee.

Take the time to provide a quiet, confidential environment and focus on the opportunities for the coming year. Although evaluation of employees is time-consuming and labor-intensive, it is an opportunity for the manager and employee to connect and revitalize their work relationship. Successful appraisals yield positive results with motivated workers.

CHRISTINE COUGHLIN

REFERENCES

Armstrong, M. (2006). *Performance management: Key strategies and practical approaches* (3rd ed.). Philadelphia: Kogan Page.

Chandra, A. (2006). Employee evaluation strategies for healthcare organizations—A general guide. *Hospital Topics: Research and Perspectives on Healthcare, 84*(2), 34–38.

de Koning, G. (2004). Evaluating employee performance (Part 2). *The Gallup Management Journal.* Retrieved July 17, 2006, from http://gmj.gallup.com

Drucker, P. F. (1999). Managing oneself. *Harvard Business Review, 77*(2), 66–74.

Jackman, J. M., & Strober, M. H. (2003). Fear of feedback. *Harvard Business Review, 81*(4), 101–107.

McGregor, D. (1957). An uneasy look at performance appraisal. *Harvard Business Review, 35*(3), 89–94.

Morgan, L. (2005). How to play to your strengths. *Harvard Business Review, 83*(1), 74–80.

Peiperl, M. (2001). Getting 360-degree feedback right. *Harvard Business Review,* 142–147.

Employee Safety

U
NDER THE WORKERS Rights Section of the Occupational Safety
and Health Act (OSHA) of 1970, all workers in the United States
have the right to a safe workplace, and OSHA requires employers
to provide a workplace that is free of serious recognized hazards and
is in compliance with the mandatory OSHA standards. Occupational
health surveillance for health care workers is targeted to specific ex-
posures (e.g., chemicals, hazardous drugs, blood-borne pathogens, air-
borne infections). A medical surveillance program should be in place to
minimize worker exposure and include appropriate elements of a hierarchy of controls (including engineering, administrative, and personal
protective equipment). Rogers (1997), a nursing expert in occupational
health, delineated five categories of safety risk hazards encountered in
health care—biological/infectious risks, chemical risks, environmental/
hazards risks, physical risks, and psychological risks. After conducting
two online surveys, one a Staffing Survey (2000) and another on Nurses'
Health and Safety Concerns (2001), the American Nurses Association
(ANA) concluded that nurses were increasingly in "harm's way" in health
care settings. In the 2001 survey, nurses reported job stress as the top
health concern, followed by back injuries, contracting HIV or hepatitis

from a needle-stick injury, becoming infected with TB or another disease, sustaining an on-the-job-assault, developing a latex allergy, and having a fatigue-related car accident after leaving work. Many of the nurses felt that unsafe working conditions interfered with their ability to deliver quality work. In response to the significant number and severity of work-related back injuries and other musculoskeletal disorders among nurses, ANA launched its highly successful *Handle with Care Campaign* (de Castro, 2004), a health care industry-wide effort to prevent back and other musculoskeletal injuries. ANA has made nurses' health, environmental, and safety issues an organizational core issue and inaugurated the Center for Environmental and Occupational Health (http://nursingworld.org/coeh/rnnoharm/). According to ANA's *Code of Ethics for Nurses*, provision 6, nurses should address concerns about the health care environment through appropriate channels and, if not successfully resolved, then it is essential to have whistleblower protections in place to ensure proper reporting of unsafe work conditions and patient safety issues.

KAREN A. BALLARD

See Also
American Nurses Association

REFERENCES

de Castro, A. B. (2004). Handle With Care®: The American Nurses Association's campaign to address work-related musculoskeletal disorders. *Online Journal of Issues in Nursing, 9*(3), 45–54.

Institute of Medicine, Committee on the Work Environment for Nurses and Patient Safety. (2004). *Keeping patients safe: Transforming the work environment of nurses.* Washington, DC: National Academies Press.

Rogers, B. (1997). As I see it: Is health care a risky business? *The American Nurse, 29,* 5–6.

Employee
Satisfaction

ONE OF THE CRITICAL conditions of organizational success is employee satisfaction. Although this particular phenomenon is true of any business enterprise, it is particularly true of health care organizations. Employee satisfaction is a cornerstone, as it were, of organizational stability and continuity of patient care. Employee satisfaction can lead to loyalty to and pride in the organization, creativity in the workplace, and mutual interchange between employer and employee; also, it can certainly influence patient satisfaction with his or her quality of care.

Employee satisfaction is important to health care organizations because it can reflect the climate of a healthy facility and a high level of organizational productivity, employee motivation, and employee performance. Satisfied employees convey a certain level of confidence to clients, which, in turn, generates a level of trust in the competence and quality of care provided by the caregiver(s) in particular, and by the organization, in general.

Over the years, professional nurses in particular have been the objects of a myriad of sociological and professional studies, including job satisfaction. This phenomenon is exemplified by the works of Aiken, Havens, and Sloane (2000), Kramer and Schmalenberg (2004), McClure, Poulin, Sovie, and Wandelt (1983), McClure and Hinshaw (2007), and the Institute of Medicine (2004).

189

The periodic and cyclical shortage of professional nurses has generated multiple approaches to remedy these shortages, such as sign-on bonuses, tuition remission or reimbursement programs for educational advancement, flexible scheduling practices, improved salary and benefits, decentralization, and changes in governance—which includes initiation of nursing practice councils and committees, all of which provides for staff input into critical decision making, as well as increased opportunities for clinical advancement (i.e., career ladders). In reexamining the characteristics of "Magnet" hospitals as published in 1983, McClure and Hinshaw (2007) reiterate the critical components of what it is that identifies those health care organizations commonly referred to as "Magnet" hospitals. These characteristics have tended to attract and retain professional nurses and certainly increase job satisfaction, even in the midst of a cyclical nursing shortage. The characteristics of "magnetism" include: nurse staffing, nursing autonomy, and control over nursing practice—all of which "require strong administrative and organizational support of the nursing staff" (McClure & Hinshaw, 2007). Clearly, the key to employee satisfaction depends largely on an administration that is open to suggestion, that demonstrates support of its employees, and that fosters an environment conducive to collaboration and creativity on the part of its employees.

M. JANICE NELSON

See Also
Magnet Hospitals

REFERENCES

Aiken, L., Havens, D., & Sloane, D. (2000). The magnet nursing services recognition program: A comparison of two groups of magnet hospitals. *American Journal of Nursing, 100*(3), 26–36.

Institute of Medicine. (2004). *Keeping patients safe: Transforming the work environment of nurses.* Washington, DC: National Academies Press.

Kramer, M., & Schmalenberg, C. (2004). Essentials of magnetic work environment: Part 1. *Nursing 2004, 36*(6), 50–54.

McClure, M. L., & Hinshaw, A. S. (2007). Spotlight on nurse staffing, autonomy, and control over practice. *American Nurse Today, 2*(4), 15–17.

McClure, M., Poulin, M., Sovie, M., & Wandelt, M. (1983). *Magnet hospitals: Attraction and retention of professional nurses.* Washington, DC: American Nurses Association.

Smith, H. L., Hood, J. N., Waldman, J. D., & Smith, V. L. (2005). Creating a favorable practice environment for nurses. *Journal of Nursing Administration, 35*(12), 525–532.

Entry Into Practice

THE TERM "ENTRY INTO PRACTICE" generally refers to the educational preparation that is required for basic practice within a profession. In nursing, however, it has become a shorthand manner for referring to the long, ongoing debate that the profession has engaged in regarding the appropriate level of education that should be required for entry into registered nurse (RN) practice.

Historically, nurses in the United States were educated in hospital schools of nursing patterned after the Nightingale Schools that were introduced in Europe during the late 19th century. By the early 20th century, a few colleges and universities were beginning programs designed to prepare nurses at the baccalaureate level, but these were not popular or numerous. Then, in the mid-20th century, the community college movement started and quickly spread across the nation; nursing became one of the earliest and most successful majors to be offered by this new form of education. For many years, the hospital schools continued to flourish as well.

Today, the large majority of the nation's nurses are prepared in community college programs, graduating with associate degrees, whereas diploma programs have declined precipitously. "RNs are seeking the BSN degree in increasing numbers. In 1980, almost 55% of registered nurses held a hospital diploma as their highest educational credential, 22% held the bachelor's degree, and 18% an associate degree, according to figures from the federal Division of Nursing. By 1996, a diploma was the highest educational credential for only 27% of RNs, while the number with bachelor's degrees had climbed to 31%, with 32% holding an associate degree" (American Association of Colleges of Nursing, 2002). Moreover, there is a growing number of universities and colleges that offer entry preparation at the Master's level (Google, 2007).

Over the years, there have been many efforts made by the profession to standardize basic nursing preparation, most of which have attempted to require at least a baccalaureate degree in order for new nurses to qualify for licensure. For example, in 1965, the American Nurses Association went on record as endorsing such a change in standards (American Nurses Association, 1965). Then, in 1975, the New York State Nurses Association attempted to have legislation introduced that would require the baccalaureate for all new RN candidates and the associate degree for all new licensed practical nurse (LPN) candidates; in spite of rigorous efforts, the bill never was introduced into the legislative body. North Dakota is the only state that was actually successful in changing their standards and required the baccalaureate degree for 17 years; however, in 2003 that change was repealed (L. Shanta, Associate Director for Education of the North Dakota Board of Nursing, personal communication, August 20, 2007). The most recent attempt at change in education for entry into nursing began again in New York State in 2004. The proposal would require that all nurses prepared at the diploma or associate degree level attain a baccalaureate degree in nursing within 10 years of their initial licensure. This idea has been explored by other states as well, but there has been substantial opposition to the plan, chiefly arising from hospital administrators and community college presidents, and it remains to be seen whether the effort will prove successful.

Of interest is the fact that a large number of developed and developing countries already require the baccalaureate degree for their nurses and a number have done so for many years. At present, this trend is spreading across Western Europe as the need for more education becomes evident among health care influentials (Spitzer & Perrenoud, 2006).

Most comparable professions report that they have gone through similar struggles whenever they have proposed an elevation of their educational standards. What is striking is the fact that nursing is the only occupation that has been unsuccessful in making such changes to date. Nonetheless, it is likely that the issue has not been put to rest and that increased pressure will again be brought to bear to raise the entry into practice issue, especially as the demand for more and better-prepared nurses becomes a reality for the delivery of 21st-century health care.

MARGARET L. MCCLURE

See Also
American Nurses Association

REFERENCES

American Association of Colleges of Nursing. (2002). *Your nursing career: A look at the facts.* Retrieved August 17, 2007, from http://www.campusrn.com/students/article.asp?news_id=892

American Nurses Association. (1965). *Educational preparation for nurse practitioners and assistants to nurses: A position paper.* New York: Author.

Google. (2007). *Entry preparation in nursing at the Master's level.* Retrieved August 17, 2007, from http://www.google.com/search?hl=en&q=entry+preparation+in+nursing+at+the+Master%E2%80%99s+level

Spitzer, A., & Perrenoud, B. (2006). Reforms in nursing education across western Europe: From agenda to practice. *Journal of Professional Nursing, 22,* 150–159.

Evidence-Based Practice

THE STRONG EMPHASIS on research within the nursing profession
is based on an implicit expectation that the results of such research
will be used to improve patient care and outcomes. Yet, interestingly, for many years no particular attention has been paid to the idea
of knowledge use and how it was to be done. Some researchers seemed
to believe that it was not for them to be concerned about what happens after they complete their work and disseminate it. Others seemed
to think that it was practicing nurses' responsibility to individually read
research, understand it, evaluate it, and figure out how to apply it to
patient situations in their practice. Unsurprisingly, this expectation did
not materialize.

In the mid-1970s, there was a spurt of discussion that appeared in
the nursing literature about the need to systematically utilize knowledge
generated through research in patient care. This may have been stimulated in part by the work being done by social scientists at the time
about approaches to "research utilization." The emphasis of these scientists tended to be on the process of change and adoption of innovations. Their examples came mostly from industry and technology, and,
most compellingly, from agriculture. They modeled agriculture extension

services and the translation function that those staffs provided to farmers, with the result that efficiencies in food production increased, fewer people were employed in food production, and the industry was able to feed the expanding population of the country.

In examining the work of these early social scientists, the fact that their discourse had a distinctly organizational dimension to knowledge application did not seem to have an impact on nursing, and people continued to believe that it was an individual nurse's responsibility to apply knowledge to practice.

It would take several decades before the issue of research utilization made a comeback, this time in the form of evidence-based practice (EBP). The profile of the current literature on EBP, however, is different, as is the climate within which the discussions are occurring. Several other health professions are engaged in major efforts to implement EBP and to teach EBP in their educational programs. As well, there is an emphasis within federal agencies on EBP, with a number of institutes within the National Institutes of Health dedicating significant amounts of funding to address issues in EBP.

Nursing has enthusiastically embraced the movement of EBP; the literature reveals that health care organizations are now dedicating highly qualified personnel teams and developing systematic strategies to facilitate the implementation of EBP on the part of their staffs. This is one of the most significant and productive movements within nursing, which has the potential of transforming the profession and the quality of care it provides the public. Several models have been developed and are now in use, including the Stetler Model of Research Utilization and the University of Iowa-Titler Model of Evidence-Based Practice to Promote Quality Care. The formation of several centers on EBP, such as the Joanna Briggs Institute (Adelaide, Australia), has been joined by Sigma Theta Tau International, and Cochrane Collaboration at York University (UK), focusing on meta-analytic studies, which has further stimulated the EBP movement in nursing both within the United States and internationally.

The Stetler Model of Research Utilization (Stetler, 2001) is divided into five phases: preparation, validation, comparative evaluation and decision making, translation or application, and evaluation. The first three phases are devoted to analysis of the research evidence, and deciding whether or not to use the research evidence in practice. The final two phases consist of the application and evaluation of the evidence in practice. The Stetler model can be applied at both institutional and individual levels. Institutions using the Stetler model can apply research findings to develop or revise policies, protocols, or other institutional initiatives (Burns & Grove, 2005). Individuals following the Stetler model can use research findings to inform practice and influence educational programs (Burns & Grove, 2005).

The Iowa Model of Evidence-Based Practice (Titler et al., 2001) was developed to provide direction to a clinical institution interested in developing evidence-based practice. The Iowa model uses an algorithm format, with multiple decision points along the path. The model begins with either problem- or knowledge-focused triggers that prompt an in-depth analysis of data available to the institution. The organization goes through a series of steps, following the algorithms of the model: evaluating and prioritizing potential research topics based on the needs of the organization, critiquing and synthesizing research evidence related to the topic, piloting a change in practice if the research evidence is sufficient, and, finally, instituting the change in practice. The Iowa model includes monitoring the impact of the change on the work environment, employees, costs, and patients (Burns & Grove, 2005).

Most research findings are not ready to be implemented into practice, nor should the findings of any single study be implemented; a variety of steps are necessary to determine the applicability of research findings (evidence) into practice within specific settings with particular populations. The nature and quality of the research need to be carefully evaluated and corroboration sought from multiple studies. With this in mind, translational research is expected to play a key role and attention is now given to approaches to translate research into forms that render findings applicable to practice.

In the recent past a major research journal published a special issue devoted to translational research. Similarly, the Agency for Healthcare Research and Quality (AHRQ) is funding studies in translation research with the aim of improving health care quality, and has played a leadership role in this regard. For example, an invitational conference was organized in 2003 with AHRQ and 11 organizations/institutions sponsoring it. The conference has been critical in setting the agenda of what needs to be accomplished to fully achieve the goals of EBP. The conference adopted a definition of translation research used by previous authors (Kovner, Elton, & Billings, 2000; Titler & Everett, 2001; Walshe & Rundall, 2001): "The scientific investigation of methods, interventions, and variables that influence adoption of evidence-based practices by individuals and organizations to improve clinical and operational decision making in health care . . . includes testing the effect of interventions on *promoting* and *sustaining* the adoption of EBPs" (Titler, 2004, p. S1). In providing an overview of the topics discussed, some of the themes considered were: assessing organizational readiness and capacity for implementing EBP; evaluation of the quality of the evidence; how to facilitate "buy-in of organizations to participate in a translation study, and conducting research on the effectiveness of a particular strategy"; consumer empowerment; the need for mid-course corrections; "use of organizational level interventions; measurement of dependent variables and study end-points" (Titler, 2004), among others.

No matter which of these models of EBP is followed, when reviewing the literature for relevant research all types of research need to be considered. Quantitative, qualitative, outcomes-focused, and intervention studies are all potentially useful, and should be evaluated for their applicability to the practice change being considered. All research studies, however, are not equal in the strength of the evidence they provide. The strength of research evidence is on a continuum, with descriptive surveys providing the weakest evidence, and meta-analyses of experimental studies providing the strongest evidence. In addition to the strength of the research evidence, the expertise of the practitioners who will be implementing the change, the values and needs of the patients who will be the recipients of the change, and, finally, the unique characteristics of the organization all need to be considered.

Nursing leaders who are interested in developing EBP may want to use an interdisciplinary approach to practice change, depending on the change being considered. For example, reducing the incidence of ventilator-associated pneumonia in mechanically ventilated, critically ill patients is an important organizational initiative. Ventilator-associated pneumonia (VAP) is a leading cause of morbidity and mortality in critically ill patients (Hilinski & Stark, 2006). Although nursing has developed evidence-based intervention bundles to reduce the incidence of VAP (Hilinski & Stark, 2006), nursing is not the sole health care profession that manages mechanically ventilated patients. Both physicians and respiratory therapists also manipulate ventilators, and therefore should be included in the development and implementation of practice changes aimed at reducing VAP.

The evidence base for many areas of nursing practice is relatively strong, whereas research evidence to assist with nursing leadership decision making is relatively weak. There is a paucity of consistent research findings available to help nursing leadership make informed decisions regarding staffing levels that optimize patient outcomes. For example, several studies have examined the relationship of hours per patient day (HPPD) to various patient outcomes (Blegen, Goode, & Reed, 1998; Cho, Ketefian, Barkauskas, & Smith, 2003; Needleman, Buerhaus, Mattke, Stewart, & Zelevinsky, 2002). Both Blegen and others and Cho and others found an unexpected positive relationship between total HPPD and the prevalence of pressure ulcers, but when Cho and others isolated RN-HPPD, they found an inverse relationship with pneumonia. Needleman and others also found an inverse relationship between RN-HPPD and pneumonia. Contradictory findings across studies suggest that more research on this topic is needed before nursing leaders can use the research evidence to make informed staffing decisions.

In summary, nursing leaders have at least two templates to choose from in helping them institute EBP. Both the Stetler and Iowa models offer guidelines for how to move EBP into an institution. Depending on the practice issue being considered, other disciplines may need to be part of the process. By promoting evidence-based practice, nursing leaders can make a powerful impact on the nursing profession and patient care.

SHAKÉ KETEFIAN
MILISA MANOJLOVICH

See Also
Agency for Healthcare Research and Quality

REFERENCES

Blegen, M. A., Goode, C., & Reed, L. (1998). Nurse staffing and patient outcomes. *Nursing Research, 47*(1), 43–50.

Burns, N., & Grove, S. K. (2005). *The practice of nursing research: Conduct, critique, and utilization* (5th ed.). St. Louis, MO: Elsevier Saunders.

Cho, S. H., Ketefian, S., Barkauskas, V. H., & Smith, D. G. (2003). The effects of nurse staffing on adverse events, morbidity, mortality, and medical costs. *Nursing Research, 52*(2), 71–79.

Hilinski, A. M., & Stark, M. L. (2006). Memory aide to reduce the incidence of ventilator-associated pneumonia. *Critical Care Nurse, 26*(5), 80–81.

Kovner, A. R., Elton, J. J., & Billings, J. (2000). Evidence-based management. *Frontiers of Health Services Management, 16*(4), 3–24.

Lewis, R. F., & Feldman, H. R. (2000). *Teaching evidence-based practice in nursing: A guide for academic and clinical settings.* New York: Springer Publishing.

Needleman, J., Buerhaus, P., Mattke, S., Stewart, M., & Zelevinsky, K. (2002). Nurse-staffing levels and the quality of care in hospitals. *New England Journal of Medicine, 346*(22), 1715–1722.

Stetler, C. B. (2001). Updating the Stetler Model of Research Utilization to facilitate evidence-based practice. *Nursing Outlook, 49*(6), 272–279.

Titler, M. G. (2004). Overview of the U.S. invitational conference "Advancing Quality Care Through Translation Research." *Worldviews on Evidence-Based Nursing, Supplement 1,* S1–S5.

Titler, M. G., & Everett, L. Q. (2001). Translating research into practice: Considerations for critical care investigators. *Critical Care Nursing Clinics of North America, 13*(4), 587–604.

Titler, M. G., Kleiber, C., Steelman, V. J., Rakel, B. A., Budreau, G., Everett, L. Q., et al. (2001). The Iowa Model of Evidence-Based Practice to promote quality care. *Critical Care Nursing Clinics of North America, 13*(4), 497–509.

Walshe, K., & Rundall, T. G. (2001). Evidence-based management: From theory to practice in health care. *The Milbank Quarterly, 79*(3), 429–457.

Executive Leadership Programs

NURSES IN EXECUTIVE PRACTICE require expertise in a broad spectrum of knowledge and skills. The American Organization of Nurse Executives (AONE) identified the competency domains required as Leadership, Business Skills and Principles, Knowledge of the Healthcare Environment, Communication and Relationship Management, and Professionalism. Formal programs are available to nurses who seek to augment their skills as executive leaders. Nationally, there are several well-established programs. The highly competitive Johnson & Johnson—Wharton Fellows Program at the University of Pennsylvania focuses on cutting-edge business and management science during an intensive 3-week session (http://www.executivefellows.net). The equally competitive Robert Wood Johnson Foundation Executive Nurse Fellows Program is a 3-year fellowship that focuses on the experience and skills necessary to be a leader in the health care system. Participants remain in their permanent jobs while completing this fellowship (http://futurehealth.ucsf.edu/Program/rwj). Both of these programs offer participants the opportunity to learn with a diverse cohort of colleagues. There are several programs that are state based. Two examples are the Midwestern Institute for Nursing Leadership, sponsored by the Illinois Organization of Nurse Leaders. The former consists of a 5-day session that includes executive decision making, strategic management, high performance teams, and change theory (http://www.ionl.org) and the latter, the Boston-based Institute for Nursing Healthcare Leadership, offers a yearly conference that stresses nursing leadership and organizational effectiveness (http://www.inhl.org). Several universities offer multidisciplinary leadership programs. Three examples are the Harvard Management Development Program (http://www.gse.harvard.edu/ppe/highered/index.html), the Leadership Development program at the University of Maryland (http://www.umuc.edu/prog/nli/ldp.html), and the Nonprofit Executive Leadership Institute at Bryn Mawr (http://www.brynmawr.edu/neli/faculty.htm).

Most leadership development programs target the individual learner and utilize small class sizes, experiential learning, and expert faculty. Given the variety of programs available, it is critical that nurse executives be clear about their individual goals, learning styles, financial resources, and time commitment in order to select the best program to meet their needs.

PAMELA AUSTIN THOMPSON

WEB REFERENCES

ExecutiveFellows.net, http://www.executivefellows.net

RWJ Executive Nurse Fellows Program, http://futurehealth.ucsf.edu/Program/rwj

Institute for Nursing Healthcare Leadership, http://www.inhl.org

Harvard Graduate School of Education, Higher Education Programs, http://www.gse.harvard.edu/ppe/highered/index.html

University of Maryland University College, National Leadership Institute, Leadership Development Program (LDP)®, http://www.umuc.edu/prog/nli/ldp.html

Bryn Mawr College, Graduate School of Social Work and Social Research, Nonprofit Executive Leadership Institute, http://www.brynmawr.edu/neli/faculty.htm

Executive Search

IN THE VERNACULAR, the term "headhunter" is used to describe the work done by an individual who searches for a qualified candidate for a specific position. According to the thesaurus the headhunter is a recruiter, or a talent scout (Kipfer, 2006). A headhunter may be a search consultant, one who has experience in the profession and subsequently uses this experience to become a consultant. Another way of describing what they do is "matchmaking." For this entry, search consultant is the term used to describe this work. The search consultant can be an independent worker or a contract worker with a search firm directly or indirectly employed by an institution. When working with applicants for a position, the consultant can take the role of mentor, career counselor, or career coach. Nursing leaders or aspiring nursing leaders may have the occasion to work with a search consultant either as an applicant or employer. Among the considerations involved in an executive search are: (1) whether or not a search firm is essential for finding the best qualified applicant, and, if so, what qualities does the employer look for when selecting a search firm; (2) what is the process used by the search consultant to find the best candidate for the position; and (3) what are the benefits of working with a search consultant. Both the applicant and the employer should expect working with a search consultant to be a positive experience.

SELECTING A SEARCH FIRM

A n institution may select from dozens of search firms. They may use word of mouth in selecting a firm, or may choose to contact an organization by searching online to learn what firms are available. Examples of Internet addresses used to identify some of these are included at the end of this entry. Posting the position in various organizational publications is also a means of advertising the position. Search firms do require a fee for their service and for this reason the institution may use them only for a specialized search. After taking into account the advantages, the administrator will determine if the institution can best be served by use of a search firm. If that is determined, the decision needs to be made about the type of firm that will best suit the needs of the institution. Some search firms work on a retainer basis and others work on a contingency basis. Large institutions may have a recruitment team on staff. Search firms that require a retainer will have an exclusive arrangement with the employing institution. They bring in applicants until the position is successfully filled. These firms receive the first part of their fee when the contract is signed, the second part when a candidate is selected, and the third part when the candidate assumes the new position. The firms that work on a contingency basis receive a fee only if the employing agency hires an applicant they bring in. A recruiter who works for the institution is called a corporate recruiter. There are search firms that specialize in health care searches and those who have a broader venue. Currently, private and corporate businesses are frequently engaging search firms for assistance in exploring the job market for the best-qualified person to fill a position.

Are search firms the most expedient way to find the best-qualified applicants? The time it takes to complete a search depends on many things, including the time of year it is started, the institution, where it is located, and how well known are its stakeholders. Freedom of interaction between the consultant and the institutional representative also influences the length of time for a search. In the last few years, many books have been written and Web sites established that give information about job searches. In spite of the vast amount of information available, many positions are filled through personal contacts. Networking is one tool, among many, that may be used in searching for the "best" applicant. Meshel and Douglas (2005), along with many others, consider networking to be an essential means of searching for a position.

Although a fee for service is required, the use of a search firm may actually save money for the institution by expediting the search, relieving the staff of the many search activities, and providing a greater pool of qualified applicants. To acquire names of applicants, the search consultant will have developed a database of well-qualified potential applicants as well as resources, such as the database of an organization or contact with persons who are in the same line of work. The work of the search consultant includes the review of all applications and referring only those who match the position profile to the stakeholders for a decision to interview or reject. Those applicants who do not match the qualifications for the position are held in the database of the consultant. Experienced search consultants know the institutions that they work with and the people who work there; they also maintain a cadre of potential persons for positions and resource persons to suggest potential qualified applicants. The fee as a search consultation comes from the institution, so they are the employer of the consultant; however, the directive comes from the institution to find the best person for the position.

SEARCH CONSULTANT PROCESS

O NE long-standing process in nursing is as follows: The search consultants will use their experience and connections as teachers or administrators, in addition to involvement in national nursing organizations, to seek the "best"-qualified applicants for a position. In addition to working with a committee of stakeholders or an institutional representative, another role of the consultant is to prepare the applicant for the position. All of this can best be done when the consultant knows the institution, the people who work there, and the kind of person needed to fill the position. To learn this, the consultant visits the institution and talks with stakeholders. After that visit, a profile of a qualified candidate is determined by the consultant and approved by the search committee or the designated representative. The search consultant will bring to the committee's attention several individuals who are qualified and appear to "fit" the position. Although the consultant provides information about the applicants to the institutional committee, it is also important that the consultant provide support so that the applicant is well prepared for the interview. The consultant suggests to the applicants issues to consider when looking at a position, for example: (1) Are the core values of the agency consistent with yours? (2) What are the personal attitudes and work style at the institution? (3) Are they congruent with yours? (4) What are the critical issues facing the institution? Applicants are reminded there are more important things they need to know about the position than salary, since this is negotiable.

The process for applying for the position is discussed with those candidates whose curriculum vitae are well done, whose experience, characteristics, and qualifications make them a good fit for the position, and who meet the position requirements. In other words, their data reflect a potential good fit (a match) with the profile of the person being sought by the institution. The consultant suggests a format for applying for the position. For example, applicants should review the position announcement and other materials that they receive. The letter of application should indicate those areas described in the position announcement where the candidates have had experience. The letter of application should be no more than two pages and should give strong evidence of the applicant's qualifications as they relate to the position. Additional information about background is provided in the resume or curriculum vita. Applications should not be encouraged from those who do not meet the basic requirements for a position.

Information obtained for the qualified applicant and provided to the committee by the search consultant include: letters of reference; results of a telephone interview conducted with the applicant; and telephone references from a list the candidate provides. Questions asked of the applicant and references are based on information learned by the consultant in discussion with the stakeholders. This information is compiled and provided to the committee as background information. If an applicant is invited to the institution for a personal interview, the consultant assists in preparing for that visit. Applicants are encouraged to learn as much as possible about the institution and the city in which it is located. They will receive the names of the members of the Search Committee and the Internet URL for the institution to learn more about the members of the Committee. The consultant will also offer suggestions to the members of the Search Committee of ways in which they can enhance the visit of the applicant.

BENEFITS OF WORKING WITH
A SEARCH CONSULTANT

W ORKING with a search consultant should be a learning experience for the applicant. Whether or not the position is attained, the experience should be a positive one. The applicant will be given information about making application for a position from the time of the first contact until a decision has been made. It should help the applicant know better what to expect in future recruitment. The applicant also should learn from interactions with stakeholders what is important in presenting oneself, which helps narrow down to greater certainty the kind of position to which they aspire. The institution benefits are related to time and cost.

The search consultant works with the committee or institutional representative in the capacity of a staff person. The consultant keeps the institutional representative informed of all information about the process and the progress of the search. The consultant systematically collects information, confirms its accuracy, and provides complete details about several applicants to the designated person or committee. The consultant also provides information and the committee makes decisions about applicants. The search consultant assists in the search from the beginning until a qualified individual signs a letter of agreement or a contract.

BILLYE J. BROWN

REFERENCES

Comeford, P. A., & Sauer, G. (2006). *Lessons from a headhunter*. Edina, MN: Beaver's Pond Press.

Kipfer, B. A. (2006). *Roget's new millennium*™ *thesaurus* (1st ed., vol. 1.3.1). Los Angeles, CA: Lexico Publishing Group.

Meshel, J. W., & Douglas, G. (2005). *One phone call away*. New York: Portfolio, Penguin Group.

Pierson, O. (2006). *The unwritten rules of the highly effective job search*. New York: McGraw-Hill.

WEB REFERENCES

Recruiters Online Network, http://www.recruitersonline.com/

Workquest.com, http://www.workquest.com/

How to Get the Best Job You Ever Had, http://www.jobmiracle.com/

The applicant may choose to post a résumé on a Web site; for example, http://www/monster.com

To find a recruiter, *Consultants News* publishes the Directory of Executive Recruiters. The URL for this group is http://www.jobjunction.com/recruiters.htm

This site lists all types of recruiters, retained, contingent, or corporate.

If you are a person who feels that you do not wish to be involved with a search firm and you want to find a job on your own, go to http://highlyeffectivejobsearch.com/

You will learn about the Pierson Method and the book about a systematic approach to job search (Pierson, 2006). It describes how one prepares to find a job.

http://www.academickeys.com/splash_flash.php

Lists academic and professional resources

Externships

A DRAMATIC DECLINE, in the number of professional nurses in the 1970s challenged nursing leaders to develop creative approaches for resolving the workforce shortage. One approach is the extern experience, which is believed to improve clinical skills that help bridge the transition from student to graduate nurse (Cantrell & Browne, 2006; Tritak, Ross, Feldman, Paregoris, & Setti, 1997). Additionally, these same individuals might be more likely to select and stay with an employer with whom they developed comfort and acceptance of the staff and the work environment. Although there are many variations in both the definition and content of extern programs, externships are generally targeted at student nurses who are in their last year of school (Cantrell & Browne, 2006) or earlier once they have had clinical experience during their academic programs. Extern programs are commonly offered in the summer and this experience may lead to a subsequent part-time position during the school year (Tritak et al., 1997).

Although extern experiences are frequently offered in medical-surgical areas, they can encompass a wide range of clinical specialties (Courtney, 2005; Dempsey & McKissick, 2006). The difference between

206

nurse extern and intern programs is that extern programs frequently do not extend academic credit while internships may provide credit for program participation (Tritak et al., 1997). Formal classes and learning experiences may be provided by organization staff on a wide range of topics, both helpful and of interest to externs. In developing an effective program, consideration needs to be given to creating an environment that is safe and supportive for the extern (Dempsey & McKissick, 2006). Although extern duties generally are similar to those of a nursing assistant, opportunities abound to advance the externs knowledge and technical skill acquisition. Observation of procedures and participation in rounds, conferences, and educational sessions all serve to enrich the extern experience. Along with providing supervision, the nurse preceptor can further the extern's critical thinking skills, organizational abilities, priority setting, and effective communication skills (Dempsey & McKissick, 2006). Supervision, outcome evaluation, and continuous, constructive feedback to the extern facilitate the transfer of theoretical knowledge to professional nursing practice. Throughout the extern experience, managers have the opportunity to assess the potential of the extern to be successful as a staff nurse and thereby reduce the likelihood of hiring someone who will not match unit or hospital needs.

Evaluation of externship programs suggests that these are successful tools for recruiting graduate nurses. A reported 50%–79% of graduate nurses accepted positions in the facility where they had been externs (Cantrell & Browne, 2006; Dempsey & McKissick, 2006; Stinson & Wilkinson, 2004). Evidence suggests that extern experience reduces the time and cost of orientation (Courtney, 2005; Dempsey & McKissick, 2006) and facilitates transition to the role of a staff nurse (Tritak et al., 1997). Self-reports from program graduates indicate that as a result of the extern experience, students have a better understanding of the role of the staff nurse, increased skill, knowledge and experience, and more self-confidence (Dempsey & McKissick, 2006; Tritak et al., 1997).

MARION BURNS TUCK

REFERENCES

Cantrell, M. A., & Browne, A. M. (2006). The impact of a nurse externship program on the transition process from graduate to registered nurse: Part III. Recruitment and retention effects. *Journal for Nurses in Staff Development, 22*(1), 11–14.

Courtney, R. J. (2005). A look at a successful perioperative nurse extern-intern program. *AORN, 81*(3), 577–578.

Dempsey, S. J., & McKissick, E. (2006). Implementation of a medical-surgical nurse extern and student nurse aide programs in critical care. *Critical Care Nursing Quarterly, 29*(3), 182–187.

Stinson, S., & Wilkinson, C. (2004). Creating a successful clinical extern program using a program planning logic model. *Journal of Nursing Staff Development, 20*(3), 140–144.

Tritak, A. B., Ross, B., Feldman, H., Paregoris, B., & Setti, K. (1997). An evaluation of a nurse extern program. *Journal of Nursing Staff Development, 13*(3), 132–135.

F

Faculty Recruitment to Academic Settings

THE NURSING PROFESSION is experiencing an acute shortage of qualified faculty to teach and conduct research in academic settings. As a result, recruitment of faculty to academic institutions is a high priority for nursing schools. Major keys to successful recruitment of faculty to academic settings are: (a) an exciting, visionary strategic plan; (b) personal contact with potential candidates; (c) an ability to generate enthusiasm in potential candidates regarding how they can be an instrumental part of the team in accomplishing the strategic plan; (d) a well organized and interesting interview schedule, (e) timely follow-up; and (f) an excellent recruitment package.

An exciting long-range strategic plan is essential for any organization (Melnyk, 2005), not only because it creates the road map for future success, but because recruitment of new faculty should match key areas of the strategic plan. Advertisements that capture the excitement of the strategic plan should be created and disseminated widely through professional journals, the *Chronicle of Higher Education,* and electronic and Web media as they are an important broad strategy to alert potential faculty to open positions. Advertisements are no substitute for and are typically not as effective in recruiting faculty as personal contacts with

211

targeted individuals, however, to explain why they were on your radar screen. Personal contacts/conversations should create an excitement in potential candidates about your school's strategic plan and end with an invitation to visit your school. For targeted senior faculty, an excellent strategy to begin to spark their interest is to invite them to your school as a visiting scholar or consultant. Immediately following the initial personal contact, mail an attractive packet of exciting information about your school with a follow-up letter.

Once potential candidates commit to an interview, they should be asked whether there are specific individuals with whom they would like to meet with during the course of their interview or places that they would like to visit (e.g., local medical centers, community agencies, interdisciplinary departments). The interview schedule should be comprised of faculty, associate deans/chairs/academic program directors, and collaborating research or clinical partners. It makes an outstanding impression on candidates for the dean to have personal individual time with them during the interview process. It also is important for the first and last individuals who meet with the candidate to be passionate about the direction of the school and be able to create excitement about their potential future on the team. Remember, you never get a second chance to make a great first impression on the candidate. Personal touches, such as placing a welcome card or small basket of fruit in the hotel room and having a faculty member meet the candidate at the airport will create lasting good impressions, even if the candidate chooses not to accept a position at your school.

All faculty recruits, whether being interviewed for clinical/teaching intensive or tenure track positions in which research is an expectation of the position, will want to know whether there are adequate supports and resources in place for them to have a successful career in teaching, research, and/or clinical practice. Potential research active faculty desire a solid research infrastructure (e.g., a research center that assists with pre- and post-award grant activities), outstanding intra- and interdisciplinary collaborators, access to clinical sites where they can obtain their samples and conduct their studies, research start-up funds with designated research space, and substantial time to conduct their research (e.g., limited teaching loads). Formal mechanisms of mentorship for teaching and research/scholarship within a school are important for all new faculty, whether in the clinical or tenure track, to assist them in being successful in the new system as well as to prevent burnout (Shirey, 2006).

Offer potential recruits good salary, or at least one that is commensurate with similar positions in the geographic region. Every year, the American Association of Colleges of Nursing (AACN) collects and publishes salary data for all tenure track and nontenure track faculty as well as for administrators in colleges of nursing (see http://www. aacn.nche.edu).

If the candidates are not familiar with the geographic location of the school, it also is a good idea to have a realtor tour them of a few living areas and provide them with information regarding the average cost of housing during the course of their visit. For stellar candidates who you are prepared to make an offer, it is important to inform them of your intent to provide them with the offer letter in the near future and have an exchange with them regarding their desired package (e.g., salary, research start-up funds, percentage of time devoted to teaching). Negotiate and save time in the hiring process by sending draft letters of offer to candidates as terms of the offer are negotiated.

Shortly following the visit, it is important to send a follow-up letter to candidates, thanking them for their time in visiting your school and informing them of your plan to be in contact with them in the near future. A quick follow-up is important, especially for those candidates for whom you will be sending offer letters, as there is heavy competition for well-qualified faculty.

BERNADETTE MAZUREK MELNYK

REFERENCES

Melnyk, B. M. (2005). Creating a vision: Motivating a change to evidence-based practice in individuals and organizations. In B. Melnyk & E. Fineout-Overholt (Eds.), *Evidence-based practice in nursing & healthcare: A guide to best practice*. Philadelphia: Lippincott, Williams & Wilkins.

Shirey, M. (2006). Stress and burnout in nursing faculty. *Nurse Educator, 31*(3), 95–97.

Faculty Retention

T HE U.S. NURSING and the nursing faculty shortages are intimately intertwined. The most frequently cited reason for denying admission to qualified prospective students is an insufficient number of nursing faculty to teach them. In 2005–2006, there were 37,514 qualified applicants turned away from U.S. baccalaureate nursing programs alone (American Association of Colleges of Nursing, 2006, Table 37, p. 79). Furthermore, nursing program administrators reported that their inability to recruit new nursing faculty is a function of several factors: insufficient funding to hire additional faculty; the inability to compete with hospitals and other practice institutions on compensation packages; the widening gap between the numbers of retiring, and new faculty and faculty resignations for reasons other than retirement such as dissatisfaction and burnout. Every nursing program should have a well-articulated nursing faculty retention program addressing what could be considered the primary drivers of faculty retention: compensation; cultural integration and career development; and advancement.

COMPENSATION

I T is a common occurrence in practice professions, such as law, medicine, and nursing that those who work in the practice arena are likely to earn much more than their counterparts in academia. Despite the fact that advanced degrees and years of experience are necessary prerequisites to a teaching career, compensation remains relatively low for nursing faculty compared to nurses in practice. It is especially disheartening to nursing faculty when the salaries of new nursing graduates in their first positions are higher than faculty salaries. As a rule of thumb, the starting salary of a new, masters prepared faculty member with clinical but little teaching experience should be 20% to 25% higher than the base salary of a new registered nurse. Compensation rates are most often driven by supply and demand factors. For example, the U.S. nursing shortage has driven staff nurses' salaries to new highs and often include sign-on and retention bonuses. The supply-demand factor is finally favoring nursing faculty because the shortage of nursing faculty is the most serious component of the U.S. nursing shortage.

CULTURAL INTEGRATION

F OR new faculty, retention begins with a substantive, formal orientation to the nursing program and the institution in which it resides. Faculty need to understand the nature of the curriculum, academic policies and procedures, the organization of the program, the school and how it fits into the college or university, as well as appropriate channels of communication and opportunities for faculty to serve on program or college/university committees. Involving veteran faculty in new faculty orientation programs facilitates collegial relationships and may lead naturally to mentor-mentee relationships if they are not already prescribed for orientation purposes. In addition to organizational and policy issues, orientation of new faculty should include an overview of student-driven issues and resources, for example, students with disabilities or students who need tutoring or counseling; and student testing policy and processes. All faculty should have the tools necessary to do their work, such as a suitable office, a computer and other technology, learning labs, and technical staff to support the teaching-learning effort. Periodic feedback from new and veteran faculty should be elicited to determine how best to improve the resources and environment. Ultimately, faculty should be led to view their work as a significant contribution to the future of the profession and ultimately to patient care.

CAREER DEVELOPMENT AND ADVANCEMENT

B OTH new and veteran faculty need clear guidelines on career development and advancement in their respective institutions. The criteria for promotion in all faculty tracks, for example, tenure or clinical educator, should be published and understood. It is the responsibility of the administrator of the unit to create a culture in which faculty can both identify and achieve their goals. Such a culture provides periodic review of faculty activities, such as teaching, advising, research, publications, and contributions to the unit or college/university. During formal reviews, faculty should be encouraged to clearly articulate their goals and to work with the unit administrator to develop strategies and opportunities to meet those goals. Advancing through the professorial ranks validates a teacher's contributions not only to student learning but also to advancing the profession and nursing knowledge. Promoting the development, reward and recognition of both new and veteran faculty will result in a high level of faculty retention.

GLORIA F. DONNELLY

See Also
American Association of Colleges of Nursing
Faculty Shortages in Registered Nurses Preparatory Programs
Global Nursing Shortage

REFERENCE

American Association of Colleges of Nursing. (2006). *Enrollment and graduations in baccalaureate and graduate nursing programs: 2005–2006*. Washington, DC: Author.

Faculty Shortages in Registered Nurses Preparatory Programs

THE NUMBER AND COMPLEXITY of issues that have merged into the "perfect storm" of the shortage of registered nurses (RNs) also have operated in the development and continuation of shortages of nursing faculty. Those dimensions have been well discussed in other venues, suffice to note that, in order to meet the increased demand for nursing services and enlarge the numbers of nurses available, nursing education must expand. A prime ingredient to the advancement of that educational mandate is the availability of a well-prepared and committed cadre of faculty; therefore, the assessment of this educational resource is vital to meeting the current crisis in availability of RNs.

There are three lenses through which the supply of faculty for programs in nursing leading to licensure as a registered nurse may be viewed. The first of these is the simple number of nurses who hold the minimal credential required by most state boards of nursing for faculty positions, namely, the Master's degree in nursing. The second approach is to summarize the extent to which individuals holding a Master's degree in nursing are prepared to fulfill a faculty role in an academic setting. And a

217

third approach is to report on the numbers of nurse faculty who hold the terminal degree commonly associated with a career in academe, that is the doctorate in nursing or a related field.

NUMBER OF NURSES HOLDING MINIMAL CREDENTIAL FOR A FACULTY POSITION

To estimate the supply of Master's prepared nurses the Preliminary Findings: 2004 National Sample Survey of Registered Nurses (Health Resources and Services Administration, 2005) was reviewed. These data estimated that there are 2,909,467 registered nurses in the country, of which 13% or 377,046 hold a Master's or doctoral degree. These would be the potential pool of faculty, being individuals who hold the minimal credential for the position. Nonetheless, a scarce 6% of these individuals actually occupy full-time faculty positions, according to the data gleaned from the American Association of Colleges of Nursing (AACN) and the National League for Nursing (NLN). In the summary of data from the AACN for 2005–2006 academic year (Fang, Wilsey-Wisniewski, & Bednash, 2006b), 11,635 full-time faculty in baccalaureate and higher degree programs are documented. This is in close agreement to the figures of the National League for Nursing (NLN, 2006), identifying 11,416 full-time faculty in such programs. In addition, the NLN data report that there are 11,166 full-time faculty in associate degree programs and 919 full-time faculty in hospital-based diploma programs. These combined sources of data reflect a full-time national cadre of nursing faculty at slightly less than 23,000.

The NLN data set also includes information on part-time faculty who appear to be proportionately distributed among the three programs, with 9,952 in baccalaureate programs, 9,015 in associate degree programs, and 367 in diploma programs, for a total 18,654 part-time faculty members. This total figure represents 5% of the total nurses who hold the Master's or the doctorate. The impact of this very large number of part-time faculty on the educational programs is beyond the scope of this section; yet, it is a piece of information that is not widely discussed or examined but that clearly effects the nature of the educational program.

EDUCATIONAL PREPARATION FOR FACULTY ROLE

EDUCATIONAL programs at the Master's and doctoral levels have experienced many stimuli for change in the last decade, none as powerful as the publication of the *Essentials of Master's Education in Nursing* by the AACN. That document had the effect of standardizing this educational level and enhancing clinical roles in advanced practice. Although this has been effective in improving many services to citizens through the expanded availability of primary care providers, and has been a major contributor to improving Master's level education, another coincidental outcome was the severe drop in programs of study at the Master's level to prepare individuals for roles in education. As Valiga (2002) has reported; in 1993 there were over 3,000 students enrolled in Master's programs preparatory to the nurse faculty role, whereas in 2001 that number had dropped to a mere 90 students.

Although interest in a career in nursing education waned, during the initial years of the 21st century, enrollment in Master's and doctoral programs across the country demonstrated consistent and substantial growth to the present level of 44,452 in Master's programs and slightly over 4,000 students in various programs of study leading to the doctorate (Fang, Wilsey-Wisniewski, & Bednash, 2006a). These education programs yield approximately 9,000 graduates per year from Master's degree programs in nursing, all of whom have multiple career options with accompanying opportunities. Despite steady growth at the level of the doctorate, the number of graduates each year has remained relatively constant at about 400. The degree to which these individuals seek careers in nursing education is greatly influenced by the ability of the educational sector to recruit these individuals and prepare them for a career in nursing education. They come to the employment arena with little or no background in teaching, curriculum, organizing learning experiences, mentoring beginning neophytes, developing an approach to content, dealing with student issues in learning, personal and professional development, and the host of other tasks incumbent in the basic faculty role. Thus, it is essential to keep in mind that although these individuals graduating from current Master's programs in the United States have considerable clinical expertise, few of these have had very much, or any, preparation for the faculty role. In 2002, the NLN examined this issue critically and developed a clear statement of needed competencies for faculty. Central to these statements was the notion that "clinical expertise was an essential, but insufficient, knowledge" base for the teaching of nursing (NLN, 2002).

NURSES WHO HOLD THE DOCTORATE

IT HAS BEEN WELL known to nurse educators that the discipline lacks the cadre of doctorally prepared faculty, which is characteristic of most academic units in higher education. In an erudite analysis, Hinshaw (2001) summarized the historical evolution of appropriately prepared nurse faculty, but noted the continued existence of less than 50% of the total nursing faculty nationally holding the preferred degree for advancement in higher education. The AACN (Fang, Wilsey-Wisniewski, & Bednash, 2006b) faculty database provides evidence that at the present time about 48% of faculty in baccalaureate and higher degree programs hold the doctorate.

Historically, nurses sought the doctorate with the intention of pursuing an academic career. At the present time, data suggest that the number of graduates from doctoral programs in nursing seeking careers outside of higher education was increasing (Bednash & Berlin, 2002). Concomitantly it is common information within schools of nursing that at least half of all doctoral students are already employed as faculty during some or all of their years of education. As a result, the numbers of students in doctoral programs cannot be "counted" as potential new recruits to higher education as they are already there.

To summarize the supply of nursing faculty, the profession has long been characterized by an academic workforce that did not meet commonly held academic standards, namely, the doctorate. In addition, despite a history of strong role preparation at the Master's level for prospective nurse faculty, recent events have decreased the availability of such preparation and fewer Master's programs in nursing education are offered. The vast majority (89%) of the total number of nurses who hold the minimal credential in nursing to qualify for a teaching position, do not work in that area. Although only 11% of all Master's and doctorally prepared nurses work either part or full time in nursing education, evidence suggests for the most part they are inadequately prepared for that role.

THE DEMAND

THE SEVERE SHORTAGE of nursing personnel at the present time and projected for the near future can only be alleviated by a dramatic infusion of new nurses to the workforce. Without a strong cadre of nurse faculty, the education sector will be unable or serious limited in its ability to meet this demand. Thus, we find ourselves now in a situation where the interest in a career in nursing has resurged at a high level across the country, but we are lacking faculty numbers to accommodate the influx. The numbers of qualified applicants being turned away from nursing programs are staggering—AACN (2006) reports 32,617 at the baccalaureate level, and the NLN reports a total of 125,037 distributed across baccalaureate—36,615, associate degree—86,680 and diploma programs—1,742.

Elements that impact the shortage of faculty, over and above the limited pool of individuals prepared to be faculty, relate to the demands of faculty positions, serious inequities between salaries in the clinical domain and those in academe for similarly prepared individuals, and opportunities for career satisfaction.

DEMANDS OF THE FACULTY ROLE

IT IS COMMONLY held notion that a faculty member in nursing must be a clinically competent nurse, a scholar with a record of evidence-based publications, a productive program of research, and an effective and efficient teacher and professional role model. This constitutes an awesome list of accomplishments to achieve. The ability of any one faculty member to be successful across this range of competencies is limited; nonetheless, criteria for promotion and tenure at most institutions require just these elements. It is little wonder then that faculty comment on stress and demands of their positions as reasons to leave higher education. The expansion of enrollment that has occurred recently adds greatly to the demands and workload of faculty.

To this list of demands on nurse faculty, the needs for professional development in that role by faculty must to be emphasized. To empower individuals who want to have a career in higher education, significant attention must be directed at facilitating new faculty, mentoring them as they develop in the role, and providing meaningful supports to them as they build their skill in pedagogy.

Inequities in salary between the clinical domain of practice and the academic arena of education are quite high, and can present even the most committed neophyte teacher with a serious dilemma. Depending on geographical areas of the country, a $20,000 higher salary for practice is common. The AACN data reflect such a difference in the lower ranks of preparation, but as the individual gains in education, to the doctoral level, those differences become even more dramatic and could even reflect a doubling of salary to leave education (Bednash & Berlin, 2002).

Most data on faculty document that there is a high degree of satisfaction found in the faculty role; however, it is also widely noted that it is a demanding and high-pressured position. Many approaches to enhancing satisfaction with the faculty role are underway. Nonetheless, the enormous challenge facing the nursing education community is being met with extraordinary commitment and vision by the 23,000 full-time faculty and 18,654 part-time faculty in the nation. These men and women provide instruction in 1,544 total basic education programs with a total enrollment of 290,309 students (NLN, 2004) and 44,452 Master's students in 364 graduate programs, and 4,000 candidates in 140 various doctoral level programs (Fang, Wilsey-Wisniewski, & Bednash, 2006a). To expand any of these enrollment figures significant increases in the numbers and preparation of the nation's nursing faculty must be pursued. An additional challenge will be to prepare faculty that reflect the diversity of the student body and patient population.

EILEEN H. ZUNGOLO

See Also
American Association of Colleges of Nursing
Faculty Recruitment to Academic Settings
Faculty Retention
National League for Nursing

REFERENCES

American Association of Colleges of Nursing. (2006). *Faculty shortages in baccalaureate and graduate nursing programs: Scope of the problem and strategies for expanding the supply.* Retrieved October 1, 2006, from http://www.aacn.nche.edu/Publications/WhitePapers/FacultyShortages.htm

Anonymous. (2006). The nursing school dilemma: Faculty shortage causes potential nursing students to be turned away. *American Academy of Ambulatory Care Nursing, 28*(1), 3.

American Association of Colleges of Nursing. (1995). *The essentials of masters education for advanced practice nursing.* Washington, DC: Author.

Bednash, G. D., & Berlin, L. E. (2002). *The shortage of doctorally prepared nursing faculty in institutions with baccalaureate and graduate nursing programs: American Association of Colleges of Nursing Perspective. National Advisory Council on Nursing Education and Practice. Second Report to the Secretary of Health and Human Services and the Congress. November 2002. Appendix E.* Retrieved August 5, 2007, from http://bhpr.hrsa.gov/nursing/nacnep.htm

Fang, D., Wilsey-Wisniewski, S. J., & Bednash, G. D. (2006a). *2005–2006 enrollment and graduations in baccalaureate and graduate programs in nursing.* Washington, DC: American Association of Colleges of Nursing.

Fang, D., Wilsey-Wisniewski, S. J., & Bednash, G. D. (2006b). *2005–2006 salaries of instructional and administrative nursing faculty in baccalaureate and graduate programs in nursing.* Washington, DC: American Association of Colleges of Nursing.

Health Resources and Services Administration. (2005). *Preliminary findings: 2004 national sample survey of registered nurses.* Retrieved October 1, 2006, from http://bhpr.hrsa.gov/healthworkforce/reports/rnpopulation/preliminaryfindings.htm

Hinshaw, A. S. (2001). A continuing challenge: The shortage of educationally prepared nursing faculty. *Online Journal of Issues in Nursing, 6,* 1. Retrieved August 5, 2007, from http://www.nursingworld.org/ojin/topic14/tpc14_3.htm

Klestzick, R. K. (2004, December 15). *Startling data from the NLN's comprehensive survey of all nursing programs evokes wake-up call.* News release retrieved October 6, 2006, from http://www.nln.org/newsreleases/datarelease05.pdf

MacDonald, J. G. (2006, October 4). Nursing schools short on teachers. *USA Today,* 7D.

National League for Nursing. (2002). *Position statement: The preparation of nurse educators.* New York: Author. Retrieved October 1, 2006, from http://www.nln.org/aboutnln/PositionStatements/prepofnursed02.htm

National League for Nursing. (2004). *Startling data from the NLN's comprehensive survey of all nursing programs evokes a wake-up call.* Retrieved on October 1, 2006, from http://www.nln.org/newsreleases/datarelease05pdf

National League for Nursing. (2006). *Nursing data review academic year 2004–2005.* New York: Author.

Valiga, T. M. (2002). *The nursing faculty shortage: National League for Nursing perspective.* National Advisory Council on Nursing Education and Practice. Second Report to the Secretary of Health and Human Services and the Congress. November 2002. Appendix D. Retrieved August 6, 2007, from http://bhpr.hrsa.gov/nursing/nacnep.htm

Failure to Rescue

F AILURE TO RESCUE (FTR) refers to situations in which hospitalized patients die following complications, particularly in instances in which their conditions were not identified and treated in a timely manner. It also refers to various methods of applying this concept to measure hospital performance. The idea behind FTR is that the likelihood of patients being saved from complications relates to the quality of surveillance of patients by staff, the speed of recognition of causes of clinical deterioration, and the timeliness of interventions to reverse it. The term "failure to rescue," as well as the original strategy for measuring rates of unsuccessful rescues using administrative data sources (specifically, hospital discharge abstracts), were both developed by Dr. Jeffrey Silber, a health services researcher at the University of Pennsylvania (Silber, Williams, Krakauer, & Schwartz, 1992), and were first used in nursing research by the Center for Health Outcomes and Policy Research, University of Pennsylvania School of Nursing. A number of different approaches to calculating FTR rates appear in the literature; research aimed at refining measures of FTR and identifying new ways to apply the concept in practice is ongoing. Guidelines and computer codes for calculating failure to rescue rates from patient discharge abstract data have been distributed by the Agency for Healthcare Research and Quality (AHRQ; see http://www.qualityindicators.ahrq.gov/psi_overview.htm) and the National Quality Forum (NQF; 2004). Failure to rescue is currently best validated for surgical patients, but the broader concept clearly has applications in other clinical populations (Clarke, 2004; Simpson, 2005).

It has been argued that FTR rates may measure quality of care as much or perhaps more than the occurrence of complications themselves (which tend to be closely linked to patients' underlying conditions). Links between FTR and nursing are felt to relate to nurses' central roles in monitoring patients and mobilizing health care teams to implement rescues (Clarke & Aiken, 2003). Organizational context as set by managers and other health care leaders (in the form of staffing levels and elements such as relations between nurses and physicians, continuing education and other resources, as well as support of clinicians' decisions by administrators) is believed to be key to successful rescues (Clarke, 2004; Clarke & Aiken, 2003). Failure to rescue rates appear to be lower in hospitals with higher ratios of nurses to patients and in those with more nurses holding higher educational credentials (Aiken, Clarke, & Sloane, 2002; Aiken, Clarke, Cheung, Sloane, & Silber, 2003; Needleman, Buerhaus, Mattke, Stewart, & Zelevinsky, 2002), as well as in teaching hospitals and those with high-technology facilities (Silber, Rosenbaum, & Roth, 1995; Silber, Williams, Krakauer, & Schwartz, 1992).

Widespread discussion of the FTR concept has led to the identification and treatment of complications, receiving much attention in the patient safety movement. One of the best known resulting approaches has been the emergence of Rapid Response Teams (mobile teams of well-trained nurses, physicians, and others who can quickly troubleshoot and intervene at the earliest signs of trouble in order to favor rescues)—these were one of the main elements of the intervention package marketed by the Institute for Healthcare Improvement's 100,000 Lives Campaign (http://www.ihi.org).

SEAN CLARKE
LINDA H. AIKEN

See Also
Agency for Healthcare Research and Quality
Institute for Healthcare Improvement
National Quality Forum
Rapid Response Teams

REFERENCES

Aiken, L. H., Clarke, S. P., Cheung, R. B., Sloane, D. M., & Silber, J. H. (2003). Education levels of hospital nurses and surgical patient mortality. *Journal of the American Medical Association, 290,* 1617–1623.

Aiken, L. H., Clarke, S. P., & Sloane, D. M. (2002). Hospital staffing, organization, and quality of care: Cross-national findings. *International Journal of Quality in Health Care, 14,* 5–13.

Aiken, L. H., Clarke, S. P., Sloane, D. M., Sochalski, J., & Silber, J. H. (2002). Hospital nurse staffing and patient mortality, nurse burnout, and job dissatisfaction. *Journal of the American Medical Association, 288,* 1987–1993.

Clarke, S. P. (2004). Failure to rescue: Lessons from missed opportunities in care. *Nursing Inquiry, 11*(2), 67–71.

Clarke, S. P., & Aiken, L. H. (2003). Failure to rescue. *American Journal of Nursing, 103*(1), 42–47.

National Quality Forum (NQF). (2004). *National voluntary consensus standards for nursing-sensitive care: An initial performance measure set.* Washington, DC: Author. Retrieved September 14, 2006, from http://www.qualityforum.org/txNCFINALpublic.pdf

Needleman, J., Buerhaus, P., Mattke, S., Stewart, M., & Zelevinsky, K. (2002). Nurse staffing and quality of care in hospitals in the United States. *New England Journal of Medicine, 346*(22), 1715–1722.

Silber, J. H., Williams, S. V., Krakauer, H., & Schwartz, J. S. (1992). Hospital and patient characteristics associated with death after surgery. A study of adverse occurrence and failure to rescue. *Medical Care, 30*(7), 615–629.

Silber, J. H., Rosenbaum, P. R., & Ross, R. N. (1995). Comparing the contributions of groups of predictors: Which outcomes vary with hospital rather than patient characteristics? *Journal of the American Statistical Association, 90,* 7–18.

Simpson, K. R. (2005). Failure to rescue: Implications for evaluating quality of care during labor and birth. *Journal of Perinatal and Neonatal Nursing, 19*(1), 24–34.

Family Educational Rights and Privacy Act of 1974 (The Buckley Amendment)

THE FAMILY EDUCATIONAL RIGHTS AND PRIVACY ACT OF 1974 (FERPA), also known as The Buckley Amendment, is a federal law that gives students rights to privacy regarding their academic and financial records. The complete document may be accessed within the Code of Federal Regulations as follows: 34CFR Part 99.1–.8 (Code of Federal Regulations, 2006). Within the Code of Federal Regulations, FERPA is divided into five subparts. Subpart A is further divided into eight additional categories that describe which educational institutions are regulated by this act, the purpose and definition, the rights of students and parents and notification procedures and legal concerns. Subpart B covers three areas regarding parental rights of inspection of records, fees for photocopying of records and specific limitations regarding record viewing. Subpart C outlines three sections related to amending academic records, requirements, and rights to a hearing. Subpart D covers 10 areas related to consent for disclosing information including record keeping, limitations, emergency or medical issues, directories, and legal concerns. Last, Subpart E identifies eight areas related to enforcement concerns including complaints, involvement of the Secretary of Education, and potential conflicts with state or local laws (FERPA, 2006). It is essential for academic faculty and administrators to understand the nuances of this federal law as it covers student's records that may include grades, advisement, clinical and theory assessments and evaluations, and potential concerns regarding unsafe clinical practice. This act provides students with access to information that is placed in their files. It also explicitly defines that only select educational personnel may access their files. The student's permission must be received in writing for any other person or party to see or read their file. If a student is financially dependent on their parents while pursuing a degree, the parents have access to these records without consent (The Buckley Amendment, 2006).

RONDA MINTZ-BINDER

REFERENCES

Code of Federal Regulations. (2006). Retrieved July 7, 2006, from http://www.gpoaccess.gov/cfr/index.html

Family Educational Rights and Privacy Act (FERPA). (2006). Retrieved July 7, 2006, from http://www.ed.gov/policy/gen/guid/fpco/pdf/ferparegs.pdf

The Buckley Amendment. (2006). Retrieved July 7, 2006, from http://www.viterbo.edu/academic/advising/buckley.htm

Financing Health Care

T HE FINANCING OF HEALTH CARE in the United States during the 20th century progressed from charitable enterprise to big business. Technological developments in the 19th century, including anesthesia, understanding germ theory through science, surgery, and medical education, along with the rapid evolution of the nursing profession, created a need for modern hospitals. Religious groups, ethnic organizations, philanthropists, women's associations, among others began and staffed hospitals in large and small communities. Among the earliest principles established for these institutions was that patients who could would pay for hospital services in the same way medical care was paid for; by fees-for-services (Stevens, 1999, pp. 30–39). From this principle evolved a role for insurance and public payments for hospital and medical care for enrolled or eligible patients; charity was displaced.

Blue Cross and Blue Shield Associations became the largest private insurance plans for financing health care for workers. Employers paid for health insurance as a benefit for employees in lieu of wage increases. Patients were asked by hospitals and doctors to "assign" the health insurance benefits to them; thus patients saw little of the financial transaction performed by these "third parties" on their behalf. Medicare and Medicaid programs followed with payments for hospitals and doctors on behalf of the elderly and the poor. Nearly all the provisions of the governmental programs were based on the fee-for-service model that Blue Cross used for hospitals and Blue Shield employed to pay physicians. The "Blues" were managed by hospitals and doctors in arrangements that insured that all costs of providing services were covered in the charges made by the hospitals to the insurance companies. Ensuring a revenue stream for hospitals and doctors, especially when the poor and elderly were covered, guaranteed growth and prosperity for all involved in providing health services. As the health services sector was not dependent on investors, much of the excess revenue was devoted to providing more and better services. Few if any births or deaths occurred in hospitals a hundred years ago and now most take place there, for example. Escalation in service provision over the course of the century led to investments in health services that were a negligible part of the gross domestic product at the start and grew to 15.3% of the 2003 GDP (National Center for Health Statistics, 2005).

The tension between the use of public and private monies for health services surfaced soon after the 1966 beginning of the public Medicare and Medicaid programs and reflected political currents that went from liberal to conservative to liberal and back again. Neither philosophy, however, had any demonstrable effect on reducing the escalation in services and their costs. Health care cost control has shifted from public to private initiatives but neither has gained sufficient support to do more than to make the shift back and forth from public to private anything more than temporary. The United States continues to spend more on health services than any other industrialized country. The government and employers have begun to shift some costs to users but even this has not slowed growth. Gaps in public and private financing for health care have resulted in 40+ million people without health care coverage, nearly 14% of the population, many members of working families. Health care financing in the United States is very problematic; yet the tendency is to employ polar opposite principles, market competition or a governmental system, in recommendations for reform. The result has been a standstill (Iglehart, 2005).

The Committee on the costs of Medical Care issued a 1932 report promoting the bundling of medical and hospitals costs and offering these services for a prepaid monthly premium (Ross, 2002). The few health maintenance organizations that followed were successful, mostly on the west coast, Kaiser and Group Health of Puget Sound, principally among them. These prepaid group plans and other so-called managed care programs were given a boost when Yale scientists founded diagnosis-related groups[1] (DRGs). DRGs facilitated the clinical interpretation of hospitals costs, melding financial and medical data and enabling the setting of all inclusive rates. In many prepaid plans, physicians continue to receive fees for services. Hospitals in the beginning of the 21st century receive flat rate payments for specified patient conditions either through Medicare or negotiations with managed care insurance carriers.

The 2004 cost of registered nurses is a significant fraction of health care costs (5.8% of NHE or $99 billion)[2] but of late they have been declining as a proportion of total National Health Expenditures (NHE). The costs of nurses and nursing, as a proportion of NHE, began to decline in 1966 with the Medicare program. As much as half of a hospital's pre-Medicare expenses were once for nurses, including nursing education. Nurse education expenses were shifted from hospitals to community colleges in the first decade after Medicare. Although more nurses were educated and employed, growth in expenses for administration, drugs, construction, and equipment, among others, far exceeded growth in the cost of nurses.

Concern for unchecked growth in NHE occupies the attention of state and federal policymakers. Nurses have opportunities to contribute to efficient and effective health care but have been hampered by limits imposed by their limited educations; most have less than a baccalaureate degree (Health Resources and Services Administration, 2005). Ambulatory mental health care has shifted away from medical care by physicians to care from therapists who are psychologists and social workers, mainly. Nurse anesthetists provide a majority of anesthesia care. These examples of what was once medical care now performed by nonphysicians suggest that similar models for primary care may potentially place well educated nurses in positions to provide initial services to patients.

The number of capable nurses, the 13% with graduate degrees (assuming all would be in practice), has severely limited such a shift away from physician care. Managed care has stimulated some of the shift from physician care to nurses in primary care. Only major investments in graduate nurse education will ensure that as many as half U.S. nurses

---

[1] John D. Thompson, RN and Robert Fetter were the Yale scientists. Thompson says he found the DRG in Nightingale's 1863, *Notes on Hospitals* (3rd ed.), that argued hospital mortality could only be compared by comparing the mortality of like cases among hospitals; Yale researchers substituted cost for mortality in their comparisons.

[2] Calculated using information from the Preliminary Findings: The Registered Nurse Population—National Sample Survey of RNs 2004. HRSA, HHS: Rockville, MD for numbers and salary data and National Center for Health Statistics (2005) Health, United States—2005. Centers for Medicare and Medicaid Services, Office of the Actuary: Washington, DC, for NHE, Table 123, pp. 365–366.

become involved in primary care. The British Medical Association advocated for patients to see nurses before they see physicians because many of the patient needs can be handled by nurses and, furthermore, physicians in the British National Health Service are not paid more for seeing more patients (Dyer, 2002). Nurses in primary care, using the framework of the International Council of Nurses, *Basic Principles of Nursing Care*, help people, sick or well, in the performance of activities they would do themselves to become independent if they had the strength, will, or knowledge (Henderson, 1997). Support, encouragement, and teaching are indeed the services many need to prevent and manage chronic illnesses. Thorpe (2005) promotes such disease prevention and health promotion as keys to reforming the U.S. health care system. Some of the most significant recent nursing research has demonstrated the capacity of nurses in keeping selected vulnerable sick people away from doctors and hospitals, with greater patient satisfaction (Brooten et al., 1986; Mishel et al., 2002; Naylor et al., 1999; Olds et al., 2002). These studies get much less application than they could in part because the results run counter to the interests of doctors and hospitals, the predominant employers of nurses.

Leaders in the nursing profession have pandered to cries of nurse shortages by preparing new entrants with beginning skills to support the existing hospital and physician dominated health system. Were there to be investments in graduate education for clinical nurses who would compete for patients, more care would be given at less cost. The advice and counsel of nurses in primary care could do the most for alleviating the shortage of nurses by using different and less invasive means for preventing and managing chronic illnesses out of hospitals. For example, a community-based nurse preventing low birth weight infants would reduce the need for the many nurses employed in neonatal intensive care units. Alternatively, a planned health system, such as the one proffered by President William and first lady Hillary Rodham Clinton in 1994, would also seek out nurses to provide primary care for the chronically ill to diminish the need for delayed, more expensive institutional care. Either effective competition or a managed government system will be necessary in the future and it makes no difference to nurses or patients which of the ideologies dominates as either can reduce cost and increase effectiveness.

Nurses are too important to be used to shore up an existing, fragmented, expensive system. Leadership is needed to see that patients have access to the services of nurses in primary care in more than token numbers. Nurses can contribute to the solution of health care financing by collaborating in the provision of primary care, as is done in Health Maintenance Organizations (HMOs), or competing with doctors and hospitals for access to patients. As it is now, nurses are seen as part of the problem of financing health care in the United States.

EDWARD J. HALLORAN

See Also
Benchmarking
Case Management
Patient Classification Systems

REFERENCES

Brooten, D., Kumar, S., Brown, L. P., Butts, P., Finkler, S. A., Bakewell-Sachs, S., et al. (1986). A randomized clinical trial of early hospital discharge and home follow-up of very-low-birth-weight infants. *New England Journal of Medicine, 315*(15), 934–939.

Dyer, O. (2002). News roundup: BMA suggests nurses could become gatekeepers of the NHS. *BMJ, 324,* 565. Retrieved March 18, 2002, from http://bmj.com/cgi/eletters/324/7337/565

Health Resources and Services Administration. (2005). *Preliminary findings: The registered nurse population—National sample survey of RNs—2004.* Rockville, MD: Author. Retrieved August 28, 2006, from http://bhpr.hrsa.gov/healthworkforce/reports/rnpopulation/preliminaryfindings.htm

Henderson, V. (1997). *ICN's basic principles of nursing care.* Geneva, Switzerland: International Council of Nurses.

Iglehart, J. K. (2005). The struggle that never ends: Reforming US health care. *Health Affairs, 24*(6), 1396–1397.

Mishel, M., Belyea, M., Germino, B., Stewart, J., Bailey, D., Robertson, C., et al. (2002). Helping patients with localized prostate carcinoma manage uncertainty and treatment side-effects: Nurse-delivered psychoeducational intervention over the telephone. *Cancer, 94*(6), 1854–1866.

National Center for Health Statistics. (2005). *Health, United States—2005.* Washington, DC: Centers for Medicare and Medicaid Services, Office of the Actuary.

Naylor, M. D., Brooten, D., Campbell, R., Jacobsen, B. S., Mezey, M. D., Paule, M. V., et al. (1999). Comprehensive discharge planning and home follow-up of hospitalized elders: A randomized clinical trial. *Journal of the American Medical Association, 281*(7), 613–620.

Olds, D., Eckenrode, J., Henderson, C., Kitzman, H., Powers, J., Cole, R., et al. (1997). Long-term effects of home visitation on maternal life course and child abuse and neglect: Fifteen year follow up of a randomized clinical trial. *Journal of the American Medical Association, 278*(8), 637–643.

Olds, D., Robinson, J., O'Brian, R., Luckey, D., Pettitt, L., Henderson, C., et al. (2002). Home visiting by paraprofessionals and by nurses: A randomized, controlled trial. *Pediatrics, 110*(3), 486–496.

Ross, J. S. (2002). Committee on the costs of medical care and the history of health insurance in the US. *Einstein Quarterly Journal of Biology and Medicine, 19,* 129–134.

Stevens, R. (1999). *In sickness and in wealth.* Baltimore: Johns Hopkins University Press.

Thorpe, K. (2005). The rise in health care spending and what to do about it. *Health Affairs, 24*(6), 1436–1445.

Financing Nursing Education

NURSING EDUCATION is financed through public and private sources and is highly varied. Therefore, it is important to determine the sources of revenue, both actual and potential. Providing adequate resources is one of the most important responsibilities of a nursing education leader.

In general for private institutions, sources of revenue include: (1) philanthropy either in operating funds (through annual gifts from donors, including alumni, to be spent that year) or from interest earned on endowments; (2) grants from private and public sources; and (3) student generated revenue through tuition and fees. In public institutions, sources of revenue include these, plus monies from state governments. It is important to know the amount and percentage from each source and the nursing leader must work to maximize funds in each category. Beyond this basic information, the leader must understand the revenue stream; for example, whether the school gets all or just a percentage of the funds generated by tuition and fees and whether these funds accrue to the school in the same year they are generated.

The art of fund-raising is beyond the scope of this entry; however, it is important that a nursing education leader acquire these skills.

Friend-making comes before fund-raising, and a leader must devote adequate time to building a support base. Annual campaigns raise funds for that year and are called operating costs, whereas endowments consist of principal (which is never spent) and interest (which is generally spent each year). Interest earned is generally divided into two parts—one added back to the principal so the corpus grows to keep up with inflation, and the other available to be spent that year. Thus, if interest earned during the year is 10%, 5% might be added back to the corpus and 5% made available for expenditure that year. In general, endowed funds are invested conservatively and returns may be below what an aggressive portfolio might earn during a given year.

There is a wide variety of grant sources and a leader must track opportunities from federal, state, and private agencies that offer competitive grant opportunities. The Division of Nursing, Bureau of Health Professions at the Department of Health and Human Services (http://bhpr.hrsa.gov/) has a long track record of offering funds for the education of nurses at all levels, including capitation grants of the late 1960s and 1970s. Likewise, a leader must be active in tracking legislation that impacts upon funds for nursing education. Research grants from public or private sources also provide funds to a school. Funds are categorized as either direct costs—salaries and so on to do the research work—and indirect costs—infrastructure costs, such as utility cost for the research space. Indirect costs may be as high as 55% of the grant or as low as 8% or in some cases they may be zero according to the funding agency. What part of the indirect costs recovered go to central administration versus the research entity (school) depends on negotiations within the university.

Ways to maximize student tuition and fees without creating an insurmountable burden on students is another challenge. Funds from state governments for public schools may come through formulas or from specific line items. Funds may be allocated to the school directly or may be funneled through the university administration. In all cases, there will no doubt be taxes or overhead deductions for central administration costs. The leader must be vigilant to negotiate the net amounts that get to the school.

There are a number of variables to be considered in analyzing a budget for an educational program. These include institutional, program, and environmental variables. Institutional variables include:

1. Type and mission of institution—for example, small liberal arts with teaching as the primary mission versus health science center with teaching, research, and service as the mission areas

2. Type of nursing program—full service (freshman-senior) versus upper division only
3. Scope of programs offered—entry-level, career ladder, graduate, and so on

Program variables include:

1. Faculty size, qualifications, workload, and salaries
2. Student enrollment and level
3. Curriculum patterns
4. Support staff size and expertise, from clerical to information technologists

Environmental variables include:

1. Political factors
2. Economic factors
3. Physical milieu
4. Accreditation requirements/status

Although there is a dearth of reliable and credible studies that calculate the cost of educating a nursing student, a figure established in 2004 was $20,000 per baccalaureate level nursing student (Starck, 2005). For conversion into current year dollars, see http://stats.bls.gov/cpi. The 2004 figure of $20,000 per student is based on a 1:10 faculty to student ratio and accounts for faculty salary, benefits, and operating costs. This is also based on a model of a faculty member spending 70% of his/her time in incoming-producing activity, including teaching, research, or practice with 30% time allowed for personal scholarship development and service to the institution and the profession, committee work, and so on. Because nursing leaders are challenged to be cost efficient and creative, it is important to design better ways to educate with the resources available. This would lead to a cost analysis to determine the cost of each degree program (BSN vs. MSN, etc.) and to determine costs within programs. For example, Health Assessment is a course that can consume a great deal of faculty time if students must be supervised in a 1:1 ratio. In one program, however, costs were reduced dramatically by getting volunteer nurses from the hospital, trained in a short orientation by the faculty, to do the end-of-course individual examinations of student performance. Another way to save resources is to maximize core courses at the graduate level as there is a tendency to develop specific courses for each specialty track, for example, a core Pharmacology course rather than a Pharmacology course for Geriatrics and every other specialty. An analysis of production costs of education can help make creative decisions about alternative ways of education. One challenge has been the move to the use of information technology in education, which requires enormous start-up and continuing costs and has yet to result in increased productivity in terms of numbers of students.

Like all things, financing nursing education is relative. Arguments can be made about the investment of education to the well-being of the economy as well as the health of society. One also can compare the cost of nursing with other disciplines within a university (Starck & Williams, 1988). Studies of the cost of education in other health related disciplines such as medicine help to establish the value of investment in nursing education; for example, 14 nurse practitioners can be educated for the cost of one physician (Gonyea, 1998).

PATRICIA L. STARCK

See Also
Philanthropy/Fund-Raising

REFERENCES

Gonyea, M. A. (1998). Assessing resource requirements and financing for health professions education. In E. R. Rubin (Ed.), *Mission management: A new synthesis* (Vol. 2, pp. 217–233). Washington, DC: Association of Academic Health Centers.

Starck, P. L. (2005). The cost of doing business in nursing education. *Journal of Professional Nursing, 21*(3), 183–190.

Starck, P. L., & Williams, W. E. (1988). What does nursing education cost? Turning the question around. *Journal of Professional Nursing, 4*(1), 38–44.

U.S. Department of Labor, Bureau of Labor Statistics. (n.d.). *Consumer price index, inflation calculator.* Retrieved June 18, 2004, from http://stats.bls.gov/cpi

Financing of Nursing Research and Research Training

NURSING RESEARCH, like other health sciences, is primarily funded through the National Institutes of Health (NIH), mainly through the National Institute of Nursing Research (NINR). A number of other nonfederal sources also fund nursing research and research training. Foundations dedicated to health issues provide research grants and research training awards to nurse investigators as well as other sources, such as professional organizations, universities, hospitals, and corporations. As research investigators grow with their research programs, different types and amounts of financing are needed. A new investigator piloting his/her research idea(s) will seek small grants funds, whereas an established investigator will seek sizeable, multiyear funding that has more limited sources. Building research centers of excellence requires another type of funding, including significant amounts and multiyear commitments. Research training and career development funding also varies widely. A central theme in the funding process is the importance of a strong match of the federal or private sources to the needs of the investigators and their research programs.

Some significant sources for financing nursing research and research training are as follows.

239

240

FINANCING OF
NURSING
RESEARCH AND
RESEARCH
TRAINING

FEDERAL

THE NATIONAL INSTITUTES OF HEALTH (NIH) (U.S. Department of Health and Human Services, HHS) provides the bulk of funds for health sciences. The National Science Foundation (NSF) funds a number of basic biological and behavioral studies. The major source of funding for nursing research is the NINR, established April 16, 1986, as one of the NIH entities (see NIH.gov Web site). Legislatively created as a National Center, it was redesignated as an Institute in June of 1993. Nursing research, however, is also funded through many other NIH entities as well, for example, the National Institute on Aging (NIA), and the National Cancer Institute (NCI). Extramural awards are provided for research and research training. Funding opportunities range from pilot grant funds (Small Grants R03) to significant amounts awarded for usually 3–5 years to support the study of important critical issues (Research Project Grants R01) to multiyear, sizeable awards to establish research Centers of Excellence (Center Grants P30, P50, P60). For a complete listing of award mechanisms (NIH, 2006a), see http://grants.nih.gov/grants/funding/funding_program.htm.

NIH funding opportunities for research training and career development awards range from pre-doctoral, individual (F31s) and institutional awards (T32s) to postdoctoral awards that can be obtained by individuals (F32s) or educational institutions (T32s). There are also funds for senior scientist awards and career development awards. See NIH (2006b) Research Training and Research Career Opportunities, http://grants.nih.gov/training/careerdevelopmentawards.htm.

FOUNDATIONS

FOUNDATIONS ARE NONPROFIT organizations established to provide funds focused on the purpose and interests of the founders and board members of the Foundation. In health care, the Robert Wood Johnson and John A. Hartford foundations are examples of nonprofit foundations funding research and research training. For example, the John A. Hartford Foundation focuses on geriatric issues and has funded nursing research centers of excellence as well as predoctoral and postdoctoral fellowships for research training. The American Nurses Foundation (ANF) funds numerous pilot projects in nursing research. The Foundation Center (http://foundationcenter.org) can be used to identify foundation funding sources.

PROFESSIONAL ASSOCIATIONS

THERE ARE PROFESSIONAL associations specific to health care professions, for example, nursing and disease conditions such as the American Heart Association, and the American Cancer Society, that sponsor

241

*Financing of
Nursing
Research and
Research
Training*

programs for research and research training, for example, Sigma Theta Tau International funds small grants through every Chapter. The Oncology Nursing Society funds pilot research in cancer care research.

EDUCATIONAL INSTITUTIONS

EDUCATIONAL INSTITUTIONS, such as universities, fund multiple pilot studies to facilitate faculty's ability to successfully compete for major federal and nonfederal grant awards. These institutions also provide numerous scholarships for research training, plus released time and sabbaticals.

HOSPITAL FINANCING

A NUMBER OF HOSPITALS finance nursing research that is of particular concern to the organization as well as the investigator. An example in nursing are the studies conducted at the University of Iowa by the Clinical Nurse Researcher employed by the hospital (Titler et al., 2001).

BUSINESS CORPORATIONS

PHARMACEUTICAL AND HEALTH care product companies invest funds in research and research training when their business purposes are also advanced by the investigations. In nursing, an example is the postdoctoral fellowships sponsored by Pfizer Incorporated.

ADA SUE HINSHAW

See Also
American Nurses Foundation
National Institute of Nursing Research
Sigma Theta Tau International

REFERENCES

Foundation Center. Retrieved August 16, 2006, from http://foundation center.org/
National Institutes of Health (NIH). (2006a). Retrieved August 14, 2006, from http://grants.nih.goJv/grants/funding/funding_program.htm
National Institutes of Health (NIH). (2006b). Retrieved August 14, 2006, from http://grants.nih.gov/training/careerdevelopmentawards.htm
Titler, M. G., Kleiber, C., Steelman, V. J., Rakel, B. A., Budreau, G., Everett, L. Q., et al. (2001) The Iowa model of evidence-based practice to promote quality care. *Critical Care Nursing Clinics of North America, 13*(4), 497–509.

Flextime

FLEXTIME IS A SYSTEM used in employee staffing and scheduling to retain employees, allowing employees to select time schedules that meet both work responsibilities and personal needs. Key features include: variable start times, such as working longer or shorter than the 8-hour shift, arriving on or leaving a unit at different times, for example, five nurses arrive at 0700 and work until 1500 or one nurse arrives at 1100 and works until 1900, and weekend programs. Leader-manager pitfalls of flextime can include disruption in continuity of patient care and communication, particularly in situations with families, over- or under-staffing, and difficulty in coordinating appropriate coverage by staff.

MARTHA J. GREENBERG

REFERENCE

American Nurses Association. (2002). *Background information and legislative maps: Nurse staffing plans and ratios*. Retrieved September 5, 2007, from http://www.nursingworld.org/HiddenDocumentVault/GOVA/Federal/2004StaffingPlansandRatios.aspx

Foundation Funding of Health Care and Nursing

F OUNDATIONS ARE DEFINED as organizations or entities that exist for the sole purpose of supporting charitable works. Foundations are often supported by the generous, philanthropic donations of individuals or families with the intention of supporting a particular mission that is of importance. For example, The John J. Barclow Foundation was developed with the sole purpose of promoting compassion and quality of life for the elderly, an issue that was of great importance to the founder, John J. Barclow, and that continues to be carried out by his family. Other foundations are supported by an endowment, which is defined as a stable account housed within a particular *institution*, such as a hospital, university, or foundation, to be used for a defined purpose. Still other foundations are supported through the collective charitable donations of a group of people with common interests, such as the Alzheimer Disease Foundation. Foundations may be privately owned and operated or public, and housed within a public charity such as the National Philanthropic Trust. Whether private or public, foundations are excellent vehicles in which a life meaning or purpose may be fulfilled, and offer private tax benefits for the donating person, family, or

243

institution. From a health care and nursing perspective, foundations provide a growing and exciting source of funding for specific health care issues.

One of the first foundations set up exclusively to support nursing was the Helene Fuld Health Trust, established in 1935. The Robert Wood Johnson Foundation has supported nursing programs since its inception, and over the years has dedicated more than $140 million to nursing projects. Other major foundations that have supported nursing and health care include the W. K. Kellogg Foundation, the Pew Charitable Trusts, the Rockefeller Foundation, the Commonwealth Fund, The Josiah Macy Foundation, and, more recently, the Bill and Melinda Gates Foundation. In addition, there are hundreds of small local, regional, and national foundations that support nursing and health care initiatives, for example, the New York–based Donald and Barbara Jonas Center for Nursing Excellence.

Key foundations that have supported nursing work include that of the Robert Wood Johnson Foundation and the Pew Charitable Trusts, which jointly in 1988 supported a multimillion dollar national project titled "Strengthening Hospital Nursing: A Program to Improve Patient Care" to provide better patient care through innovative, hospital-wide restructuring; the John A. Hartford Foundation support of geriatric nursing initiatives through several education and research projects; and the Independence Foundation, which funded endowed professorships at 10 private schools of nursing.

Foundations that support health care and nursing are generally organizations with a particular purpose, such as enhancing research about a particular disease or promoting a certain type of care. The missions may be broad, such as that of the Gustavus and Louise Pfeiffer Research Foundation for the general improvement of the public health through the advancement and promotion of medicine and pharmacy, or more specific such as the Lance Armstrong Foundation, which aims to educate and empower cancer survivors. Thus it is important in seeking foundation funding that health care and nursing professionals target foundations with similar missions. In this way, relationships may be built that provide a continued source of support for important research and work in health care. In developing such relationships and grant applications, it is also important to be aware that although these foundations often fund health care, they may not have nurses and health care providers on the review board for applications. Consequently, it is important that nursing and health care jargon be avoided and the project under review explained in a manner that all populations will understand. Finally, from an ethical perspective, the researcher may have greater experience in identifying consent and approval issues than the foundation. Thus, great attention must be made to adhering to ethical nursing standards for research, regardless of foundation requirements.

MEREDITH WALLACE
JOYCE J. FITZPATRICK

See Also
Philanthropy/Fund-Raising

REFERENCE

Roelofs, J. (2003). *Foundations and public policy: The mask of pluralism.* Albany, NY: State University of New York Press.

WEB REFERENCES

National Philanthrapic Trust, http://www.nptrust.org/
Foundations.org, www.foundations.org
Foundation Center, www.fdncenter.org
Council on Foundations, www.cof.org
Association of Small Foundations, www.smallfoundations.org
Network Solutions, www.nnh.org/NewNNH/foundations.htm
Grantmakers in Health, www.gih.org

Franklin, Martha Minerva

MARTHA MINERVA FRANKLIN was born in Connecticut in 1870; she died in 1968 at the age of 98 (Carnegie, 1995). The only black student in her class, Franklin graduated from the nurses' training school at Women's Hospital in Philadelphia in 1897 (Carnegie, 1995). Franklin was among the first to actively campaign for black equality in nursing, for equitable availability of jobs in nursing, and for equitable treatment in the various nursing organizations. Black nurses wanted to organize; as a result, groups began to form at the local level to discuss the issues of segregation and discrimination. As a party of one, Franklin single-handedly polled 1,500 black nurses to garner their opinion about a national assembly to address these same issues (Carnegie, 1995). The National Association for Colored Graduate Nurses (NACGN) evolved from this initiative in 1908. The primary goals of this neophyte organization included the promotion of standards and welfare of all trained nurses, and the development of strategies to abolish racial discrimination within the profession of nursing. In 1951, the NACGN was integrated into the American Nurses Association. Franklin was inducted posthumously into the American Nurses Association Hall of Fame in 1976.

M. JANICE NELSON

See Also
American Nurses Association
ANA Hall of Fame
National Black Nurses Association, Inc.

REFERENCES

American Nurses Association. (2006). *1976 inductee: Martha Minerva Franklin, 1870–1968*. Retrieved March 22, 2006, from http://nursingworld.org/hof/franmm.htm

Carnegie, M. E. (1995). *The path we tread: Blacks in nursing worldwide* (3rd ed.). New York: National League for Nursing Press.

G

Gender and Leadership

TOMORROW BELONGS TO WOMEN forecasts Tom Peters in one of his latest works on leadership. Peters realizes, as others have, that women's talents are much better suited to the new service economy of the 21st century than men's are. Because of gender differences in the way they process the world around them, many experts believe that women are better at a lot of the skills that matter in leadership (Peters, 2005). For instance, relationship skills are vital to the new breed of transformational leaders. Leaders have an uncanny ability to "connect" with followers and, often, other leaders. Trust is a crucial ingredient, as are empathy and emotional intelligence. These are areas in which women excel. Women have a talent with relationships and often can read all the guideposts and relationship barometers that tell you whether you're on the right track (Peters, 2005). Women have a greater capacity to read body language or nonverbal cues (Peters, 2005). They generally have greater emotional sensitivity, intuition and empathy, and generally are more patient and have the ability to do many things simultaneously. Undoubtedly, many of us have noticed that emotionally sensitive traits like these are more prevalent—in general—in women than men. Now there is science to back up this claim.

Fairly dramatic differences in the reactions of the brains of the men and women have been found (Gur et al., 1999). Female brains show reactions that span eight times greater an area in the brain than that of male subjects in the limbic or emotional seat of the brain. Findings have led to the same conclusion: the thoughts and emotional processes of men and women are fundamentally different in a number of ways. Men's thinking is more compartmentalized, whereas women's is more integrated.

Research on feminine cognition reveals the ability to move more gracefully from intellect to intuition and from linear to nonlinear thought than men. This is the reason why women—our wives and our mothers and the female leaders—are so good at multi-tasking, the ability to do many different things at once. Their male counterparts, brilliant though they may be in their fields, are not as able to juggle many activities simultaneously.

UNBROKEN WHOLENESS: IT'S BECOMING A 'WOMAN'S WORLD'

THESE NEW SCIENTIFIC findings are very significant for leadership when you consider new findings in physics that herald a fundamental shift in our scientific worldview. The shift changes our perspective from a mechanical, compartmentalized Cartesian view to a worldview of unbroken wholeness in which everything is linked and interrelated. Just as Newtonian science and its dependence on mechanical force has produced a "masculine world," the new physics and its dependence on the power inherent in relationship and connection herald the advent of a world that values things that are "feminine" in essence. We have long favored the separateness of the individual self over connection to others, leaning more toward an autonomous life of work than toward the interdependence of love and connection toward each other. And all that is slowly changing. Somehow through interaction, subatomic particles are briefly summoned out of a world of potentiality and possibility into the solid world of tangible things and events. At this level, all is interconnected. How we subjectively experience events, interactions and our inner self is "observer created"—created by us (Hawkens, 2003).

The exploitation of nature has gone hand in hand with the exploitation of women, who have been identified with nature throughout the ages. Francis Bacon, the father of the scientific method, was predisposed to leave women out of the picture. Bacon said of science that it is like a "Woman to be brought into submission and bound and conquered as a slave," leaving an indelible black mark on female ways of knowing (Shearer, 1997). The objective reality that we were all brought up to believe in has proven to be illusive. Space and time are relative. People do not perceive distance and time in exactly the same way. In fact, relative space and time have been shown to be quite subjective; everyone has a different opinion about what they see. In the meantime, the thinking of men like Bacon has created a world that is preoccupied with control and obsessed with carving things into pieces and maintaining boundaries in order to achieve control. As a result, the high values we place on separation, independence, and autonomy have always been taken as fact, and not simply the views of the thought leaders of science at the time.

As Harvard psychologist Carol Gilligan (1993)—known for discovering that female development centers around connection, not separation—states, "The dissociation between thoughts and feelings, suppressing what one knows, the use of one's voice to cover rather than convey one's inner world, so that relationships no longer provide channels for exploring the connections between one's inner life and the world of others," is characteristic of our masculine-minded culture. As the new millennium becomes a more feminine world, our interdependence will create a new understanding of the power of relationships. Gilligan (1993) said, "You cannot take a life out of history," as she discovered that Erik Erikson's well-known theory of *human* development was really a conception of *male* development. His well-known stages of development were centered on separation and autonomy, because the study of the male, as well as mechanistic worldviews, was the norm in science. Scientific discoveries do not exist in a vacuum either, but reflect the beliefs and values of the people in a society, including men like Erikson.

It is no accident that as a new scientific paradigm reveals a world with a new respect for the feminine, the sheer demographic power of baby boomer women in society gives them unprecedented influence. Baby boomer women have ushered in major social reforms including childbearing, reproductive choice, and reforms in women's health, such as the inclusion of women in clinical trials. They represent nearly 25% of the population, and they are the most educated cohort of women in society that there have ever been. Currently, there are one million perimenopausal baby boomer women who have brought menopause and reproductive rights out of the closet.

It has been a task for women to provide leadership throughout history and "Go on believing in life when there was almost no hope," in the words of Margaret Meade. Now science is emerging as the powerful context for a new age of women leaders. Women have always shown love and compassion. The movement in science and the urge toward the feminine are bound to make female leadership the tsunami of the millennium.

PAM MARALDO

REFERENCES

Erikson, E. H. (1963). *Childhood and society*. New York: W. W. Norton & Company.

Gilligan, C. (1993). *In a different voice*. Cambridge, MA: Harvard University Press.

Gur, R. C., Turetsky, B. I., Matsui, M., Yan, M., Bilker, W., Hugett, P., et al. (1999). Sex differences in brain gray and white matter in healthy young adults: Correlations with cognitive performance. *Journal of Neuroscience, 19*(10), 4065–4072.

Hawkens, D. R. (2003). *Reality and subjectivity*. Sedona, AZ: Veritas Publishing.

Peters, T. (2005). *Excerpt from "Re-imagine."* Retrieved August 20, 2006, from http://www.usatoday.com/money/books/2003-12-05-reimagine-excerpt_x.htm

Shearer, A. (1997). *Athene*. New York: Penguin Books.

Global Nursing Shortage

THE GLOBAL NURSING shortage impacts nearly every country and has spawned both competition and cooperation among countries desperate for registered nurses. This reaction by the international community has led to an increase in both the migration and existing shortage of nurses (Thobaben et al., 2005). "The global nurse shortage impacts healthcare delivery in every corner of the world and will require interventions from all sectors of society" (Rosenkoetter, 2005). The reasons for the shortage are complex and involve numerous factors, but in the United States they focus primarily on a high-stress work environment, an aging nursing workforce as well as an aging population, past decreases in nursing school enrollments, a multiplicity of attractive educational and career opportunities for women, the flawed image of nursing, and the increasing demand for nursing services and advanced degrees. Not all of these issues, however, are specific to the United States. The International Council of Nurses (ICN) has issued *The Global Shortage of Registered Nurses: An Overview of Issues and Actions* (2004) and suggests, among other things, that all countries must address the issue of the ratio of nurses to patients. International recruitment, especially from low-income countries that have inadequate nurse to patient ratios, has nevertheless significantly

255

increased. The practice of high-income countries recruiting nurses from less-developed countries that are in need of nurses to address their own health care shortages not only has complicated the shortage but also has created serious ethical dilemmas.

Recruitment from low-income countries is being increasingly scrutinized. International health care leaders are questioning whether it is ever justified to recruit foreign educated nurses from developing countries that are sorely in need of health care providers. Yet nurses have the right to pursue economic and professional career options in more advantaged countries such as the United States, the United Kingdom, Ireland, Norway, and Australia, also called "destination countries" by the World Health Organization (WHO) (Buchan & Sochalski, 2004, p. 587). In doing so, however, those less advantaged countries decrease their own supply of nurses. By pursuing advanced education in the United States or the United Kingdom, for example, nurses have the opportunity to return to their home countries with new knowledge and skills that they can invest in those health care systems and enhance the quality of life of patients and families (Bannon & Roodman, 2004). But the reality is that there is no guarantee that they will return to their home countries, and no data exist that track their migration to, and length of stay in, destination countries (Buchan & Sochalski, 2004).

This conundrum generates additional questions and concerns that nurses in leadership positions need to address when they embark on a program of international recruitment. Should foreign-educated nurses be encouraged to stay in the United States, or should they return to their own countries when their recruitment contracts have ended? If their employment in a high-income country contributes to their families' incomes at home, should they be required to return home after their employment contract is over? Which country has the priority and what are the implications for the migrating nurse in these situations? Additionally, foreign educated nurses may have difficulty with the new culture, the language, and the legal requirements, and may encounter strains on their families in their new country. Hospitals in particular need to provide enculturation programs to assist these nurses with their adjustment, as well as with the patient care they provide, the language, and their social interactions. The ethical considerations in these dilemmas need to be addressed and the time has arrived for nurse recruitment to be the domain of hospital ethics committees.

A study on international nurse mobility (ICN, 2003) sponsored by the WHO, ICN, and the Royal College of Nursing suggests that inadequate working conditions and aggressive recruiting have created "push-pull" forces that foster unhealthy international nurse migration patterns. On the one hand, nurses are needed in the country sponsoring the recruitment; on the other hand, nurses are needed in the countries from which they are being recruited. Although the migrating nurse worsens a "brain-drain" and health care shortage in their own countries when they practice abroad, their incomes often subsidize their families, and indirectly, the economy of their communities, as well as contributing to a better quality of life. In response, "the World Health Organization is exploring policy options for recruiting, managing, and retaining the health workforce in varied labor markets ... [by] ... developing global evidence-based ethical recruitment policies for all of its member states" (Rosenkoetter, 2005).

In the United States, the American Academy of Nurses' Expert Panel on Global Health and Nursing has also studied the complex interrelated factors involved in the shortage, and has issued a *White Paper on Global Nursing and Health* (Rosenkoetter, 2005). Recognizing that a global problem calls for global collaboration in creating solutions, its 13 recommended actions focus on the Academy's key role in fostering dialogue, sharing ideas, and disseminating viable solutions among nurse leaders internationally.

The challenge now for "resourced-countries" is to develop national policies on self-sufficiency. Nurse leaders in health care systems and professional organizations can meet this challenge by participating in the development of policies on the ethical recruitment, retention, and enculturation of foreign nurses, while developing strategies that support their return to their homelands with new practice skills and advanced education. One such strategy is the agreement between the United Kingdom and South Africa, allowing health care professionals to work in each other's countries for only a specified length of time before they must return home. These nurses return home, then, with new skills and resources that benefit their own country and its health system (Sheer, 2006). Another strategy to manage outward migration is the regional collaboration of the Pan American Health Organization (PAHO), nursing organizations, businesses, universities, and governmental agencies in the Caribbean to prevent the ad hoc recruitment of nurses in a region where the average nurse vacancy rate is now approximately 40%. This managed migration model calls for a regulated recruitment, a structured process, incentives to encourage return migration in an agreed-on time frame, and ongoing dialogue between destination and source countries to ensure a more beneficial process (Salmon & Yan, 2005).

Recruiting nurses from other countries today involves not just seeking out those nurses but also the obligation to understand and adequately appreciate the legal and financial implications of migration to the United States. These nurses must now complete the VisaScreen™ and have the more recent advantage of taking the NCLEX-RN® in international locations, including Hong Kong, London (UK), and Seoul, Korea. The process is expensive, especially for nurses who come from low-income countries, and can easily exceed U.S. $2,500. In addition, there are the costs for relocation, including international travel, language courses, courses to upgrade nursing knowledge and skills, housing, and insurance. The nurse leader may decide to assume the responsibility for all or some of these costs. This increases the financial burden of recruitment considerably and may not always be a fiscally responsible decision.

Finding solutions to the global nursing shortage requires a multidimensional approach not only to the global need for nurses and skilled health care providers but also to solving the problems that have caused the shortage. To that end, nurse leaders can, and should play a pivotal role in decisive strategy and policy development, and in advocating for the regulation and monitoring of international recruitment. By promoting integrated transnational investigations of the causes for the global shortage and facilitating the development of multinational solutions, nurse leaders in the United States can be at the forefront of addressing a critical issue in global health care.

MARLENE M. ROSENKOETTER
DEENA A. NARDI

See Also
Commission on Graduates of Foreign Nursing Schools
World Health Organization

REFERENCES

Bannon, A., & Roodman, D. (2004). Partners for development? *Perspectives in Health, 9*(2), 14–21.

Buchan, J., & Sochalski, J. (2004). The migration of nurses: Trends and policies. *Bulletin of the World Health Organization, 82*(8), 587–594.

International Council of Nurses (ICN). (2003). *International nurse mobility: Trends and policy implications.* Retrieved August 5, 2007, from http://www.icn.ch/Int_Nurse_mobility%20final.pdf

International Council of Nurses (ICN). (2004). *The global shortage of registered nurses: An overview of issues and action.* Retrieved August 5, 2007, from http://www.icn.ch./global/shortage.pdf

Rosenkoetter, M. (2005). White paper on global nursing and health. *American Academy of Nursing, Expert Panel on Global Nursing and Health.* Retrieved August 5, 2007, from http://www.aannet.org/committees/ep_global/white_paper.pdf

Salmon, M., & Yan, J. (2005, July 5–10). *The Caribbean context: Prelude to regional strategies.* Paper presented at the International Nurse Migration: Bellagio Conference. Retrieved August 5, 2007, from http://www.academyhealth.org/international/nursemigration/salmon.ppt

Sheer, B. (2006). *Highlights of the 4th ICN International Nurse Practitioner/Advanced Practice Nursing Network conference.* Retrieved August 5, 2007, from http://www.medscape.com/viewarticle/540557?rss

Thobaben, M., Roberts, D., Badir, A., Wang, H., Murayama, H., Murashima, S., et al. (2005). Exploring nursing education in the People's Republic of China, Japan, and Turkey. *Contemporary Nurse, 19*(1–2), 5–16.

H

Hall, Lydia E.

LYDIA ELOISE HALL was born in 1906 and died in 1969. Hall is considered to be one of the early nurse theorists who promulgated the notion that therapeutic use of self and good nursing care are the chief therapies for chronically ill patients. In the late 1960s, Hall postulated her "Core, Care, and Cure" nursing practice model, which presupposes that individuals can be conceptualized in three separate domains: the body (care), the illness (cure), and the person (core) (Ahrens, 2006). Hall believed that the "Care" component was exclusive to nursing, whereas "Cure" is in the realm of the physician but shared by the nurse who assists the patient or families to deal with physician prescriptions. The "Core" is a shared discipline domain involving psychologists, clergy, social workers, and the like. Hall enacted her theory at the Loeb Center for Nursing and Rehabilitation in New York City, which she established and directed from 1963 to 1969 (American Nurses Association, 2006). Hall was inducted posthumously into the American Nurses Association Hall of Fame in 1984. Additional information regarding Lydia Hall can be accessed on the Web at http://www.enursescribe.com/Lydia_Hall.htm.

M. JANICE NELSON

REFERENCES

Ahrens, W. (2006). *Lydia Eloise Hall.* Retrieved May 12, 2006, from http://www.nurses.info/nursing_theory_person_hall_lydia.htm

American Nurses Association. (2006). *Lydia Eloise Hall (1906–1969) 1984 inductee.* Retrieved August 30, 2007, from http://www.nursingworld.org/FunctionalMenuCategories/AboutANA/WhereWeComeFrom_1/Hallof Fame/19761984/hallle5544.aspx

Touhy, T. A., & Birnbach, N. (2001). Lydia Hall, the care, core, and cure model. In M. Parker (Ed.), *Nursing theories and nursing practice* (pp. 132–142). Philadelphia: F. A. Davis.

Health Care Systems

N THE broadest sense, "health care systems" reflect the totality of the health care industry and delivery system—from the patients who receive care, to the providers who manage the care of patients, to the suppliers of equipment and pharmaceuticals used in caring for patients, to the insurers who pay for care, to the decision makers who set local, state, and national policies that guide the delivery of health care (Finkler, Kovner, & Jones, 2007). When used in this macro-level manner, health care systems encompass the structures and processes for delivery and financing of care, as well as the outcomes of care delivery. Important considerations at this macro-level are the economic, political, and regulatory environments. These considerations influence structural aspects of health care systems financing, and the financing of health care systems (including public and private sources) influences the structures and processes of care delivery and ultimately, the outcomes of care delivered.

"Health care systems" also can be viewed at a micro-level to reflect a single organizational entity—which may include one or more organizations—that provides an array of health care services (Bazzoli, Shortell, Dubbs, Chan, & Kralovec, 1999; Dubbs, Bazzoli, Shortell, & Kralovec, 2004). Bazzoli and colleagues distinguish health *systems* from

265

health *networks*, primarily based on the issue of ownership: health care systems have a single owner and represent a tightly connected organizational arrangement, whereas networks have two or more owners and organizations within the network are loosely connected. The authors also use the term "health systems" versus "health care systems," yet "health systems" necessarily implies that care is delivered within the organizational arrangement. The macro-level health care systems described here influence the micro-level health care systems through policy making and financing, which in turn influence specific organizational arrangements.

Interestingly, "health care systems" is becoming known as a specific area of study in business, nursing, and health care leadership. For example, the Wharton School of Business at the University of Pennsylvania (2007) has a Department of Health Care Systems that prepares undergraduate and graduate students with knowledge of health care economics and financing, managing health care organizations, and health policy to work in the health care systems described earlier and in health care–related fields (http://www.wharton.upenn.edu/faculty/acad_depts/hcmgdept.cfm). Health care systems faculty conducts research that supports this area of study, such as examining health care payment systems, health care management strategies, and health care policy making.

Schools of nursing also offer graduate programs in "health care systems." The development of these programs reflects a comprehensive view of potential nursing leadership roles that expands beyond the traditional nursing administration programs. For example, the University of Rochester (n.d.) offers a program of graduate study in health care systems that focuses on health promotion and disaster preparedness. The University of North Carolina at Chapel Hill (2007) also offers a health care systems program of graduate study focusing on nursing administration, education, informatics, and quality improvement. Other similar programs are offered in schools of nursing across the United States (see, for example, the University of Minnesota School of Nursing [2005] and the University of Texas Health Science Center at San Antonio [2007]). These programs have the shared characteristics of preparing nursing leaders with advanced knowledge of the structures, processes, and outcomes of health care systems and particularly the environments within which nursing and health care is delivered. Faculty who teach in these programs conduct research to support this area of study, such as examining models of nursing and health care delivery, nursing workforce issues, and the organization and delivery of nursing and health care—all of which affect and are affected by the health care systems described earlier and within which nursing and health care services are provided.

Health care systems have relevance for nursing leaders because they must distinguish between the various usages to appreciate the associated points of reference and the characteristics of each; however, there are more practical reasons for nursing leaders to possess a clear understanding of the differing usages of the term health care systems. Nurses are increasingly called on to fill leadership roles in both micro- and macro-level health care systems. These nursing leaders must first possess a solid understanding of the intricate relationships among key participants at the macro-level of health care systems. Understanding these relationships provides a context for positioning nursing and nursing leadership roles and opportunities within health care systems.

Second, nursing leaders must understand health care systems at the micro-level to appreciate important characteristics of the system, such as its structure, processes, and outcomes, as well as its culture, resilience, and weaknesses or vulnerabilities in the health care system (Carthey, de Leval, & Reason, 2001). This level of understanding also allows nursing leaders to promote learning within health care systems (Reason, Carthey, & de Leval, 2001). Third, an understanding of the health care system at both the macro- and micro-levels is necessary to understand how the systems and individuals within them behave. For example, micro-level health care systems may take certain actions that influence the practices of individuals within them because of health care systems decision making at the macro level (Finkler, Kovner, & Jones, 2007).

Finally, given that health care systems is fast becoming recognized as an area of study within nursing, business, and health care, nursing leaders must understand this area of study in order to successfully deploy and manage nurses and other health professionals who possess this training. This more comprehensive educational view encompasses critical economic, political, regulatory, and management aspects of health care and holds the promise of preparing nursing leaders with the knowledge, skills, and abilities to bring change and innovations to health care systems and care environments of the future.

CHERYL BLAND JONES

REFERENCES

Bazzoli, G. J., Shortell, S. M., Dubbs, N., Chan, C., & Kralovec, P. (1999). A taxonomy of health networks and systems: Bringing order out of chaos. *Health Services Research, 33*(6), 1683–1717.

Carthey, J., de Leval, M. R., & Reason, J. T. (2001). Institutional resilience in health care systems. *Quality and Safety in Health Care, 10*(1), 29–32.

Dubbs, N. L., Bazzoli, G. J., Shortell, S. M., & Kralovec, P. D. (2004). Reexamining organizational configurations: An update, validation, and expansion of the taxonomy of health networks and systems. *Health Services Research, 39*(1), 207–220.

Finkler, S. A., Kovner, C. T., & Jones, C. B. (2007). *Financial management for nurse managers and executives.* St. Louis, MO: W. B. Saunders.

Reason, J. T., Carthey, J., & de Leval, M. R. (2001). Diagnosing "vulnerable system syndrome": An essential prerequisite to effective risk management. *Quality in Health Care, 10*(4, Suppl II), 21–25.

University of Minnesota School of Nursing. (2005). *Area of study: Nursing and healthcare systems administration.* Retrieved August 19, 2007, from http://www.nursing.umn.edu/MS/ProspectiveStudents/AreasStudy/NursingAdmin/home.html

University of North Carolina at Chapel Hill School of Nursing. (2007). *MSN: Health care systems.* Retrieved August 19, 2007, from http://nursing.unc.edu/degree/msn/hcs.html

University of Rochester School of Nursing. (n.d.). *Leadership programs.* Retrieved August 19, 2007, from http://www.son.rochester.edu/son/prospective-students/programs/leadership/leadership

University of Texas Health Science Center at San Antonio School of Nursing. (2007). *Nurse managers & leaders: Administration in community & health care systems in nursing.* Retrieved August 19, 2007, from http://nursing.uthscsa.edu/grad/achcs.shtml

Wharton School of Business at the University of Pennsylvania. (2007). *Academic department: Health care systems.* Retrieved August 19, 2007, from http://www.wharton.upenn.edu/faculty/acad_depts/hcmgdept.cfm

Health Policy

NURSING IS PROFOUNDLY affected by the actions and decisions of legislative bodies, government agencies, payers, and others whose decisions and actions shape the environment where nurses practice. Federal, state, and local legislatures, government agencies and courts, along with private payers and accrediting bodies, determine or influence such varied issues as: the type of health care coverage and services to which patients are entitled; which professionals are authorized to provide those services; what kinds of standards clinicians, health care organizations, and systems need to meet; how much these providers receive in payment for their services; when care can be withheld; what kinds of privacy rights patients are entitled to; and a range of other issues. Some matters that have traditionally been within the province of individual hospitals are now debated in the policy arena, such as when nurses can be required to work overtime or whether hospitals must adhere to specific standards for nurse staffing levels.

Mason, Leavitt, and Chaffee (2002) describe policy as "encompass[ing] the choices that a society, segment of society or organization makes regarding its goals and priorities and the ways it will allocate its resources to attain those goals" (p. 8). More generally, *health policy* refers to rules, actions, and decisions by government and private bodies—which affect the delivery of health care and the processes by which health care takes place. Much of the study of health policy focuses on the roles of government bodies and officials—that is, *public policy*—but the actions of some private groups, such as large health plans and private accrediting organizations—also have an important impact on health care delivery.

THE IMPORTANCE OF UNDERSTANDING POLICY

A LTHOUGH it would be unrealistic (and unnecessary) to expect all nurse leaders to be experts in health policy, it is increasingly important to have a working knowledge of contemporary and anticipated changes in policy, as well as the processes by which these changes occur. This is important so that nurse leaders can understand and respond to changes in health care, help to explain these changes to those whom they lead, and so these leaders can help to determine strategies for seeking to shape further change. Arguably, all nurses ultimately should achieve "policy literacy" (Malone, 2005)—they should have some understanding of the external policy-related factors that have an impact on their practice and their patients and they should have at least a basic knowledge of relevant policy-making processes. If every nurse should be at least "policy literate," then nurse leaders should have sufficient familiarity with policy issues and processes to inform and guide their actions as leaders.

KNOWLEDGEABLE USE OF EXPERTS

P OLICY expertise often involves complex concepts and issues that require the consultation and guidance of experts. Nursing organizations and health care systems, for instance, often use professional lobbyists to assist in understanding proposed legislation or regulations and to formulate appropriate responses. Making optimal use of such experts, however, requires some degree of knowledge on the part of nurse leaders—not only to guide their own decision making but also to integrate their clinical, management, or professional expertise with the knowledge provided by policy experts. To cite another example, health care delivery organizations and systems may use internal and external experts to understand changes in reimbursement and to make decisions about the reallocation of resources based on those changes. Without a sufficient understanding of those changes, however, it is difficult for nurse leaders to participate fully in such decisions and to ensure that sufficient resources are allocated to nursing services. Similarly, without some understanding of changes in scope of practice legislation and reimbursement policies for advanced practice nurses, it is difficult for nurse leaders in health care delivery organizations to engage in discussions with medical staff and other leaders regarding appropriate utilization of nurse practitioners and clinical nurse specialists in ambulatory, emergency, or inpatient services.

HEALTH POLICY TRAINING AND EDUCATION

A LTHOUGH traditionally advanced nursing education has not included significant policy content (Mechanic & Reinhard, 2002), policy-focused courses are increasingly common in nursing masters and doctoral programs. Increasingly, academic programs that prepare nurses for leadership roles include content on health policy. The American Association of Colleges of Nursing (AACN) has identified health care policy, organization of the health care delivery system, and health care financing as part of the core content for clinical masters programs in nursing (AACN, 1996).

Although a basic understanding of policy and policy making should be part of the knowledge base of all nursing leaders, the profession also needs leaders whose primary expertise focuses on health policy. Such policy leadership is necessary to help guide nursing and its organizations in responding to changes in the policy environment and to develop increased capacity to analyze and shape health policy. There are many nurses for whom policy-related activities are a significant part of their practice (Gebbie, Wakefield, & Kerfoot, 2000). Nurses have advanced into roles as policy leaders through a variety of routes. Some have served as elected or appointed government officials. Others have served as key staff to members of Congress or state legislators. Others have developed policy expertise through leading volunteer or staff roles in professional associations. Increasingly, many nurses have received specialized academic and training programs in health policy. Several nurse leaders, for example, have completed The Robert Wood Johnson Health Policy Fellowship program, which trains mid-career health professionals through didactic and practical experience in Washington, DC, including the opportunity to work directly with a member of Congress.

Some graduate programs provide a specific focus on health policy. The University of California–San Francisco offers nursing Master's and PhD programs in health policy (Harrington, Crider, Benner, & Malone, 2005), whereas the specific focus of the nursing PhD program at the University of Massachusetts Boston is on health policy (Ellenbecker, Fawcett, & Glazer, 2006). Other graduate programs include substantial policy content within a broader framework, such as Columbia University's Doctor of Nursing Science (DNSc) program, the PhD program at Virginia Mason University and the Master's program in management, policy, and leadership at Yale University (Yale School of Nursing, n.d.). Johns Hopkins offers programs through its Institute for Policy Studies (http://ips.jhu.edu), which has an international fellows program and George Mason University has a Graduate Health Systems Management Degree with a Health Policy Analysis Concentration and holds an annual Washington Health Policy Institute (http://www.gmu.edu/departments/chpre/news-events/news-events.html) that includes didactic studies and an opportunity to discuss a variety of issues with members of Congress. Many nurse leaders have received advanced education in health policy through academic programs outside of nursing, including Master's and doctoral degrees in public health, public administration, public policy, and social policy.

OTHER AVENUES FOR HEALTH POLICY KNOWLEDGE

OTHER avenues exist for nurse leaders to increase their knowledge and understanding of health policy. Most large nursing organizations include current legislative and other public policy–related information on their Web sites; these include the Web sites of the American Nurses Association (http://www.nursingworld.org), National League for Nursing (http://www.nln.org), the American Association of Colleges of Nursing (http://www.aacn.nche.edu), and large specialty organizations including the Association of periOperative Registered Nurses (http://www.aorn.org), American Association of Critical-Care Nurses (http://www.aacn.org), American Organization of Nurse Executives (http://www.aone.org), the Emergency Nurses Association (http://www.ena.org), the American College of Nurse Practitioners (http://www.acnpweb.org), American Academy of Nurse Practitioners (http://www.aanp.org), the American College of Nurse Midwives (http://www.acnm.org), and the American Association of Nurse Anesthetists (http://www.aana.com). This is, of course, not a complete list. Many unions and state organizations, including state nurses associations, include similar information. The Nightingale Policy Group (http://www.npg.org), formed in 2006 by nurses with substantial experience working in health policy, also seeks to develop a range of information resources to increase policy knowledge and expertise in nursing.

In addition, several nursing publications include policy-related information, research, or analysis. The *American Journal of Nursing,* for instance, regularly includes policy-focused articles and columns. *Policy, Politics & Nursing Practice* (edited by this author) focuses specifically on the relationships between health policy and nursing. The *Online Journal of Issues in Nursing* also includes a significant focus on policy issues.

DAVID M. KEEPNEWS

See Also
American Association of Colleges of Nursing
American Nurses Association
American Organization of Nurse Executives
National League for Nursing

REFERENCES

American Association of Colleges of Nursing. (1996). *Essentials of masters education in health policy*. Washington, DC: Author.

Ellenbecker, C. H., Fawcett, J., & Glazer, G. (2006). A nursing PhD specialty in health policy: University of Massachusetts Boston. *Policy, Politics & Nursing Practice, 6*(4), 229–235.

Gebbie, K. M., Wakefield, M., & Kerfoot, K. (2000). Nursing and health policy. *Journal of Nursing Scholarship, 32*(3), 307–315.

Harrington, C., Crider, M. C., Benner, P. E., & Malone, R. E. (2005). Advanced nursing training in health policy: Designing and implementing a new program. *Policy, Politics & Nursing Practice, 6*(2), 99–108.

Malone, R. E. (2005). Assessing the policy environment. *Policy, Politics & Nursing Practice, 6*(2), 135–143.

Mason, D. J., Leavitt, J. K., & Chaffee, M. W. (2002). Policy and politics: A framework for action. In *Policy & politics in nursing and health care* (4th ed., Ch. 1). St. Louis, MO: Saunders.

Mechanic, D., & Reinhard, S. C. (2002). Contributions of nurses to health policy: Challenges and opportunities. *Nursing and Health Policy Review, 1*(1), 7–15.

Yale School of Nursing. (n.d.). *Masters in nursing management, policy and leadership*. Retrieved October 11, 2006, from http://nursing.yale.edu/Academics/Masters/NMPL/

Health Resources and Services Administration

T HE HEALTH RESOURCES AND SERVICES ADMINISTRATION (HRSA) was created in 1982 when two parent agencies, the Health Resources Administration and the Health Services Administration combined. The HRSA is an agency within the U.S. Department of Health and Human Services and is the principal federal division aimed at improving health care access to vulnerable and special needs populations (HRSA, 2006a). Five bureaus and 12 offices are coordinated through HRSA, thereby offering specialized grants to medical and nursing professionals across the United States and to U.S. territories. The HIV/AIDS Bureau gives medical treatment and support programs to roughly 600,000 low-income Americans. The Bureau of Primary Health Care financially supports 3,700 health centers that provide health care services to 14 billion low-income and uninsured Americans (HRSA, 2006b).

Known as the nation's access division, HRSA has seven broad goals that underscore their focus on the underserved and medically vulnerable: (a) to offer better medical care access; (b) to improve health related outcomes; (c) to enhance the quality of medical care; (d) to eradicate health related inequalities; (e) to enhance community health; (f) to increase the response to health-related emergencies; and (g) to attain superior management styles (HRSA, 2006a).

The HRSA grant availability is announced two ways: (a) HRSA Preview through the HRSA Web site, (b) Grants.gov Web site. Through these online resources, the program title and number, related governing agency, purpose, top funding priorities, review criteria, available monies, application deadline, and project timeline are published for each funding option (HRSA, 2006c). As of 2006 the required grant submission procedure for this agency is through their online system.

RONDA MINTZ-BINDER

REFERENCES

Health Resources and Services Administration. (2006a). *About HRSA.* Retrieved July 6, 2006, from http://www.hrsa.gov/about/default.htm

Health Resources and Services Administration. (2006b). *HRSA: America's health care safety net.* Retrieved July 6, 2006, from http://www.hrsa.gov/about/overview/hrsaoverview_files/outline.htm

Health Resources and Services Administration. (2006c). *HRSA grant preview.* Retrieved July 6, 2006, from http://www.hrsa.gov/

Henderson, Virginia A.

VIRGINIA AVENEL HENDERSON was born on November 30, 1897, in Kansas City, Missouri, and died on March 19, 1996, at the age of 99. Henderson graduated in 1921 with a diploma from the Army School of Nursing in Washington, DC. She received her baccalaureate and master's degrees from Teachers College (TC), Columbia University. She subsequently became a member of the faculty and taught for 14 years at TC. Henderson held many accomplished positions including cofounder of the Interagency Council on Information Resources in Nursing (ICIRN), cofounder of the New England Regional Council on Library Resources for Nursing, and first chairperson of the *International Index* Editorial Advisory Committee. She also compiled the *Nursing Studies Index*. Henderson created a definition of nursing that was internationally accepted and clearly delineated the field of nursing from the field of medicine. Henderson was one of the first nurses to elucidate that nursing was not just merely following physician's orders but could be utilized as a therapeutic mechanism in and of itself. Henderson produced the first *Annotated Index of Nursing Research* while on faculty at Yale University. Consequently, she incited a research movement in the field that led to recognition of nursing as a professional and

276

respected occupation. Henderson was involved in developing holistic and humane nursing practices associated with the delivery of nursing care. She was an innovator in identifying key concepts, such as continuity of care, patient advocacy, multidisciplinary scholarship, outcomes orientation, and health promotion (Allen, 1997). Henderson was a member of the International Council of Nurses. She was inducted posthumously into the American Nurses Association Hall of Fame in 1996. Additional information on Henderson can be accessed on the Web at http://www.sandiego.edu/nursing/theory/henderson.htm.

M. JANICE NELSON

REFERENCES

Allen, M. (1997). *Tribute to Virginia Avernal Henderson, 1897–1996 from the Interagency Council on Information Resources for Nursing (ICIRN)*. Retrieved March 22, 2006, from http://www.sandiego.edu/nursing/theory/henderson.htm

American Nurses Association. (2007). *Virginia A. Henderson (1897–1996) 1996 inductee*. Retrieved August 30, 2007, from http://www.nursingworld.org/FunctionalMenuCategories/AboutANA/WhereWeComeFrom_1/HallofFame/19962000Inductees/hendva5545.aspx

Virginia Commonwealth University. (2004). *Virginia Avenel Henderson of the Virginia Nursing Hall of Fame*. Retrieved March 22, 2006, from http://www.enursescribe.com/henderson.htm/Summary

Human Dignity and Ethical Decisions in Nursing

ETHICAL DILEMMAS in health care today present new and complex issues for the profession of nursing. In leadership roles as administrator, clinician, researcher, and educator, nurses are in a strategic position to protect and defend the dignity and freedom of the patient or health care proxy who often must make difficult treatment decisions. Since the early Christian era, nursing has a long and illustrious history in responding to the dynamics of the society and culture, which threaten the dignity of the human person, be it illness, discrimination, allocation of resources, access to health services, or the existence of unjust social policies. Defending and protecting the dignity of the human person is nursing's indelible and irrefutable commitment to caring for persons living a world order in which the intrinsic dignity of the human person may be at risk.

THE DOCTRINE OF HUMAN DIGNITY

THROUGH the doctrine of intrinsic human dignity, the central moral principle in health care, we can come to a fuller understanding of the ethical issues in nursing and how our responses to them affirm the dignity of the person. Immanuel Kant, a German philosopher, has been credited with providing the current understanding of human dignity. In his *Metaphysics of Morals*, Kant states:

> A human being is regarded as a person, that is, as the subject of a morally practical reason, is exalted above any price; for as a person he is not to be valued merely as a means to the ends of others or even to his own ends, but as an end in himself, that is, he possesses a dignity (an absolute inner worth) by which he exacts respect for himself from all other rational beings in the world. (Gregor, 1996, p. 186)

This absolute inner worth is intrinsic dignity; that exalted level of value that is present simply because the person is human. No authority of any kind, of any nation, of any laws, or any illness, or station in life can ever obliterate intrinsic dignity from character of the human person.

A MODEL FOR MAKING ETHICAL DECISIONS

S EVERAL philosophical and theological frameworks, models for ethical decision making, and professional codes of ethics are well established in the professional literature and are readily applied in nursing practice. Although the nursing profession does not advocate for one distinctive framework, the American Nurses Association's (ANA) Code of Ethics (2001) is the most frequently cited. Its very first article states:

> The nurse, in all professional relationships, practices with compassion and respect for the inherent dignity, worth and uniqueness of every individual, unrestricted by considerations of social or economic status, personal attributes, or the nature of health problems. (ANA, p. 7)

Complementing an ethical framework and its methodological application in nursing is the nursing process, which provides a systematic method for identifying health care and nursing needs of patients to bring resolution to them. The examination of actual and potential ethical issues in health care and nursing that impact on the patient, family, community, organization, or society benefits from the same rigorous investigation and analysis found in the nursing process. Commitment to evidence-based practice and to caring for the whole person (and not the disease alone) requires that the identification and analysis of ethical issues in patient care be systematically integrated into every step of the nursing process.

The following protocol, designed by the ethicists at the Center for Clinical Bioethics at Georgetown University (1991), focuses on the protection and affirmation of the dignity of the patient and the clinician as ethical issues in health care are examined and resolved. The steps of the protocol, applicable also to the analysis and resolution of organizational ethical issues, are briefly outlined here:

1. What are the facts with this patient: diagnosis; prognosis; therapeutic options; chronology of the occurrence of clinical events; the biography of the patient (age, gender, family, career, etc.); decisional capacity and informed consent; who is the decision maker—patient or health care proxy; the current clinical setting; time constraints (critical status; decision makers); and the existence of an advance directive and a health care proxy who is competent and understands the role;

2. What are the issues with this patient: are the issues ethical in nature; are there problems in communication or differences in clinical opinions and treatment protocols; are there resource allocation issues that may interfere with care, that is, third-party reimbursement; are there conflicts among the ethical principles of the patient, the family, the nurse, attending physician, the health care facility;

3. What is the good for this patient: the patient's biomedical good (technically good act identified by clinicians and decided by patient or health care surrogate); the patient's perception of his/her own good at the time and in the particular circumstances of the clinical decision; the good of the patient as a human person capable of reasoned choices (freedom; dignity; autonomy self-determination); the patient's ultimate good (value and meaning of life; suffering; God; family; society);

4. What are the goods and interests of other parties: family; community; society; the law; policies of health care institutions/clinical settings; members of the health care team;

5. How do the issues stand vis-à-vis the issues in comparable cases: is this case analogous to others; has some moral consensus been achieved in the analogous cases; are there ethical precedents, legal precedents; in terms of the facts, the issues, and the framing of the issues, how well does this particular case fit any paradigmatic cases?

6. The prudential question—what to decide?: In synthesizing the data from these questions and moving toward a proposed intervention two critical questions emerge: (1) *What can be done for this patient?* and (2) *What should be done for this patient?* Medical science, clinical research and innovative technology continue to advance at a phenomenal pace. Today, the lives of persons with life-threatening

chronic illnesses can be extended. For example, certain forms of carcinomas once considered fatal now successfully respond to treatment. With advanced technology, much *can be done* to treat specific illness. The question that is paramount in analyzing the needs and resolving ethical dilemmas of the whole person is what *should be done* for this patient—what is both the technically good and morally right action for *this patient*. The answer to this question requires a careful review of all of data accumulated in the course of the analysis. Critical to this analysis is the centrality of the human person and the good that he identifies as important to him as a person with intrinsic dignity and worth.

7. Evaluation: once decisions are made, an assessment of the integrity of the process should be carefully reviewed.

CHALLENGES IN MAKING ETHICAL DECISIONS

N URSING leaders are in a strategic position to support patients and health care proxies who may confront difficult treatment decisions. To be unwilling to enter into the experience of the patient moves the nurse to the position of technician and abandons the patient at a time when she/he is most vulnerable and in need of support. With an increase in the vulnerability of the patient, the dignity of the person is once again at great risk. There are times, however, when the choices of the patient, family, nurse, physician, the health care organization, or managed care group are in conflict. Ethics consultations that are grounded in protecting and defending human dignity of the person who is sick can often resolve conflicts satisfactorily.

Today we are confronted with threats to human dignity through euthanasia, physician-assisted suicide, malnutrition, assisted nutrition and hydration, persistent vegetative states and postcoma unresponsiveness, in the terminally ill, the mentally and physically challenged, those stigmatized by cancer, AIDS, and substance use, those who have had abortions, women, children, and the elderly, persons of color, the homeless, minorities, single parents, those who have limited access to health services, legislation that is unresponsive to human need, and a national health care system that is driven by the commoditization of the human person.

Regardless of the reason for one's illness or his decisional capacity, a living person is never less than fully human. The application of the doctrine of human dignity requires nurses and all others who participate in ethical decisions to continually re-examine the direction of their moral compass and focus on the question *"what should be done for this patient?"* How this challenge is embraced and applied in light of caring for persons diminished in any way by reason of illness, will speak loudly about our

282

HUMAN
DIGNITY AND
ETHICAL
DECISIONS IN
NURSING

faithfulness to nursing's intrinsic, indelible and irrefutable commitment to protecting human dignity.

BRO. IGNATIUS PERKINS

REFERENCES

American Nurses Association. (2001). *Code of ethics for nurses with interpretative statements*. Washington, DC: Author.

Center for Clinical Bioethics. (1991). *The ethics workup*. Washington, DC: Center for Clinical Bioethics, Georgetown University Medical Center.

Gregor, M. (Ed.). (1996). *Immanuel Kant: The metaphysics of morals*. New York: Cambridge University Press.

Human Resource Management

ONE OF THE MOST IMPORTANT roles of the nurse leader is that of Human Resource Manager. Understanding key concepts of recruitment, selection, retention, developing, promoting, and terminating are core competencies of the nurse leader. The way an organization manages its human resources is increasingly recognized as centrally important to the execution of its strategy (Hambrick, Frederickson, Korn, & Ferry, 1989). In addition to strategic implications, Lado and Wilson (1994) concluded that human resource strategies may be an especially important source of sustained competitive advantage.

NURSE RECRUITMENT

A FORMAL nurse recruitment plan should be developed and reviewed at least annually by the nurse leader. According to Pattan (1992), the following elements should be included in a nurse recruitment plan:

1. A supply and demand analysis.
2. Clear objectives for the plan.

3. Strategies to accomplish the objectives.
4. An annual recruitment budget.
5. Operational plans to implement strategies.
6. A feedback process to take corrective action.

In addition to a solid recruitment plan, the nurse leader should implement marketing strategies to increase the pool of qualified nursing applicants. Typically, marketing to nurses is focused on many things, such as job profile, organizational culture, working locations and conditions, the reputation of the institution, and compensation (Pattan, 1991). One of the best methods for recruiting is the use of existing employees. Word-of-mouth recruiting supplemented with incentive programs for employee referrals is a cost-effective and highly successful means of recruiting staff.

CANDIDATE SELECTION

T HE typical selection process includes the interview, an offer by the employer, acceptance by the employee, and, in some cases, the execution of an employment contract. Before scheduling the interview, the nurse leader should review an applicant's resume and application. On verifying that the applicant meets the minimum requirements of the role, such as licensure and certification, careful attention should be given to the applicant's employment history. Be aware of gaps in employment and be sure to question about gaps during the interview process. After carefully reviewing the application, the nurse leader should begin preparing for the interview. Hiring managers should elicit the input of those with whom the candidate will be working on a daily basis, including support staff and physicians. Many organizations have implemented structured peer interview processes and include the peer interview as a key component of employee selection. Before implementing this process, the nurse leader should work with human resource professionals to provide adequate training to staff on the appropriate methods for conducting interviews. It is critically important that front-line staff who participate in peer interviews understand the laws related to interviews and especially what is appropriate to ask a candidate.

Following the interview, the nurse leader should prepare a formal offer for the prospective employee. In some organizations, the offer is managed by the human resources representative. Either way, it is always a good practice to consult with human resource professionals before making final offers of employment. The formal offer is best provided face-to-face or over the phone and then immediately followed up in writing. At minimum, the offer should include: the job title, the shift the employee will be working, details about compensation and benefits, any pre-employment requirements such as employee health screening, and a start date. It is good management practice to ask the applicant to acknowledge and accept the offer by signing a copy of the offer letter and returning it to the hiring nurse leader. A copy of the signed offer letter should be placed in the employee's permanent human resource file. Finally, as hospitals have increased the number of new graduate training programs, it is becoming more common to have new graduate nurses execute employment contracts. Typical contracts include a sliding scale repayment program in the event the new graduate leaves the organization prior to the end of an agreed-on time frame, generally 1 to 2 years for example, in the case where the nurse completes an internship program.

EMPLOYEE RETENTION

T HE retention of competent nurses is a major problem of the health care system in the United States. A study by Spitzer-Lehmann (1990) indicated that nurses stayed in their jobs: when they received peer support, participated in professional practice activities, received tuition reimbursement, and had input into decision making; when communication was open; and when medical staff was supportive. In 1983, an American Academy of Nursing study described both nurse administrators and staff nurses as agreeing on which factors attracted nurses to become and remain employees of the hospital. These hospitals were labeled *Magnet Hospitals*. Today, Magnet Hospitals are national leaders not only in nurse retention but also in nurse sensitive patient outcomes. Jones-Schenk (2001) cited the multidimensional value provided to nurses in Magnet organizations. These later became known as the 14 forces of magnetism:

1. Quality of nursing leadership
2. Organizational structure
3. Management style
4. Personnel policies and programs
5. Quality of care
6. Professional models of care
7. Level of autonomy
8. Quality assurance
9. Consultation and resources
10. Community and the hospital
11. Nurses as teachers
12. Image of nursing

13. Nurse-physician relationships
14. Professional career development

These variables should be considered in any well-developed retention program. It is important to remember that retention begins with the initial contact with the organization and is rooted in a solid orientation program.

DEVELOPING AND PROMOTING EMPLOYEES

P ROFESSIONAL career development and coaching are integral parts of the nurse leader's role. The first step in developing and promoting is assisting the nurse in assessing his or her interests, skills, and values. Next, the nurse compares the results of this assessment with open and available positions. Although it is always preferable to keep great employees in one's own organization, appropriate opportunities may only be available outside the organization and the nurse leader should support nurses who wish to advance in this manner.

In addition to a traditional promotion, many organizations have re-instituted clinical ladder programs. A clinical ladder is a horizontal development system based on specific criteria used to develop, evaluate, and promote nurses who are in direct care providing roles. Furthermore, clinical ladder programs in larger organizations are tending toward specialized tracks for clinical practice, education, administration, and research. The clinical ladder framework provides a solid model for the development and promotion of staff. The model can be adapted to other types of development, such as management promotions. The most important factor in establishing a solid promotion and development program is proactive succession planning. Succession planning is a formal process where senior leaders look at current and potential vacancies and assess the internal talent pool for potential development and/or promotion opportunities.

TERMINATION OF EMPLOYEES

F IRING an employee is an unpleasant, but sometimes necessary, part of the nurse leader's job. Before considering termination, frontline managers should consult with superiors and human resource professionals to ensure all policies and procedures have been consistently followed. Clear documentation should exist demonstrating that a progressive discipline process, moving from coaching, to written, to suspension or final written warning has taken place. In rare instances, an employee's conduct may be so egregious that progressive discipline may not be appropriate and termination is the first and only step in the disciplinary process.

Planning is key to a successful termination session. The nurse leader should plan well ahead of the session and take the following steps:

1. Discuss the termination with human resources, superiors, and union representatives if applicable.
2. Plan the session at a time when a witness is available. Never terminate an employee without a witness. The witness should be a human resources representative or another manager in the organization. This person should cosign the termination document to indicate his or her presence in the meeting.
3. Prepare detailed documentation in accordance with your organization's policies.
4. Be open, honest, and direct in your communication with the employee. If you are nervous about the meeting, practice with another manager before the session.
5. Be prepared for any reaction (Dumville [1993] identified four stages of employee reaction to termination: shock with physical symptoms, rejection, emotion, and withdrawal).
6. Provide the employee with a signed copy of the termination documentation and your organization's grievance policy.

SUMMARY

M ANAGING human resources is a key core competency for the nurse leader and can be one of the most rewarding aspects of the role. Not only is the function important in creating a positive culture for employees, recent studies show a link between the management of human resources and patient mortality in acute care hospitals. A study by West and others (2002) demonstrated this link. Specifically, their work noted that the sophistication and extensiveness of appraisal and training for hospital employees and the percentage of employees working in teams in the hospital were all significantly associated with measures of patient mortality.

JEFFREY N. DOUCETTE

See Also
Clinical Ladder
Magnet Hospitals
Orientation and Staff Development

REFERENCES

American Academy of Nursing Task Force on Nursing Practice in Hospitals. (1983). *Magnet hospitals: Attraction and retention of professional nurses.* Kansas City, MO: American Nurses Association.

Dumville, J. C. (1993). Delivering the mortal blow. *Supervision, 54*(4), 6–7.

Hambrick, D. C., Frederickson, L. B., Korn, B., & Ferry, R. M. (1989). Preparing today's leaders for tomorrow's realities. *Personnel, 8,* 23–26.

Jones-Schenk, J. (2001). How magnets attract nurses. *Nursing Management, 33*(1), 41–44.

Lado, A., & Wilson, M. (1994). Human resource systems and sustained competitive advantage: A competency-based perspective. *Academy of Management Review, 19,* 699–727.

Pattan, J. E. (1991). Nurse recruitment: From selling to marketing. *Journal of Nursing Administration, 21*(9), 16–20.

Pattan, J. E. (1992). Developing a nurse recruitment plan. *Journal of Nursing Administration, 22*(1), 33–39.

Spitzer-Lehmann, R. (1990). Recruitment and retention of our greatest asset. *Nursing Administration Quarterly, 14*(4), 66–69.

West, M., Borrill, C., Dawson, J., Scully, J., Carter, M., Anelay, S., et al. (2002). The link between the management of employees and patient mortality in acute hospitals. *International Journal of Human Resource Management, 13*(8), 1299–1310.

I

Image of Nursing

NURSES ARE THE LIAISONS of the health care system. They act as advocates and health educators for patients, families, and communities. One of the pivotal roles of the nurse is to be a patient advocate to protect the interests of patients when they are unable to advocate for themselves because of illness or inadequate health knowledge. Two government reports, one by the U.S. Bureau of Labor Statistics (2001) and the other by the U.S. Department of Health and Human Services (2000) entitled "National Sample Survey," shed light on the image of nursing. They found that nursing was an ethical, trustworthy, and caring profession. These reports were released to present a positive image of the nursing profession, but they did not reflect the true public image of nursing (Murray, 2002).

The various ways nurses are portrayed in the media and text does not reflect the value of the profession in our society. According to Turow and Gans (2002), fictional TV significantly influences the state of our health care system and policy options for improving the delivery of care. In some instances, physicians are depicted on TV as controlling and providing care that nurses or other health professionals actually do in reality (Buresh & Gordon, 2001). This disastrously impacts the image of accurate care giving. Nurses have limited meaningful impact in Hollywood and have endured regressive, inaccurate images for decades (Kalisch, B. J. & Kalisch, P. A., 1983, 1984; Kalisch, P. A. & Kalisch, B. J., 1982, 1985, 1987). In 2001, The Center for Nursing Advocacy (www.nursingadvocacy.org) was formed as a watchdog group to "increase public understanding of the central, front-line role nurses play in modern health care. The focus of the Center is to promote more accurate, balanced and frequent media portrayals of nurses and increase the media's use of nurses as expert sources" (The Center for Nursing Advocacy, 2006). According to the mission statement, the center focuses "its efforts on improving the portrayal of nurses in the media, especially Hollywood, since television and films are so influential" (The Center for Nursing Advocacy, 2006).

The media image of nurses as portrayed on popular medical television shows depicts nurses as handmaidens to physicians. The nurses on such programs are retrieving charts and laboratory data for the powerful and confident physicians. This portrayal is detrimental to recruitment efforts and will not attract young adults on their quest for a career (Murray, 2002). In a study of primary and secondary school students, most respondents wrongly described nursing as a girl's job, a technical job "like shop," and an inappropriate career for private school students (JWT Communications, 2000).

Although some physicians have a good sense of nursing, many do not. A physician's actions seem to reflect a self-absorbed culture of medicine. This culture equates medicine with health care and rarely questions society's traditional assumptions. Nurses cannot be expected to be immune to the effect of the media. The ill treatment of nurses in the media leads to decreased morale and pride, which in turns encourages cynicism and creates a world where nurses tend not to stand up for themselves or their patients (Gordon, 2006).

When members of the public seek out health care, the general term used for any female caring for their needs is "nurse," whether it is an individual who bathes patients, draws their blood, or delivers their meals. Actually, the nurse is the lifeline to the whole professional team. The nurse customizes a plan of care to address the medical and emotional needs of patients. Nurses must do a better job of educating the public to preserve their professional status. This can be done in a sensitive way by ensuring that nurses are known as nurses either through their attire or their words. Nonnurse health care workers have to make it clear that they are not nurses (Zwerdling, 2003).

Although images of nursing in media are generally inaccurate, the future holds suggestions for changing that image. According to Raymond (2004), "chuck the cartoon jackets unless you're in pediatrics," and develop a uniform of "solid well-tailored scrubs" with a "starched white lab coat," "nursing pins and honors," and a "name badge with last name and degrees." "Nursing image equals nursing power" (Buresh & Gordon, 2001). These small steps can change the face of the image of nursing.

DOLORES FAZZINO
LYN M. PUHEK
LISA SACCO
JOYCE J. FITZPATRICK

REFERENCES

Bureau of Labor Statistics, U.S. Department of Labor. (2001). *Occupational outlook handbook, 2006-07 edition, registered nurses.* Retrieved June 26, 2006, from http://stats.bls.gov/oco/ocos083.htm

Buresh, B., & Gordon, S. (2001). *From silence to voice.* Retrieved from http://www.nursingadvocacy.org/news/2001_silence_to_voice.html

Gordon, S. (2006). *How does the media affect real life nursing?* Retrieved July 8, 2006, from http://www.nursingadvocacy.org/faq/media_affects_nursing.html

JWT Communications. (2000). *Memo to nurses for a healthier tomorrow on focus group studies of 1,800 school children in 10 cities.* Retrieved October 14, 2006, from http://www.nursingadvocacy.org/research/lit/jwt_memo1.html

Kalisch, B. J., & Kalisch, P. A. (1983). Heroine out of focus: Media images of Florence Nightingale. Part II film, radio, and television dramatizations. *Nursing & Health Care, 4*(5), 270–278.

Kalisch, B. J., & Kalisch, P. A. (1984). The Dionne quintuplets legacy: Establishing the "good doctor and his loyal nurse" image in American culture. *Nursing & Health Care, 5*(5), 242–251.

Kalisch, P. A., & Kalisch, B. J. (1982). The image of the nurse in motion pictures. *American Journal of Nursing, 82*(4), 605–611.

Kalisch, P. A., & Kalisch, B. J. (1985). When Americans called for Dr. Kildare images of physicians and nurses in the Dr. Kildare and Dr. Gillespie movie 1937–1947. *Medical Heritage, 1*(5), 348–363.

Kalisch, P. A., & Kalisch, B. J. (1987). *The changing image of the nurse.* Menlo Park, CA: Addison-Wesley.

Murray, M. K. (2002). The nursing shortage. *Journal of Nursing Administration, 32*(2), 79–84.

Raymond, P. (2004, June 1). Nursing image = nursing power [Special issue]. *The Sacramento Bee.* Retrieved from http://www.reallifehealthcare.com

The Center for Nursing Advocacy. (2006). *How does the media affect how people think?* Retrieved June 26, 2006, from http://www.nursingadvocacy.org

Turow, J., & Gans, R. (2002, July). *As seen on TV: Health policy issues in TV's media dramas* (Report No. 3231). Kaiser Family Foundation. Retrieved from http://www.kff.org/entmedia/3231-index.cfm

U.S. Department of Health and Human Services. (2000). *National sample survey*. Washington, DC: Bureau of Health Professions Division of Nursing.

Zwerdling, M. (2003). *Postcards of nursing: A worldwide tribute*. Philadelphia: Lippincott.

Informed Consent (Research)

I NFORMED CONSENT is an essential ethical requirement for research that involves human subjects. It is an individual's voluntary consent to participate in a research study and is given after receiving and understanding essential information about the research. This consent may be for adults themselves or for children.

REGULATIONS FOR THE PROTECTION OF HUMAN SUBJECTS

THE NUREMBERG CODE was developed in 1949 (The Nuremberg Code, 1949) and provides guidelines that help to evaluate the consent process. It was the basis for the Declaration of Helsinki, adopted in 1964, and has undergone many revisions by the World Medical Association since its adoption (World Medical Association Declaration of Helsinki). The Declaration of Helsinki details ethical principles related to the protection of the life, privacy, health and dignity of the human subject. In 1973, the Department of Health, Education, and Welfare developed regulations for the protection of human subjects, specifically protections for persons with limited capacity to give consent. In 1978, the National Commission for the Protection of Human Subjects of Biomedical and Behavioral Research

295

was formed. This commission identified three ethical principles that are important when conducting human subjects' research: respect for persons, beneficence, and justice. The commission prepared and submitted the Belmont Report (The National Commission for the Protection of Human Subjects of Biomedical and Behavioral Research, 1979) to the Department of Heath and Human Services (HHS), which contained guidelines for research based on these three principles.

Following submission of the Belmont Report, HHS developed a set of regulations, Code of Federal Regulations Title 45, Part 46 Protection of Human Subjects (U.S. Department of Health and Human Services, 2005), which contain a set of guidelines related to the requirements and documentation of informed consent. They are updated regularly; the last update was in 2005. The Office for Human Research Protection (OHRP) is responsible for interpreting and overseeing the implementation of these regulations.

VULNERABLE INDIVIDUALS

THERE ARE A NUMBER of individuals that are considered "vulnerable" with regard to giving consent for participation in a research study. This category includes those individuals with legal or mental incompetence or diminished autonomy, or those confined to an institution. They need additional protections because of their decreased ability or inability to give informed consent. Children (minors), mentally impaired patients, and unconscious patients are deemed legally and mentally incompetent to give informed consent. They lack the ability to understand information about a research study and are unable therefore to make informed decisions about participating in or withdrawing from such a study. Children and their involvement in the informed consent process vary depending on the age of the child. Usually children up to the age of 7 years of age are not involved in the consent process. Instead, the parents or guardians give the consent. Once the child is 7 years of age, the child can usually assent to participate in the research study. Assent means that the child gives affirmative agreement to participate in the research. Older children should be more involved in decisions regarding their participation in research studies. The HHS guidelines recommend getting the assent of the child, if the child is capable, along with the consent of the parent or guardian.

There are adults who because of mental illness, cognitive impairment, or being in a comatose state are incapable of giving consent. In these circumstances, the researcher must get consent from the individual's family and his/her legal representative to give consent on behalf of the person to be a participant in the research study. The inclusion of individuals with diminished autonomy in a research study is more acceptable if the research is therapeutic rather than nontherapeutic, and both vulnerable and nonvulnerable groups are included in the research study. In addition, it is expected that all aspects of the consent process are strictly followed to ensure the participant's rights. Prisoners who are confined to institutions are designated as having diminished autonomy under Federal Law. They might feel coerced to participate because they fear negative consequences if they refuse to participate in the research. Hospitalized patients are a vulnerable population because of their illness and being confined to a health care setting. They may feel obliged to participate in the research as they fear their care may be otherwise compromised. Other vulnerable individuals include employees, students, illiterate subjects, those who do not speak English, and those mentally capable to give consent but physically unable to sign the consent document. Pregnant women, human fetuses, and neonates are also classified as vulnerable.

THE INFORMED CONSENT DOCUMENT

INFORMED CONSENT DOCUMENTS must include the eight basic elements of informed consent provided in the Code of Federal Regulations Title 45, Part 46 Protection of Human Subjects (U.S. Department of Health and Human Services, 2005). There are six additional elements of informed consent that may be required depending on the research (U.S. Department of Health and Human Services, 2005). These elements provide an excellent framework for informed consent documents for all human subjects' research. The detailed information on the elements for the consent document in this section is taken from the Code of Federal Regulations Title 45, Part 46 Protection of Human Subjects (U.S. Department of Health and Human Services, 2005).

Each subject must be given information related to each of the eight basic elements of informed consent as follows:

1. A research statement must be provided that clearly identifies that this is a research study. This research statement must include: a statement that the study involves research, an explanation of the purposes of the research and the expected duration of the subject's participation, a description of the procedures involved in the research, and identification of any procedures that are experiments.
2. Any foreseeable risks and discomforts must be clearly described.
3. The benefits must be detailed, clearly describing any benefits to the subject or others that may reasonably be expected from the research;
4. Alternative procedures or courses of treatment, if any, that might be advantageous to the subject must be identified.
5. A statement describing the extent, if any, to which confidentiality of records identifying the subject will be maintained;

6. Research involving more than minimal risk must have an explanation as to whether any compensation and any medical treatments are available if injury occurs and, if so, what they consist of, or where further information may be obtained;

7. An explanation of whom to contact for answers to pertinent questions about the research and research subjects' rights, and whom to contact in the event of a research-related injury to the subject.

8. A statement that participation is voluntary, refusal to participate will involve no penalty or loss of benefits to which the subject is otherwise entitled and the subject may discontinue participation at any time without penalty or loss of benefits to which the subject is otherwise entitled.

In addition, there are the Six Additional Elements of Informed Consent that may be required in the consent document. Additional information that will have an impact on a subject's willingness to voluntarily participate in the research; and protects the subject's rights and welfare in a meaningful way should be included. The six additional elements are as follows:

1. A statement that the particular treatment or procedure may involve risks to the subject (or to the embryo or fetus, if the subject is or may become pregnant) that are currently unforeseeable;

2. Anticipated circumstances under which the subject's participation may be terminated by the investigator without regard to the subject's consent;

3. Any additional costs to the subject that may result from participation in the research;

4. The consequences of a subject's decision to withdraw from the research and procedures for orderly termination of participation by the subject;

5. A statement that significant new findings developed during the course of the research, which may relate to the subject's willingness to continue participation will be provided to the subject.

6. The approximate number of subjects involved in the study.

LANGUAGE OF THE INFORMED CONSENT DOCUMENT

THE INFORMED CONSENT document must be in a language understandable to the participant or his/her legally authorized representative (U.S. Department of Health and Human Services, 2005). It must be written in language that is at the appropriate reading and comprehension level for the targeted population. It must be in lay language and should not include technical language that would not be understandable to all potential subjects.

OBTAINING INFORMED CONSENT FOR RESEARCH

INDIVIDUALS MUST BE given detailed information about the research in order to decide whether or not they wish to participate or continue to participate in a research study. This includes information on all aspects of the study, including the risks and benefits. The informed consent process should include opportunities to allow potential subjects to ask questions. The researchers also must keep the subjects informed of any new information that may affect their willingness to remain in the study. This is particularly important in longitudinal studies.

The signature section on the currently approved and Institutional Review Board (IRB) date-stamped informed consent documents must be signed by the subject or individual giving consent. The person obtaining consent must both sign and print his or her name on the document also. A copy of the signed informed consent documents must be given to the subject or his or her legally authorized representative. If an unsigned copy is given to the subject it must be an exact copy of the signed consent form.

The principal investigator for an IRB-approved study is ultimately responsible for the conduct of the research study including all aspects of the informed consent process. All persons who will be obtaining consent must have a certificate in human subjects' protections. The IRB requires that documentation of informed consent be obtained from all subjects unless alternate procedures are approved by the IRB.

MARY T. QUINN GRIFFIN

REFERENCES

The National Commission for the Protection of Human Subjects of Biomedical and Behavioral Research. (1979). *The Belmont report: Ethical principles and guidelines for the protection of human subjects of research.* Retrieved May 24, 2007, from http://ohsr.od.nih.gov/guidelines/belmont.html

The Nuremberg Code. (1949). Retrieved May 24, 2007, from http://ohsr.od.nih.gov/guidelines/nuremberg.html

U.S. Department of Health and Human Services. (2005). *Protection of human subjects: Code of Federal Regulations, Title 45, Part 46.* Retrieved May 24, 2007, from http://www.hhs.gov/ohrp/humansubjects/guidance/45cfr46.htm

World Medical Association Declaration of Helsinki. (n.d.). *Ethical principles for medical research involving human subjects.* Retrieved May 24, 2007, from http://www.wma.net/e/policy/b3.htm

Informed Patient Consent and the Patient Self-Determination Act

T HE PRINCIPLE OF AUTONOMY, or the right to self-determination, is preserved in health care by ethical mandates and legislative rulings. *Informed patient consent* and the *Patient Self-Determination Act* (*PSDA*) are grounded in the principles of autonomy and empower the patient to be an active and informed participant in health care. Patient autonomy moved to the forefront in health care during the latter half of the 20th century. Advances in technology expanded the boundaries of medical care. The potential to sustain a patient's life indefinitely was realized. These advancements, however, did not come without costs. Monetary considerations and quality of life issues were topics of debate in ethical, political, and social forums. As the physician's beneficiary role was questioned, courts were petitioned on behalf of the autonomous voice of the patient (Baker, 2002; Berg, Appelbaum, Lidz, & Parker, 2001; Cantor, 2001; Kellum & Dacey, 2006). It was within this climate that the concept of informed patient consent was meaningfully defined and the PSDA was passed. Informed patient consent and the PSDA promote patient autonomy. Health care providers play an important role in their success.

Informed patient consent refers to a process of open communication between the patient and the health care professional through which information is shared, questions are raised, and values are clarified. The goal of this process is to enhance the patient's ability to make an informed decision about participation in a newly proposed or continuing medical intervention. Essential elements of this process, as identified by Beauchamp and Childress (2001), include (a) competence, or decision-making capacity, (b) disclosure, (c) understanding, (d) voluntariness, and (e) consent. Each of these is recognized legally, but state law is more prescriptive about disclosure. The types of information generally required to be disclosed are the nature and purpose of the proposed intervention, its risks and benefits, and any available alternatives. It has been reasonably argued that disclosure should also address the intervention's probability of success and any provider-specific information that is relevant (Annas, 2004; Berg et al., 2001).

The courts judge adequacy of the disclosure by three standards. The *professional community standard* recognizes what a typical physician would disclose in similar circumstances. The *reasonable person standard* acknowledges what another person of sound reasoning would want to know given the circumstances. The *subjective standard* requires the physician to use experience and judgment to tailor the information to the individual patient's needs. Although the latter is the preferable moral standard of disclosure, it is difficult to implement clinically and to evaluate legally (Beauchamp & Childress, 2001; Berg et al., 2001).

The process of informed patient consent requires the patient to have decision-making capacity, and decision-making capacity assumes comprehension. Effort should be made to enhance the patient's understanding of the information disclosed as it relates to personal values and goals. If it is determined that the patient lacks decision-making capacity, the informed consent process should be initiated with an identified surrogate decision maker (Annas, 2004; Beauchamp & Childress, 2001). The actual consent or authorization by the patient to participate in the proposed medical intervention must be voluntary. This implies that the patient consents freely, without controlling influences (Beauchamp & Childress, 2001). Some situations do not lend themselves to obtaining informed patient consent and are recognized as exceptions to the legal doctrine. These include circumstances of medical emergencies, when therapeutic privilege is exercised, and when the patient waives his or her right to participate in this process (Berg et al., 2001). To promote the interest of the patient, components of the informed consent process, and the patient's decision to consent or to refuse participation in the medical intervention, should be documented in the medical record. Consent forms are not required but can be used (Berg et al.).

The PSDA is a federal law that passed in 1990 and became effective on December 1, 1991. The PSDA also sets forth regulations about the patient's role in treatment decisions. These apply to health care agencies receiving any federal funding. There are four provisions mandated by the PSDA: (a) provide written information to adults, upon admission, of their right under state law to make decisions about their medical care; (b) ask all adults if they have an advance directive and document the response accordingly in the medical record; (c) do not discriminate against any adult based upon whether the adult has an advance directive; and (d) educate the staff of the health care agency or program and the community at large about advance directives (Brown, 2003).

Although the original intentions of the PSDA were to empower patients to make decisions about their own medical treatment and to promote the use of advance directives, the means to achieve these goals were not well articulated. As a result, there has been limited success in implementing the PSDA. This has been attributed to low literacy levels of patients, ethnic influences, hesitancy to discuss death and dying by patients and physicians, medical uncertainties, vagueness of advance directives, and the limited time and knowledge of providers to engage in meaningful discussions with patients (Baker, 2002; Brown, 2003; Cantor, 2001; Duffy, Jackson, Schim, Ronis, & Fowler, 2006).

DIANE M. GENGO

REFERENCES

Annas, G. J. (2004). *The rights of patients: The authoritative ACLU guide to the rights of patients* (3rd ed.). Carbondale: Southern Illinois University Press.

Baker, M. E. (2002). Economic, political and ethnic influences on end-of-life decision-making: A decade in review. *Journal of Health and Social Policy, 14*(3), 27–39.

Beauchamp, T. L., & Childress, J. F. (2001). *Principles of biomedical ethics* (5th ed.). New York: Oxford University Press.

Berg, J. W., Appelbaum, P. S., Lidz, C. W., & Parker, L. S. (2001). *Informed consent: Legal theory and clinical practice* (2nd ed.). New York: Oxford University Press.

Brown, B. A. (2003). The history of advance directives: A literature review. *Journal of Gerontological Nursing, 29*(9), 4–14.

Cantor, N. L. (2001). Twenty-five years after *Quinlan*: A review of the jurisprudence of death and dying. *Journal of Law, Medicine & Ethics, 29*(2), 182–196.

Duffy, S. A., Jackson, F. C., Schim, S. M., Ronis, D. L., & Fowler, K. E. (2006). Racial/ethnic preferences, sex preferences, and perceived discrimination related to end-of-life care. *Journal of the American Geriatrics Society, 54,* 150–157.

Kellum, J. A., & Dacey, M. J. (2006). *Ethics in the intensive care unit: Informed consent; withholding and withdrawal of life support; and requests for futile therapies.* Retrieved September 25, 2006, from http://uptodateonline.com

Institute for Healthcare Improvement

FOUNDED IN 1991, the Institute for Healthcare Improvement (IHI) is a not-for-profit organization located in Cambridge, Massachusetts, whose mission is to "lead the improvement of healthcare throughout the world" through education, research, and demonstration projects (Institute for Healthcare Improvement, 2007). The current president, CEO and cofounder is Donald M. Berwick, MD, MPP, an international expert on health care performance improvement who has lectured and published extensively regarding quality improvement models and health care policy. One of Berwick's well-known publications, *Escape Fire: Lessons for the Future of Healthcare* (Berwick, 2002), is an essay that describes gaps in the safety and quality of U.S. health care, and he exhorts the public and providers to create a sense of urgency for fundamental reform. Berwick names the reform approach "escape fire," a metaphor that is drawn from a term that firefighters use for a deliberately burned piece of land, which, in an emergency, can create a safe haven from an oncoming blaze. This platform of "escape fire" has defined the work of IHI, which calls for fundamental redesign of health care processes so that in a new system of care "the possibility of invention and the opportunity to make sense . . . will open not only routes of escape, but vistas of achievement, that the old order could never have imagined" (Berwick, 2002, p. 55).

IHI aims to achieve improvement in the "lives of patients, the health of communities, and the joy of the healthcare workforce" (Institute for Healthcare Improvement, 2007), and proposes to accomplish this by focusing their programs and products on the six aims for improving 21st century health care systems identified in the Institute of Medicine report, *Crossing the Quality Chasm: A New Health System for the 21st Century*. These six aims are: safety, effectiveness, patient-centeredness, timeliness, efficiency, and equity (Committee on the Quality of Healthcare in America, 2001, pp. 39–40).

IHI offers programs on a variety of health care topics in formats that include conference calls, live Web-based knowledge exchange programs, professional development seminars, workshops and conferences, collaborative innovation and learning communities, and on-demand Web-based events. It also publishes a series of monographs and "white papers" on innovation and performance improvement topics, many of which are available without charge to registered IHI.org community users. Registration as a community user or member includes a number of benefits, including use of "Improvement Tracker" to document improvement projects, connection with experts and peers from around the world, participation in discussion groups, and access to download interactive improvement tools. IHI annually hosts a National Forum on Quality Improvement in Healthcare that draws over 5,000 health care leaders from around the world who participate in plenary sessions and more than 100 workshops.

IHI's history includes six phases of events that have shaped this quality improvement journey: awareness, education, collaborative improvement, redesign, movement, and full scale (Institute of Healthcare Improvement, 2007). The current phase of "full scale" involves changing mainstream practice standards by ensuring widespread deployment. Two visible IHI campaigns from the "full scale" phase have significantly influenced patient safety initiatives in the United States. The first is the 100,000 Lives Campaign, which has disseminated improvement tools throughout the American health care system, beginning in 2004. This campaign aimed to enlist thousands of U.S. hospitals in a commitment to deploy interventions that had been proven to prevent unnecessary death. These interventions include the following:

* Deploy rapid response teams
* Deliver reliable, evidence-based care for acute myocardial infarction
* Prevent adverse drug events (ADEs)

* Prevent central line infections
* Prevent surgical site infections
* Prevent ventilator-associated pneumonia

In December 2006, IHI announced the 5 Million Lives Campaign. The goal of this effort is to engage 4,000 U.S. hospitals to implement 12 interventions intended to prevent five million incidents of patient harm over a 24-month period ending December 9, 2008. In addition to the six interventions from the 100,000 Lives Campaign, six new interventions were identified:

* Prevent harm from high-alert medications
* Reduce surgical complications
* Prevent pressure ulcers
* Reduce Methicillin-resistant *Staphlococcus Aureus* (MRSA) infection
* Deliver reliable, evidence-based care for congestive heart failure
* Get boards on board by defining and spreading the best-known leveraged processes for hospital boards of directors

Another example of an IHI initiative that is focused exclusively on nursing care and nursing practice is a partnership developed in 2001 with The Robert Wood Johnson Foundation (2007). This program, Transforming Care at the Bedside, or TCAB, seeks to empower nurses to redesign work processes on hospital medical-surgical units in order to improve the reliability of patient care.

In summary, since the 1990s, there has been an increasing focus on quality and safety in nursing and health care, enabled by several national commissions that documented concerns with the U.S. health care system (Committee on the Quality of Healthcare in America, 2001; Institute of Medicine, 2003; Institute of Medicine, Board on Healthcare Services, 2004; Kohn, Corrigan, & Donaldson, 2000). The Institute for Healthcare Improvement has established a visible international profile and reputation for setting standards that have transformed knowledge and reformed systems for improved performance and results for patients, families, and communities.

THOMAS D. SMITH

REFERENCES

Berwick, D. M. (2002). *Escape fire: Lessons for the future of healthcare.* New York: The Commonwealth Fund.

Committee on the Quality of Healthcare in America. (2001). *Crossing the quality chasm: A new health system for the 21st century.* Washington, DC: National Academies Press.

Institute for Healthcare Improvement. (2007). *About us.* Retrieved July 13, 2007, from http://www.ihi.org/ihi/about

Institute of Medicine. (2003). *Health professions education: A bridge to quality.* Washington, DC: National Academies Press.

Institute of Medicine, Board on Health Care Services. (2004). *Committee on the work environment for nurses and patient safety.* Washington, DC: National Academies Press.

Kohn, L. T., Corrigan, J. M., & Donaldson, M. S. (Eds.). (2000). *To err is human: Building a safer health system.* Washington, DC: National Academies Press.

Robert Wood Johnson Foundation. (2007). *New partnership spreads TCAB successes nationwide.* Retrieved July 13, 2007, from http://www.rwjf.org/newsroom/featureDetail.jsp?featureID=2621&type=3&pid=&c+EMC

Institute of Medicine

T HE NATIONAL ACADEMY OF SCIENCES was created by President Abraham Lincoln on March 3, 1863, to "investigate, examine, experiment, and report upon any subject of science or art" whenever called upon by the government. That institution was expanded to include the National Research Council (1916), the National Academy of Engineering (1964), and the Institute of Medicine (1970), and those four entities are now collectively known as The National Academies. The Institute of Medicine (IOM) is the body specifically charged by Congress with providing advice on the scientific and technological matters that help shape health policy. Committed to the improvement of health, the IOM has adopted processes that ensure the provision of unbiased, evidence-based, and authoritative information. Reports that synthesize and analyze the state of the science are regularly issued by expert committees peopled by member and nonmember experts. IOM is an honorific membership organization, over 1,500 strong in 2006. Though most members are physicians, an interdisciplinary perspective is valued, and about 60 members are nurses (http://www.iom.edu).

The IOM is important to nursing leadership because it is a venue through which nurse experts can join other health care professions in evaluating what is known on a particular topic and what next steps need to be taken to improve practice, fund additional research, and/or develop new policy guidelines. The resulting reports provide excellent summaries of the state of the science on various topics; see the reports section of IOM's Web site for a complete listing (http://www.iom.edu). For example, Greiner and Knebel (2003) issued a report on the five core competencies that all health care professionals will need in the 21st century and another one on the importance of nursing leadership in creating environments that keep patients safe (Page, 2004). The IOM's Board on Health Policy Educational Programs and Fellowships also sponsors midcareer and senior-career opportunities available to nurses, e.g., the Robert Wood Johnson Health Policy Fellowship and the IOM/ANF/AAN Distinguished Nurse Scholar Program (for details go to http://www.iom.edu/CMS/2953.aspx).

ANGELA BARRON MCBRIDE

REFERENCES

Greiner, A. C., & Knebel, E. (Eds.). (2003). *Health professions education: A bridge to quality*. Washington, DC: The National Academies Press.

Page, A. (Ed.). (2004). *Keeping patients safe: Transforming the work environment of nurses*. Washington, DC: The National Academies Press.

Interdisciplinary Leadership in Nursing

EXPERT REPORTS AND COMMISSIONS addressing the challenges facing the U.S. health care system in the 21st century implore the leadership of health care professions to develop strategies for interdisciplinary research, education, and practice. Interdisciplinary competence is seen as one of the keystones of providing the highest quality of health care to the nation. The Pew Health Professions Commission (1998) noted that an interdisciplinary model of care could best manage the care of both acutely and chronically ill patients because "... the expertise and instincts of a number of trained health practitioners are brought to bear in an environment that values brainstorming, consultation, and collaboration." More recently, the Institute of Medicine (Greiner & Knebel, 2003) convened over 150 health care leaders and experts to develop strategies for restructuring clinical education for the 21st century. Among the five core competencies, they recommended that future students and working professionals have experience "working as part of interdisciplinary teams" (Greiner & Knebel). Similarly, the President's New Freedom Commission on Mental Health (2003) suggests that a solution to the current fragmentation of mental health care in the United States is expanded use of collaborative care models that promote interdisciplinary partnerships.

Each of the core mental health professions, including nursing, is challenged to play a leadership role that supports widespread implementation of collaborative care models in primary health care settings.

Over the past decade, several foundations have promoted the development of interdisciplinary collaboration by providing valuable support to interdisciplinary training programs. For example, the John A. Hartford Foundation in New York funded the Geriatric Interdisciplinary Team Training (GITT) Program to encourage interdisciplinary training among health professionals. Data from this program indicate that knowledge and attitudes related to interdisciplinary roles can be improved through such training, thereby promoting quality and cost-effective clinical outcomes (Fulmer et al., 2005). There is also evidence to support the idea that expanding screening and interdisciplinary care models, such as the Collaborative Care Model for treating late life depression in primary care settings, reduces the prevalence and severity of depression symptoms or results in complete remission, leading to higher satisfaction with depression treatment (Unutzer et al., 2002).

The essence of interdisciplinary leadership is predicated upon expertise in some area of knowledge that is valued by and valuable to a range of disciplines. Nursing leadership has long recognized interdisciplinary practice, education, and research as both necessary and beneficial to good patient care. The American Nursing Association's (ANA) Social Policy Statement (Ervin & McNamara, 2003) identifies nursing's scope of practice as one that "... overlaps those of other professions involved in health care ... and members of various professions cooperate by sharing knowledge, techniques, and ideas about how to deliver quality health care." Virtually every major document that guides professional practice at the registered nurse and advanced practice levels promotes the importance of interdisciplinary leadership in improving patient outcomes, including the American Association of Colleges of Nursing (AACN) Essentials of Baccalaureate and Master's Education (www.aacn.nche.edu), the National Organization of Nurse Practitioner Facilities (NONPF) Competencies (www.nonpf.com), and the ANA Scope and Standards of Clinical Nursing Practice (www.nursingworld.org).

In recent years, interdisciplinary leadership by the nursing profession has gained momentum with, for example, a nurse-president of the American Heart Association, a nurse-president of the American Diabetes Association, a nurse-president of the American Public Health Association, a nurse-president of the Society of Behavioral Medicine, and a nurse-president of the Gerontological Society of America. These leadership inroads recognize the importance of nursing in promoting and sustaining national initiatives. Nurse leaders are voted into leadership positions because they are demonstrated experts in the specialty areas addressed by the organizations noted. There are, however, barriers to sustaining interdisciplinary leadership, among these the lack of commitment to interdisciplinary education by professional schools. Without regulatory or other incentives by accrediting bodies or funders to encourage professional schools to redesign curriculum requirements, schools may not emphasize or even provide room for interdisciplinary courses or activities. Therefore, professional educational silos continue, and students do not have the opportunity to understand the history and theory of practice of other professions, to develop interdisciplinary communication skills, or to gain experience with how interdisciplinary practice improves patient outcomes.

The hierarchical nature of health delivery settings also serves to reinforce and replicate the professional separateness. Although there are, in most settings, daily incidences of collaboration and teamwork among professions, it usually is due more to individual preferences and style rather than to institutional policy. The teamwork that may exist at senior management levels of nursing and medicine is not always replicated at the point of patient care delivery. At the patient care level, nurses and physicians more commonly meet, make rounds, and have clinical conferences separately. Traditions related to how each profession organizes daily practice and the schedules and routines of the service delivery setting make it impossible to have, for example, one interdisciplinary conference to start the day.

As entrenched as these barriers to interdisciplinary education, research, and practice seem, the nursing leadership in universities and colleges has unique opportunities to develop models of interdisciplinary collaboration and circumvent if not overcome them. For example, academic nursing leaders can agree to new models by pointing to the shared goals of academia—to produce new knowledge, test new ideas and models, translate them into practice, and transfer a commitment to collaboration to the next generation of health professionals. Realistic action plans can gain support for (a) collaborative teaching within existing professional curricula using equitable revenue sharing models, (b) collaborative research in areas of shared clinical interests that capitalize on "low lying fruit," those areas of similar expertise and interest that reflect synergy across disciplines, and (c) collaborative faculty practices that demonstrate how multiple health professions contribute to quality and cost-effective patient outcomes.

Academic nursing leaders must communicate the values, expertise, and knowledge base of nursing throughout the university to increase the visibility and create an understanding of how nursing makes value-added contributions to the health care team. Academic nursing leaders also must convince the general university leadership that support for strong interdisciplinary collaboration in the health professions strengthens each profession's educational program and thus raises the visibility and status of the entire academic health science endeavor.

Beyond academics, our practice leaders can do much to influence interdisciplinarity as well. Chief nurse officers can and do lead important interdisciplinary committees across an array of health care settings and should do all that is possible to learn essential leadership lessons from their experiences to advance the development of leadership competencies in the next generation of nurse leaders. For example, leadership development using a mentor–mentee model can be a powerful influence for advancing the interdisciplinary leadership skill set for these future academic, practice, and research leaders in their settings.

In the health policy arena, nurses who are experts have led interdisciplinary programs with major foundations and government agencies. For example, Dr. Shirley Chater headed the Social Security Administration during President William Jefferson Clinton's first term, Sheila Burke was Chief of Staff to then Senator Robert Dole, Virginia Trotter Betts was an Undersecretary of Health and Human Services and is currently the Commissioner of TennCare, and Vice Admiral Richard H. Carmona, the former Surgeon General, started his health care career as a nurse. Each time examples of nurses who are leaders in health policy arenas are noted, the scope of their interdisciplinary influence must be recognized and new lessons must be learned from the exercise of their content expertise and political savvy and skill.

In the 21st century, there is an urgent need to confront the challenges of providing affordable high-quality health care, caring for the increasing number of elderly, and adopting more complex technology into patient care. Nursing leadership can respond by taking immediate and aggressive steps to reinforce existing interdisciplinary efforts and to develop new models. The nursing profession is strategically positioned to lead interdisciplinary efforts in education, practice, and research settings. Indeed, it is imperative to do so to improve patient care and to meet the population's health needs in the coming decades.

HILA RICHARDSON
JUDITH HABER
TERRY FULMER

REFERENCES

Ervin, N. E., & McNamara, A. M. (2003). Nursing's social policy statement 2003. *Nursing's Social Policy Statement Revision Task Force, 2001–2003*. Silver Spring, Md. The Publishing Program of American Nurses Association.

Fulmer, T., Hyer, K., Flaherty, E., Mezey, M., Whitelaw, N., Jacobs, M. O., et al. (2005). Geriatric interdisciplinary team training program: Evaluation results. *Journal of Aging and Health, 17*(4), 525–534.

Greiner, A., & Knebel, E. (Eds.). (2003). *Health professions education: A bridge to quality*. Washington, DC: National Academies Press.

New Freedom Commission on Mental Health. (2003). *Achieving the promise: Transforming mental health care in America. Final report* (DHHS Publication No. SMA-03-3832). Rockville, MD.

Pew Health Professions Commission. (1998). *Recreating health professional practice for a new century. The fourth report of the Pew Health Professions Commission.* Retrieved September 20, 2006, from http://www.futurehealth.ucsf.edu/pdf_files/rept4.pdf

Unutzer, J., Katon, W., Callahan, C. M., Williams, J. W., Jr., Hunkeler, E., Harpole, L., et al. (2002). Collaborative care management of late-life depression in the primary care setting: A randomized controlled trial. *Journal of American Medical Association, 288,* 2836–2845.

International Council of Nurses (ICN)

THE INTERNATIONAL COUNCIL OF NURSES (ICN) was founded in 1899 as an organization to represent nurses and their interests worldwide. ICN goals are as follows: (a) align nurses on a global level, (b) continue to internationally advance the profession of nursing, and (c) maintain a strong influence within health policy (ICN, 2006b). Within the ICN federation, 128 national nurse organizations represent their respective countries and thereby millions of nurses around the world.

ICN is the international voice of nurses through global efforts focused on three primary programs: professional practice, regulation, and social economic welfare (ICN, 2006a). Professional practice includes leadership development, the International Classification of Nursing Practice (ICNP), and linkages to national and international organizations, such as World Health Organization (WHO), UNICEF, and the International Red Cross (ICN, 2006c). Within the leadership component, ICN offers a *Leadership for Change* focus consisting of five modules presented to course participants over a 2-year period of time. The regulation focus ensures high standards for education and practice globally. ICN works with WHO to promote regulatory standards for nursing (ICN, 2006d). The social economic welfare focus is targeted toward equitable and reasonable compensation

316

I n t e r n a t i o n a l
C o u n c i l o f
N u r s e s (I C N)

with appropriate work benefits for nurses. ICN also represents nursing within the International Labour Organization to consistently protect nursing and nurses' workplace issues (ICN, 2006e).

In 2006 ICN issued a news release in support of a United Nations Agency for Women that would directly address gender equality with a specific focus on women's rights related to domestic violence, HIV/AIDS, and poverty. ICN bulletins and newsletters are published in the official ICN languages (English, French, and Spanish) and are available on the ICN Web site (http://www.icn.ch). The bulletins cover leadership, regulations, research, socioeconomic news, nurse practitioner/advanced practice issues, and ICNP.

RONDA MINTZ-BINDER
JOYCE J. FITZPATRICK

REFERENCES

International Council of Nurses. (2006a). *Frequently asked questions.* Retrieved July 5, 2006, from http://www.icn.ch/faqs.htm

International Council of Nurses. (2006b). *ICN's membership structure in the new millennium.* Retrieved July 5, 2006, from http://www.icn.ch/membership_structure.pdf

International Council of Nurses. (2006c). *ICN professional practice.* Retrieved July 5, 2006, from http://www.icn.ch/professional.htm

International Council of Nurses. (2006d). *ICN regulation.* Retrieved July 5, 2006, from http://www.icn.ch/reghistory.htm

International Council of Nurses. (2006e). *ICN socio-economic welfare.* Retrieved July 5, 2006, from http://www.icn.ch/sew.htm

International Leadership in Nursing

EFFECTIVE LEADERS IN NURSING demonstrate an understanding of health care systems, are visionary, think strategically, plan effectively, contribute to policy development, manage change, and work effectively in teams. The effective nurse leader understands resource management, marketing, and media skills, communicates effectively, negotiates, and motivates and influences others (International Council of Nurses [ICN], 2006). Nurses who use these skills to effect change across national boundaries are international leaders.

Leadership through international nursing organizations brings health concerns to the global arena. International leaders in nursing focus on health planning and decision making, professional development of nurses, promoting the contributions of nurses in health care, promoting nurse entrepreneurship, defining nursing roles and scope of practice, and promoting the legislative involvement of nurses in their home countries. They seek to increase nursing influence globally by building cooperative coalitions to effect change in local communities. Significant and ongoing issues of concern among global nursing groups have been gender disparity and working conditions for women.

317

Global issues facing nurse leaders are of wide scope and are being approached and critically evaluated in a cohesive and structured manner. Leading the way are impassioned and strong members of many international organizations. For example, the International Council of Nurses (ICN, 2006) represents nursing worldwide to advance the profession of nursing and to influence health policy. The Florence Nightingale International Foundation (FNIF) supports the objectives of the ICN. Activated in 1929, the memorial works with member associations to increase the influence of nursing globally for the health of people in general (FNIF, 2005). Sigma Theta Tau International Honor Society of Nursing (STTI) supports the learning, knowledge, and professional development of nurses and has created a global community of nurse leaders that influences the world through education, service, and social responsibility (STTI, 2005).

Three significant international issues of concern have been the global shortage of nurses, international migration of nurses, and health sector reform and organizational restructuring. To address the issue of a global nursing shortage, *Global Nursing Review Initiative: Policy Options and Solutions* (FNIF, 2005) was written by members of the ICN and FNIF, with support through the Burdett Trust for Nursing. Members included representatives from the Nursing and Midwifery Council from the United Kingdom, the World Bank Institute, National Institute of Health based in the Philippines, The Democratic Nursing Organization of South Africa, the Pan American Health Organization, Ghana Health Service, Norwegian Agency for Development Cooperation, Victorian Order of Nurses, Norwegian Agency for Development Cooperation, World Health Organization of South-East Asia, International Labour Office, and representatives of the World Health Organization from Geneva, Switzerland. Multiple issue papers, consultations with government leaders, an international summit focusing on the Global Nursing Workforce, regulation development, and project publications have come forth in the last 2 years (FNIF, 2005).

As part of the global nursing shortage, critical challenges that affect world regions have been identified. The HIV/AIDS challenge, most prominent in sub-Saharan Africa, is one example. HIV/AIDS creates an increasing demand for health services yet reduces health team availability and functioning as mortality rates and absenteeism among health care workers increase. Due to the HIV/AIDS crisis, the nursing workforce challenge in sub-Saharan Africa is by far the most serious in comparison to any other geographical zone in the world (ICN, 2004). Internal and international migration has been another critical challenge. As recruitment of international nurses to the United States increases, there is a concomitant drain of nursing personnel from developing countries. Developed and financially stable countries are successfully recruiting younger and newly educated nurses, which negatively affects the quality and level of nursing care in smaller, unstable, and less developed countries (ICN, 2004). Improved monitoring of the flow of the international nursing labor workforce is essential to addressing global workforce issues. Yet another critical challenge is facilitating health sector reform and organizational restructuring occurring in many countries worldwide. Cost control, quality improvement, and a stronger and more efficient workforce are key factors related to reform and restructuring (ICN, 2004). Stronger education and training, motivation, involvement of staff, and planning can be used to address the need for reform.

RONDA MINTZ-BINDER
KIM L. CARNAHAN LEWIS
JOYCE J. FITZPATRICK

See Also
Health Policy
International Council of Nurses
Florence Nightingale
Sigma Theta Tau International

REFERENCES

Florence Nightingale International Foundation. (2005). *Project Communique 3. Global nursing review initiative: Policy options and solutions.* Retrieved June 16, 2006, from http://www.fnif.org/communique03_05.htm

International Council of Nurses. (2004). *Global shortage of registered nurses: An overview of issues and actions.* Retrieved June 16, 2006, from http://www.icn.ch/global/shortage.pdf

International Council of Nurses. (2006). *Leadership for change.* Retrieved June 21, 2006, from http://www.icn.ch/leadchange.htm

Sigma Theta Tau International Honor Society of Nursing. (2005). *Policy position statement.* Retrieved June 20, 2006, from http://www.nursingsociety.org/

Internships

THE MERRIAM-WEBSTER DICTIONARY defines "intern" as an advanced student or graduate usually in a professional field gaining supervised practical experience. Interns are primarily college or university students or other young adults. An internship may be paid, unpaid, or partially paid. Internships offer benefits that may include work experience, networking opportunities, instruction, and mentorship.

Nurse mentors play a pivotal role in fostering confidence and enhancing professional growth. The peer mentoring process involves a commitment to shared learning (Tourigny & Pulich, 2005), with individuals accountable for critical thinking, skills development, and cultural sensitivity. The mentoring process in internships is characterized by a focus on professional advancement. In many health care organizations, student nurse interns are given a one-to-one educational opportunity to experience nursing while being mentored. They learn technical, time management, priority setting, and communication and assessment skills, as well as management of a full assignment of patients with multiple diagnoses. The intern becomes accountable as an employee on the hospital staff and transitions from being one student among many to a member of the health care team. The intern is able to form continuing relationships with the staff as well as with patients and families.

The student nurse-mentor relationship focuses on planning, collaborating, and coaching. The mentor serves as a role model and "reality check" as the intern observes his/her practice. These ties nurture the student's desire for experience and identify strengths and weaknesses (Evers, 2000). The interns are paired with mentors who consider them as protégés. Hence, the mentor provides feedback by confirming when a protégé is doing well, by helping a protégé exercise social judgment, and by following formally recognized organizational norms (Tourigny & Pulich, 2005). The process allows for a focus on patient/family education and theoretical frameworks.

The internship program is an excellent bridge between academia and clinical practice in a hospital setting. In short, peer mentoring provides a nurturing climate for personal growth of the interns (Walter & Glass, 2000) and is an integral part of nursing recruitment and retention.

MICHAEL E. IMPOLLONIA
KAREN W. LAUFER
KATHLEEN R. PARISIEN

REFERENCES

Evers, C. (2000). Helping new nurses succeed. *Gastroenterology Nursing, 23*(6), 288–289.

Tourigny, L., & Pulich, M. (2005). A critical examination of formal and informal mentoring among nurses. *The Health Care Manager, 24*(1), 68–76.

Walter, R., & Glass, N. (2000). An experience of peer mentoring with student nurses: Enhancement of personal and professional growth. *Journal of Nursing Education, 39*, 155–160.

ADDITIONAL REFERENCES

Busen, N. H., & Engebretson, J. (1999). Mentoring in advanced practice nursing: The use of metaphor in concept exploration. *The Internet Journal of Advanced Nursing Practice, 2*(2).

Cullen, L., & Titler, M. G. (2004). Promoting evidence-based practice: An internship for staff nurses. *Worldviews on Evidence-Based Nursing, 4*, 215–233.

Dracup, K., & Bryan-Brown, C. (2004). From novice to expert to mentor: Shaping the future. *American Journal of Critical Care, 13*, 448–450.

Kupier, R. A. (2004). Nursing reflections from journalizing during a perioperative internship. *AORN Journal, 79,* 195–218.

Sweitzer, F., & King, M. A. (2003). *The successful internship: Transformation and empowerment in experimental learning.* Belmont, CA: Wadsworth.

Vance, C., & Olson, R. K. (Eds.). (1998). *The mentor connection in nursing.* New York: Springer Publishing.

L

Lambertsen,
Eleanor C.

E LEANOR C. LAMBERTSEN'S life spanned from 1915 until 1998. Lambertsen began her nursing career as a staff nurse at Overlook Hospital, Summit, New Jersey. She progressed to be the Director of the School of Nursing and started her long interest in nursing education. Lambertsen earned her Bachelor's, Master's, and doctoral degrees at Teachers College (TC), Columbia University (Nursing World News, 1998). Lambertsen demonstrated a vibrant and focused interest in developing nursing education programs throughout the country. She served as Director of the Division of Nursing of the American Hospital Association, as Dean of the Cornell University/New York Hospital School of Nursing, as Senior Associate Director of Nursing at New York Hospital, and as Director of the Division of Health Services, Sciences, and Education while concomitantly serving as Helen Hartley Professor of Nursing Education and Chair of the Department of Nursing at TC. Lambertsen participated in many organizations including the American Nurses Association and the American Medical Association; she served as secretary for the National Commission for the Study of Nursing and Nursing Education. Lambertsen was a member of the Surgeon General's Consulting Group that spearheaded the first Nurse Training Act, which was a source of significant

325

federal funding for nursing education. Lambertsen was a prolific writer and carried a regular column in *Modern Healthcare*, the official organ of the American Hospital Association. Additionally, she published a series of professional publications that are housed in the Eleanor C. Lambertsen Pamphlet Collection in the Center for the History of Nursing of the School of Nursing at the University of Pennsylvania. She spearheaded the concept of team nursing as a model for the practice of nursing. Her experiences in education and service enabled Lambertsen to educate the public on the value of nursing education, on the need to change the then current structure of hospital nursing services, and on the administration and future of nursing education (Nursing World News, 1998).

M. JANICE NELSON

See Also
American Nurses Association

REFERENCES

New York Times. (1998). *Lambertsen, Eleanor C., Ed.D., R.N. New York Times paid notice: Deaths.* Retrieved March 24, 2006, from http://www.query.nytimes.com/gst/fullpage.htm

Nursing World News. (1998). *Former ANF president dies.* In University of Pennsylvania (Ed.), *Lambertsen, Eleanor C., papers, 1915–1977, BC2.* Retrieved March 24, 2006, from http://www.nursing.upenn.edu/history/collections/lamberts.htm

Leadership
Development

LEADERSHIP DEVELOPMENT implies learning experiences, processes, and devices that enable individuals to influence the thoughts or actions of another or others toward some specified purpose or goals. This means that leadership development is an aspect of human maturation that is essential for competent and effective leadership. Therefore, it is heralded as a key priority for enhancing the performance and achievements of individuals, groups, and organizations. In recent years, there has been a rapid emergence of leadership development programs and related training initiatives within academic institutions, health services systems, professional associations, and a wide array of freestanding groups and organizations (http://www.leadershipdevelopment.com).

The curriculum of most nursing schools and colleges provides content on leadership. There are Master of Science in Nursing (MSN) programs that offer a minor or concentration in leadership. In some cases, there are programs leading to a Master of Science Degree in Nursing Leadership focused on such areas as Public Health, Long Term Care, Complex Health Care Organizations, and Advanced Practice. National nursing professional organizations and nursing service organizations in health care systems offer short-term training courses, workshops or institutes to advance the leadership development of nurse executives, educators, and clinical practitioners. Business schools around the country offer a wide range of leadership development opportunities and resources. Many offer regularly scheduled seminars, courses, or workshops for middle and senior managers from private, public, and nonprofit sectors. In addition, leadership development programs are offered by numerous other enterprises that profess to strengthen the capacity of individuals and organizations. In several cases, the programs are based on specific models of leadership. Popular among them are *Servant Leadership* (http://www.greenleaf.org) and *Transformational Leadership* (http://www.tcslearning.com).

Perspectives of leadership development evolve from conceptions of the meaning and nature of leadership. Very often, leadership is conceived as the function of a single individual (i.e., a leader) within a group or organization. In numerous cases, this narrow conception of leadership is apparent in the descriptions of courses, programs, and other initiatives intended to enhance leadership capabilities. This reflects a limited perspective of what leadership development entails. In these cases, efforts are focused on preparing individuals for effective performance as *a leader*—absent comparable attention to their preparation for effective performance as a *follower*. Also missing are indications of the interactive and mutually dependent relationship between leaders and followers, which can enhance or undermine effective performance in these leadership roles. Furthermore, the principles and model approaches in these cases are inattentive to the impact of social, political, collective, and other contexts on the performance, achievement, and productivity of leaders and followers.

This tendency to equate *leader* development with *leadership* development compromises efforts to build the leadership capacity of groups and organizations. It is suggested that support for programs or other training initiatives that reflect this tendency has been a misallocation of resources (Iles & Preece, 2006). The most enlightening and productive leadership development approaches are those in which a broad conception of leadership is apparent. For example, the term "leadership" is used to refer to a mechanism, process, or modality for achieving some specified purpose or goals—not to refer to the purpose or goals, per se. The program or special initiative purports to prepare individuals for competent and effective performance in leadership roles—not merely to prepare leaders. Special attention is given to the interactive and mutually dependent relationships of leaders and followers; the nature and significance of authority, power, and related issues or problems that are ubiquitous in human groups and organizations, and the nature and significance of contextual factors that can enhance or inhibit effective leadership.

Comprehensive models for leadership development display the features described above. There are no apparent indications of the tendency to equate *leader* development with *leadership* development or to confuse leadership with management. They give due attention to the play of group dynamics, interpersonal relationships, and intrapersonal processes on the performance of leaders and followers. They are purported to offer opportunities for individuals to obtain the kind of learning that attends the personal qualities, knowledge, and capabilities deemed essential for effective performance in leadership roles. The objectives are to promote the kind of learning that comes from direct experience of fact and situation, reflective and abstract thinking, and integrative and reflective practice. They have been described as "learning *for* leadership," "learning *about* leadership," and "learning *to succeed* in leadership roles," respectively (Dumas, 2006). The modes of instruction are necessarily experiential as well as didactic. Although it is difficult to find all these features in a single leadership development program, close approximations are apparent in the offerings of such organizations as the A. K. Rice Institute (http://www.uvm.edu/~mkessler/akrice/index.html); the Center for Creative Leadership (http://www.ccl.org); the National Training Laboratories (http://www.ntl.org); and the James MacGregor Burns Academy of Leadership (http://www.academy.umd.edu).

RHETAUGH GRAVES DUMAS*

REFERENCES

Aroian, J., & Dienemann, J. A. (2005). Practice oriented leadership education. In H. R. Feldman & M. Greenberg (Eds.), *Educating nurses for leadership*. New York: Springer Publishing.

Bessent, H. (2006). *The soul of leadership*. Battle Creek, MI: The W. K. Kellogg Foundation.

Bolden, R. (2004). Leadership and performance. In *What is leadership? Southwest research report*. Exeter, UK: Centre for Leadership Studies, Exeter University. Retrieved June 2, 2006, from www.leadershipsouthwest.com

Cleveland, H. (1985). *The knowledge executive: Leadership in an information society*. New York: E. P. Dutton.

Dumas, R. G. (1990). Leaders and followers. *Journal of National Black Nurses' Association, 4*(2), 3–8.

Dumas, R. G. (2006). *Leadership: An enlightened perspective*. Unpublished manuscript. University of Michigan, School of Nursing.

---

* A noted leader in her own right, Dr. Dumas died several months after submitting this entry, but prior to its publication.

Feldman, H. R., & Greenberg, M. J. (Eds.). (2005). *Educating nurses for leadership.* New York: Springer Publishing.

Iles, P., & Preece, D. (2006). Developing leaders or developing leadership? *Leadership, 2*(3), 317–340.

McBride, A. (1999). Breakthroughs in nursing education: Looking back looking forward. *Nursing Outlook, 47*(3), 114–119.

Rigolosi, E. L. (2005). *Management and leadership in nursing and health care* (2nd ed.). New York: Springer Publishing.

WEB REFERENCES

Leadership Development, http://www.leadershipdevelopment.com

Greenleaf, http://www.greenleaf.org

TCSlearning.com, http://www.tcslearning.com

A. K. Rice Institute, http://www.uvm.edu/~mkessler/akrice/index.html

Center for Creative Leadership, http://www.ccl.org

NTL Institute, http://www.ntl.org

The James MacGregor Burns Academy of Leadership, http://www.academy.umd.edu

Leadership in Practice Settings

L EADERSHIP IN PRACTICE SETTINGS refers to the skill sets that facilitate care delivery, or to the roles of leadership in various positions that informally or formally constitute an agency's leadership structure. Leadership skill sets are best described by primary sources such as Kouzes and Posner (1997) in their text on evidence-based practice. The best practices of leadership are characterized as: (1) challenging the process; (2) inspiring a shared vision; (3) enabling others to act; (4) modeling the way; and (5) encouraging the heart. A writer and speaker whose work has greatly influenced organizational development in nursing is Tim Porter-O'Grady. Leadership using these concepts ultimately is embodied in shared governance structures that may be as formalized as elected bodies of staff who determine practice.

The role of leadership in patient care settings ranges from clinical leadership at the bedside encounter to the leadership/management of the chief nursing officer (CNO). Leadership principles must be exercised by the nurse providing direct care that both delivers and integrates the plan of care with the patient and family, by the charge nurse coordinating the activities of the unit during a shift, and by the formal leader of a division of patient care units.

331

Novice leadership skills are expected of new graduates, with mutual understanding that an organization provides support and development of the following skills: prioritization, time management, communication, interdisciplinary collaboration, patient/family education, and delegation and follow-up with ancillary care staff. Recognition of the need to further develop the leadership role of new graduates is evidenced in the various curricula that have been developed for nurse internship or residency programs.

Leadership of a group of nurses during a shift involves the ability to facilitate patient flow, to allocate human resources (nursing staff) that match patient needs based on acuity and goals of care, and to effectively communicate the "hand-off" to the next leader. The nurse manager position, as the 24-hour leader, is the single most critical position in most organizations. This formal leader is responsible for the hiring, development, and termination of nursing staff, fiscal performance of the unit, and quality outcomes of patients and staff. The development of nurse managers is a national priority. A breadth of resources is available on this topic (American Organization of Nurse Executives, 2007). Additional nursing leaders essential to patient safety, staff support, and agency operations are supervisors or nurse administrators who are both nursing and hospital/facility representatives on evenings, nights, and weekends. These unsung nursing leaders form the arms around the living delivery system of patient care.

The Chief Nurse Executive (CNE or CNO) provides the direction, vision, advocacy, and resources for nursing. This role is complex, demanding, and requires a portfolio of both leadership and management skills. The CNO must possess and demonstrate an understanding of the discipline of nursing practice, financial, change, performance and outcomes management, quality drivers, information technology, regulatory compliance, the value of evidence based practice and research, cultural diversity, ethics, interdisciplinary collaboration, and governance. The CNO of an excellent organization inspires passion about nursing, care delivery, healthy work environments, and a culture of patient safety.

SUSAN BOWAR-FERRES

See Also
American Organization of Nurse Executives
Shared Governance Is Structure Not Process
Staff Retention

REFERENCES

American Nurses Association. (2004). *Scope & standards of nurse administrators.* Washington, DC: Author.

American Nurses Credentialing Center. (2005). *Magnet recognition program.* Washington, DC: Author.

American Organization of Nurse Executives. (2007). *Nurse manager leadership collaborative.* Retrieved August 20, 2007, from http://www.aone.org/aone/resource/NMLC/nmlc.html

Kouzes, J. M., & Posner, B. Z. (1997). *The leadership challenge.* San Francisco: Jossey-Bass.

McClure, M. L., Poulin, M. A., Sovie, M. D., & Wandelt, M. A. (1983). *Magnet hospitals: Attraction & retention of professional nurses.* Kansas City, MO: American Academy of Nursing.

Krueger Wilson, C., & Porter-O'Grady, T. (1999). *Leading the revolution in healthcare.* Gaithersburg, MD: Aspen Publications.

Page, A. (Ed.). (2004). *Keeping patients safe: Transforming the work environment of nurses.* Washington, DC: The National Academies Press.

WEB REFERENCES

American Nurses Association, http://www.ana.org

American Nurses Credentialing Center, http://www.nursecredentialing.org

ExecutiveFellows.net, http://www.executivefellows.net

Leadership Traits

N HIS CLASSIC BOOK *On Becoming a Leader* (1994), Dr. Warren Bennis stated that "managers are people who do things right, while leaders are people who do the right thing." Being a leader, as distinct from a manager, requires certain attributes or leadership traits. Controversy has existed as to whether these traits are inborn or are acquired. The main categories of useful leadership characteristics are moral and ethical values, technical competence, knowledge and conceptual skill, a desire to be a leader, personality, and people skills. These traits encompass an intellectual and emotional ability to envision and to communicate that vision, an ability to establish successful interpersonal relationships, and the ability to use power to influence.

Leaders must have in-depth knowledge in the field in which they lead, an ability for abstract thinking, a history of achieving results, an ability to communicate, motivate, and delegate, and an ability to cultivate talent in others, good judgment, and good character. Leaders are able to motivate others, use highly developed knowledge and technical skill, and lead change. Some are inspirational, or charismatic; all need to be clear communicators who show commitment and compassion. A leader must be willing, trustworthy, and just. Moral leadership is critical; one must do *good*, in as honest and courageous a way as possible. Leadership means to be vulnerable, to take risks and to be willing to accept mistakes.

Many different descriptions of leadership abound, including relational, servant, transactional, transformational, directive, supportive, participative, achievement-oriented, charismatic, and quantum. Quantum leadership is based on the concepts inherent in chaos theory, which states that the environment is constantly shifting and becoming more complex, everything is interconnected and that roles are fluid and outcome-oriented (Porter-O'Grady & Malloch, 2003, p. 20).

The current thinking of what constitutes a good leader is a departure from the past when the focus was on control and command. Today's leader, who is transformational, needs to have a healthy quotient of Emotional Intelligence (EI) and the desire and confidence to empower others. Persons who are successful leaders have self-awareness, the capacity to self-reflect, insight, and empathy. The importance of these traits was emphasized in the late 1990s when "emotional intelligence" (EI) was identified by Goleman (1998) in the book *Working with Emotional Intelligence,* as a critical skill necessary for effective leadership.

The term "transformational leadership" was first coined by Burns, in his seminal work, *Leadership* (1978). Transformational leadership builds on complexity theory and these leaders are described as having vision, self-confidence, self-direction, honesty, energy, loyalty, commitment, and the ability to develop and implement a vision while empowering followers (Barker, Sullivan, & Emery, 2006; Finkelman, 2006). Burns looked at the leadership styles of famous political leaders such as Mahatma Gandhi, Franklin Delano Roosevelt, and John Fitzgerald Kennedy. Leaders must have purposes that are positive and productive and followers whose needs are met and satisfied and thus motivated to high levels of performance (Barker et al., 2006).

To be successful and transformative, one needs to be in a transformational culture where working with change becomes the norm, a way of life, and the expectation is that the transformational leader will enable others to develop their leadership potential. Transformation can only happen in the context of an interactive relationship.

Nursing leadership in today's world, with its rapidly changing health care environment, requires talent and skills necessary to keep up with and stay ahead of the curve. The Institute of Medicine report, *Keeping Patients Safe: Transforming the Work Environment of Nurses* (2003), underscores this belief as a way to increase safety and reduce errors. Transformational leadership that recognizes the interdependence between a chaotic environment and a visionary leader is required to be successful. The multiplicity of demands and the rapidity of change require the successful leader to have the necessary traits to know how to manage effectively in a chaotic environment.

MARILYN JAFFE-RUIZ

See Also
Change
Complex Adaptive Systems (Chaos Theory)
Emotional Intelligence
Power and Leadership

REFERENCES

Barker, A. M., Sullivan, D. T., & Emery, M. J. (2006). *Leadership competencies for clinical managers*. Boston: Jones and Bartlett.

Bass, B., & Avalio, B. (1994). *Improving organizational effectiveness through transformational leadership*. Thousand Oaks, CA: Sage.

Bennis, W. (1994). *On becoming a leader*. Reading, MA: Perseus Books.

Burns, J. M. (1978). *Leadership*. New York: Harper and Row.

Curtin, L. (2001). Guest editorial: EQ is more important now than ever before. *Seminars for Nurse Manager, 9*(4), 203–205.

Dunham-Taylor, J. (2000). Nurse executive transformational leadership found in participative organizations. *Journal of Nursing Administration, 30*(5), 241–250.

Finkelman, A. (2006). *Leadership and management in nursing*. Upper Saddle River, NJ: Prentice Hall.

Goleman, D. (1998). *Working with emotional intelligence*. New York: Bantam Books.

Hassmiller, S. B. (2006). Are you the best leader you can be? *American Journal of Nursing, 106*(2), 67–69.

Hesselbein, F., & Johnson, R. (2002). *A leader to leader guide on mission and leadership*. San Francisco: Jossey-Bass.

Institute of Medicine. (2003). *Keeping patients safe: Transforming the work environment for nurses*. Washington, DC: Author.

Malloch, K., & Porter-O'Grady, T. (2005). *The quantum leader: Applications for the new world of work*. Sudbury, MA: Jones and Bartlett.

Porter-O'Grady, T., & Malloch, K. (2003). *Quantum leadership*. Sudbury, MA: Jones and Bartlett.

Swearingen, S., & Liberman, A. (2004). Nursing leadership: Serving those who serve others. *Health Care Manager, 23*(2), 100–109.

The Leapfrog Group

T HE LEAPFROG GROUP was officially launched in November of 2000 amid discussions sparked by the 1999 Institute of Medicine's report, *To Err is Human: Building a Safer Health System.* The report brought to light serious concerns regarding errors in U.S. hospitals, which may account for as many as 98,000 deaths annually. The report went on to recommend many potential solutions, one of which is for large employers to utilize their purchasing power to exert market pressures on hospitals to pay more attention to quality standards (Kohn, Corrigan, & Donaldson, 1999). According to the organization's Web site, The Leapfrog Group is "a member supported program aimed at mobilizing employer purchasing power to alert America's health industry that big leaps in health care safety, quality and customer value will be recognized and rewarded" (Leapfrog Group, n.d.a, para. 1). The foundation of The Leapfrog Group was made possible through funding from the Business Roundtable, and the members constitute several Fortune 500 companies representing more than 37 million Americans in 50 states (Leapfrog Group, n.d.a).

The data collected by The Leapfrog Group are based on hospitals' self-reporting and is completely voluntary. The Leapfrog Group Hospital

337

Quality and Safety Survey is the tool utilized and it is most applicable to urban-acute care hospitals, although any hospital is invited to participate. The data are then posted on a monthly basis for the public and employers to view when making decisions regarding care (Leapfrog Group, n.d.b). The over 1,960 hospitals that participate in the survey encompass thirty-one regions of the United States (Leapfrog Group, n.d.a).

The leaps in quality and safety that have been defined and tracked by The Leapfrog Group to date include Computer Physician Order Entry (CPOE), Evidence-Based Hospital Referral (EHR), Intensive Care Unit (ICU) Physician Staffing, and The Leapfrog Safe Practices Score. The CPOE indicator shows the extent to which the hospital has adopted a CPOE system, whether it is utilized across the organization or only in some parts of the organization. EHR refers to a hospital's volume and outcomes associated with certain high-risk surgeries or medical conditions, such as coronary artery bypass graft or pancreatic resection. Intensive Care Unit Physician staffing refers to the utilization of *intensivists*, which are physicians with specialized training in critical care. Lastly, The Leapfrog Safe Practices Score is based on the 2003 report from The National Quality Forum, *Safe Practices for Better Healthcare: A Consensus Report*. This report highlights specific actions that can bring about a safer practice environment, such as only utilizing standard abbreviations. Hospitals report if they have adopted such practices and to what extent. Health care consumers can visit The Leapfrog Group website and compare hospitals on the criteria explained above. This provides the individual consumer with outcome and safety based data on which to make their decisions about care.

The Leapfrog Hospital Rewards Program is "a pay-for-performance program to recognize and reward hospitals for their performance in both the quality and efficiency of inpatient care" (Leapfrog Group, n.d.c, para.1). The rewards may be in the form of a bonus payment, higher reimbursement rates, public recognition, or increased patient market share. According to a study by the Center for Studying Health System Change (HSC) in Washington, DC, however, most hospital executives report difficulty implementing the safety practices because of financial constraints and limited financial incentives post-implementation ("Few Hospitals are Close to Filling Leapfrog Goals," 2004). The Leapfrog Group creates guidelines and tools to determine appropriate incentives, yet it remains up to the employers or insurance companies to be willing to provide these financial incentives.

The impact of implementing the safety initiatives outlined by the Leapfrog Group is subject to varying support in the literature. Although some of the initiatives, such as the standards of care for the patient suffering acute myocardial infarction, are supported by a great deal of research and backed by the American Heart Association, others have less reliable data supporting their implementation. A recent study found in *Critical Care Medicine* created a model to analyze the financial implications of staffing ICUs with intensivists. The findings indicate an average cost savings of $510,000 to $3.3 million for a 6- to 18-bed ICU. However, a limitation of this study is its partial funding by the Business Roundtable, which also sponsors The Leapfrog Group (Pronovost et al., 2006). Additionally, issues are at play with the operations of initiatives such as CPOE. There is very little known about the impacts of verbal orders and RNs entering orders into CPOE as a courtesy to physicians. The health care industry needs to ensure its practices and improvement initiatives are founded on evidence-based care.

Another key component when discussing The Leapfrog Group initiatives is the consideration of nurses' impact on patient safety and quality standards. The three goals currently outlined by The Leapfrog Group have very little to do with direct nursing care. Nursing leaders voice the need to look at the nursing shortage and quantify its impact on patient safety and outcomes (Wynd, 2002). Several studies are finding that "a number of medical, cardiac, and respiratory complications and length of stay [are] directly related to nursing care" (Hudon, 2003, p. 236). How nursing contributes to patient safety is not clearly understood by the public or by the members of The Leapfrog Group. A great deal of this is a result of limited nursing research indicating clear, measurable impacts on patient safety.

The Leapfrog Group has certainly been successful in heightening the awareness of patient safety issues in hospitals for both consumers and providers; however, the implementation is lagging mainly as a result of fiscal barriers and some uncertainty regarding patient safety and outcomes estimates. The Leapfrog Group safety initiatives would benefit from more research to quantify the impacts of their implementation. The nursing profession needs to clearly define and measure its impact on patient safety in order to be become a larger part of the equation. Only then will The Leapfrog Group, consumers, and employers be able to grasp the significance of nursing on patient safety and outcomes.

STACY HUTTON JOHNSON

See Also
Evidence-Based Practice
Institute for Healthcare Improvement
National Quality Forum

REFERENCES

Few hospitals are close to filling Leapfrog goals. (2004, April 1). *Healthcare Risk Management*, 45.

Hudon, P. S. (2003). Leapfrog standards: Implications for nursing practice. *Nursing Economic$, 21,* 233–236.

Kohn, L. T., Corrigan, J., & Donaldson, M. S. (1999). *To err is human: Building a safer healthcare system.* Washington, DC: National Academies Press.

Leapfrog Group. (n.d.a). *Leapfrog Group fact sheet.* Retrieved September 28, 2006, from http://www.leapfroggroup.org/about_us/leapfrog-factsheet

Leapfrog Group. (n.d.b). *How Leapfrog works.* Retrieved September 28, 2006, from http://www.leapfroggroup.org/about_us/how_leapfrog_works

Leapfrog Group. (n.d.c). *Leapfrog hospital rewards program.* Retrieved September 28, 2006, from https://leapfrog.medstat.com/hrp/index.asp

Pronovost, P. J., Needham, D. M., Waters, H., Birkmeyer, C. M., Calinawan, R. B., Birkmeyer, J. D., et al. (2006). Intensive care unit physician staffing: Financial modeling of the Leapfrog standard. *Critical Care Medicine, 34*(2), S18–S24.

The National Quality Forum. (2003). *Safe practices for better healthcare: A consensus report.* Retrieved October 3, 2006, from http://www.qualityforum.org/txsafeexecsumm+order6-8-03PUBLIC.pdf

Wynd, C. (2002). AONE's leadership exchange: Leapfrog Group jumps over nursing. *Nursing Management, 33(12),* 20.

Legal Nurse
Consulting

A **LEGAL NURSE CONSULTANT** combines nursing expertise with specialized training to assist attorneys with medical-related cases. Legal nurse consultants come from every nursing specialty and apply their nursing knowledge and skills to all kinds of health care and nursing issues. The legal nurse consultant is a full-fledged professional member of the litigation team. The attorney is the expert on legal issues and the legal nurse consultant is the expert on nursing, the health care system, and medical record documentation. Few attorneys know how to review medical records or understand the health care issues important to medical malpractice and personal injury lawsuits.

Using a legal nurse consultant is far more cost-effective for the attorney than using an MD expert, yet legal nurse consultants have a better grasp of the medical records. Because they spend much of their time educating patients, legal nurse consultants are also superbly qualified to educate attorneys on medical terminology, disease processes, and the health care system in general. The legal nurse consultant's expertise saves the attorney time and money, and benefits the legal system by promoting fair and just resolution of medical-related cases.

TYPES OF CASES LEGAL NURSE CONSULTANTS CONSULT ON

L EGAL nurse consultants consult on a myriad of cases, from simple back injury cases caused by auto accidents, to complex cases, such as brain injury in a newborn.

MEDICAL AND NURSING MALPRACTICE CASES

THESE CASES INVOLVE the professional negligence of a health care provider or facility. Every year, 98,000–195,000 people in hospitals die from medical negligence. On average, every day hospitals experience one medication error per patient. Medical malpractice litigation pervades practically every nursing specialty. A legal nurse consultant's role in these types of cases is to research standards of care that apply and point out any deviations from or adherences to the applicable standards.

GENERAL NEGLIGENCE CASES

THESE ARE NONPROFESSIONAL negligence cases, such as an auto accident, slip and fall in a grocery store, amusement park ride death, and so on. The legal nurse consultant helps the attorney understand the extent of the injuries and examine whether or not they were caused by that incident.

PRODUCT LIABILITY CASES

THESE CASES INVOLVE allegedly defective products, such as medical devices, pharmaceuticals, and nonmedical devices. Legal nurse consultants have worked on many headline cases in the news, for example, Fen-Phen, Vioxx, Fosamax, and implantable defibrillators. Nonmedical cases include defective automobiles, washing machines, or hair dryers. A legal nurse consultant's role in such cases is to identify whether or not the defective product caused the alleged injuries.

TOXIC TORT AND ENVIRONMENTAL CASES

THESE CASES INVOLVE injuries as a result of exposure to toxins and chemicals, such as dumping of toxic sludge into a residential community and contamination of groundwater by a manufacturing plant. The role of the legal nurse consultant is to help identify whether or not the alleged toxins caused the injuries or deaths.

WORKERS' COMPENSATION AND WORKPLACE INJURY CASES

THESE CASES INCLUDE any job-related injury, for example, repetitive motion injuries such as carpal tunnel syndrome, back injury, and body part amputations.

CRIMINAL CASES

A CRIME IS ANY ACT that society has deemed contrary to the public good. Legal nurse consultants work on criminal cases ranging from driving under the influence (DUI) to homicide to elder abuse.

ANY CASE IN WHICH HEALTH, ILLNESS, AND INJURY IS AT ISSUE

PROBATE OR MEDICARE fraud, and custody battles are examples of other types of cases where legal nurse consultants provide a variety of services to attorneys, for example:

* Interpret medical records
* Review medical and nursing literature
* Identify standards of care
* Assist with discovery
* Detect tampering within medical records
* Help assess injuries
* Identify causation issues and contributing factors
* Point out potential defendants
* Locate and work with expert witnesses
* Interview and prepare clients, key witnesses, and experts
* Prepare questions for deposition or trial examination
* Prepare exhibits and other demonstrative evidence

Legal nurse consultants may consult with attorneys behind the scenes or testify as expert witnesses. In addition to working with plaintiff and defense attorneys, legal nurse consultants work with insurance companies, utilization review firms, government agencies, private corporations and hospitals, both as staff members and as independent consultants.

THE LEGAL NURSE CONSULTANTS' IMPACT ON THE LEGAL SYSTEM

A S REPRESENTATIVES of the nursing profession, legal nurse consultants uphold the standards of care for the entire health care community. By giving their objective opinions on the merits of cases and deviations from recognized standards, they help to improve the quality of nursing practice. A legal nurse consultant's opinions also contribute to the effectiveness of the legal system and are often critical in reaching a fair and just outcome for all parties. As a result, the legal nurse consultant plays an invaluable role on the litigation team. Another contribution legal nurse consultants make is identifying fraudulent and nonmeritorious claims, thus helping to defend against such claims or keep them out of the system. By making all parties aware of the documented facts and research connected with a case, legal nurse consultants help to ensure that the legal system uses this information properly and without distortion.

LEGAL NURSE CONSULTING CERTIFICATION AND CAREER OPTIONS

N URSES wishing to enter the field of legal nurse consulting undergo training and certification. The Certified Legal Nurse Consultant^{CM} (CLNC®) certification is the official certification of the *National Alliance of Certified Legal Nurse Consultants* (*NACLNC®*) and is available through the Vickie Milazzo Institute (http://www.legalnurse.com). With approximately 6,000 members, the *NACLNC®* is the largest and most recognized association of legal nurse consultants.

The legal nurse consulting profession affords nurses of all ages and experience levels an option for establishing a satisfying and profitable part-time or full-time career. Registered nurses (RNs) are best prepared to enter the field with at least 3–5 years of clinical experience. Certified Legal Nurse Consultants^{CM} typically earn fees of $150 per hour by using their nursing expertise in this unique and exciting way. The field of legal nurse consulting is rapidly growing in popularity with attorneys, as well as with RNs, and was voted one of the 10 hottest jobs for 2007 by CareerBuilder.com.

VICKIE L. MILAZZO

See Also
Consultation
Malpractice

WEB REFERENCES

Core Curriculum for Legal Nurse Consulting®—available from Amazon.com
Legal Nurse Consulting Ezine—FREE subscription available at LNCEzine.com
CLNC® Success Stories, Third Edition—available on Amazon.com
Preview Your New Life as a CLNC® Consultant DVD—available at Legal-Nurse.com
National Alliance of Certified Legal Nurse Consultants – NACLNC.org

Leone, Lucille Petry

LUCILLE PETRY LEONE was born in 1902 in Frog Heaven, Ohio and died in San Francisco, California in January 2000 (American Association for the History of Nursing, 2007). She earned her Bachelor of Arts degree from the University of Delaware, a diploma in nursing from the Johns Hopkins School of Nursing, and Master of Arts degree from Teachers College, Columbia University (American Nurses Association, 2000). Petry Leone was involved in the development of the U.S. Nurse Corps and was given the responsibility to oversee the nursing care provided to American soldiers during World War II (Johns Hopkins School of Nursing, n.d.). Petry Leone served as president of the National League for Nursing; she was chief nursing officer and director of nursing education for the United States Public Health Service. She also served as technical expert on nursing for the World Health Organization, and served as Director of the U.S. Cadet Nurse Program during World War II. Petry Leone was the first woman to attain the rank of Assistant Surgeon General of the United States; she also attained the rank of Brigadier General. Lucille Petry Leone was prominent in the move for more governmental support for health care. The Cadet Nurse Corps program initiated by her not only filled a vital need to recruit and train nurses in time of war, but it also eliminated the need to draft nurses into service during World War II. Petry Leone paved the way for a new understanding of educational organization and the future of nursing education. She was instrumental in persuading public health nurses to aspire for positions of power, and she was largely responsible for improving nursing relationships with the federal government

M. JANICE NELSON

See Also
American Nurses Association
National League for Nursing

REFERENCES

American Association for the History of Nursing. (2007). *Archived obituaries*. Retrieved August 19, 2007, from http://www.aahn.org/obituaries.html

American Nurses Association. (2000). *Nursing pioneer dies*. Retrieved March 20, 2006, from http://www.nursingworld.org/news/nwst01.00.htm

Johns Hopkins School of Nursing. (n.d.). *History of the Johns Hopkins School of Nursing*. Retrieved March 20, 2006, from http://www.hopkinsmedicine.org/about/history/history8.html

Licensure

IN **THE UNITED STATES,** the legal authorization to practice certain professions is a state's right and controlled by each state's relevant statutes (laws), rules, and regulations. The privilege to practice the profession of nursing as a registered professional nurse (RN) (independent licensure) or a licensed practical/licensed vocational nurse (LPN/LVN) (dependent licensure requiring supervision of practice) and, in some states, as an advanced practice registered nurse (APRN), is separately authorized by each state, territory, and commonwealth. In 1903, the first statutes (registration laws) governing the practice of nursing were passed in North Carolina, New Jersey, New York, and Virginia. It would be the mid-1930s before states successfully passed Nurse Practice Acts requiring licensure by the state of all those who would practice the profession of nursing (Driscoll, 1976).

Once licensed as an RN or LP/VN, one is "never not a nurse," and it is a privilege granted by the state to practice the profession of nursing, not a right of ownership. Nurses who in their personal lives are charged or convicted of tax evasion, driving while under the influence or intoxicated, committing acts of civil disobedience, or who are convicted of other types of misdemeanors or felonies are usually reported to the state oversight agency. Depending on the state's laws and regulations, this may result in an interruption of practice privileges by either temporary or permanent loss of licensure.

Licensure is a state's legal mechanism for protecting the public from harm and ensuring that an individual has the basic competence to practice nursing (RN or LP/VN). Only those so authorized can use the credentials (title protection). Most states require that an applicant for licensure have completed a course of study from an approved school of nursing or, if from a foreign country, can demonstrate equivalency of education. States also require successful passage of the NCLEX-RN or NCLEX-PN for licensure; there is a single national pass rate and the examinations are electronically administered unless an applicant requests a modification based upon a recognized disability. States may have additional state-specific qualifying criteria such as child abuse, domestic violence, HIV/AIDS, and pain management education; compliance with social laws such as payment of student loans, alimony, or state fines; and being of "good moral character" with no outstanding felony or misdemeanor charges/convictions (Daly, Sandra, Jackson, Lambert, & Lambert, 2005). Once licensed, the state expects that a nurse will remain professionally committed to meeting any new educational requirements, maintaining appropriate competence in practice and refraining from acts of professional misconduct.

When moving to a new state, an RN or LPN must apply for licensure to practice in that state; this process is known as "endorsement" and can differ among states. One may hold licensure in as many states or territories that one wants as long as the nurse meets the requirements to maintain the license or places it on inactive status according to the regulations of the particular state. The nurse who is licensed in multiple states is required to know the different state nurse practice acts and any variations in scope of practice among the states of licensure. Most states have an ongoing registration process (2 or 3 years) that requires nurses practicing in the state to register their licenses by paying a fee and bringing personal information up-to-date with the state's oversight agency. Some states require that RNs who are also advanced practice registered nurses (APRNs), specializing as nurse anesthetists (CRNA), nurse midwives (CNM), nurse practitioners (NP), or clinical nurse specialists (CNS), obtain a second license from the state to practice in such a role. The uniformity that exists in RN and LPN licensure does not exist with regard to APRNs and, therefore, some states strictly regulate the authorization to practice, whereas other states require no separate permission to practice in these roles. The National Council of State Boards of Nursing (NCSBN) has attempted to institute a second mandatory licensure process with an examination to address the APRN role. NCSBN has addressed the differences in state licensure laws for RNs, LPNs and APRNs by promoting two types of voluntary licensure compacts for the states (similar in theory to the national driver's license compact). These are known as the Multistate RN/LPN Licensure Compact and the APRN Licensure Compact (http://www.ncsbn.org). Both compacts have met with mixed responses from the states because of a variety of issues such as negative opinions from state attorneys general on legality, loss of revenue streams to the state and oversight agency, concerns about discipline issues, and the public's ability to have recourse when dissatisfied with a nurse's practice.

KAREN A. BALLARD

See Also
Advanced Practice Registered Nurses
The National Council of State Boards of Nursing, Inc. (NCSBN)

REFERENCES

Daly, J., Sandra, S., Jackson, D., Lambert, V., & Lambert, C. E. (2005). *Professional issues Concepts, issues and challenges*. New York: Springer Publishing.

Driscoll, V. M. (1976). *Legitimizing the profession of nursing: The distinct mission of the New York State Nurses Association*. Schenectady, NY: The Foundation of the New York State Nurses Association.

National Council of State Boards of Nursing. (2007). *Nurse licensure compact— About*. Retrieved September 2, 2006, from www.ncsbn.org/156.htm

Living Legends

I N 1994, THE BOARD OF DIRECTORS of the American Academy of Nursing (AAN) created the "Living Legend" (LL) Program to honor Fellows who were leaders among leaders. Not only was there a perceived need for such a senior-level recognition program, but there were two organizational problems that this initiative was expected to address: many of the most distinguished (and older) Fellows were no longer attending meetings because they did not know the younger Fellows who also did not know them. Thus, the LL Program was meant to serve as a history lesson and to strengthen intergenerational leadership by highlighting the achievements of pioneering role models.

To be eligible for this recognition, Fellows must have been active in the AAN for 15 or more years, must have made extraordinary and sustained contributions to nursing and health, and must have transitioned from the formal work role, even though they continue to influence the profession. The first two cohorts (1994 and 1995) honored legendary figures in all aspects of the profession: Faye Abdellah, Myrtle Aydelotte, Mary Elizabeth Carnegie, Luther Christman, Rheba de Tornyay, Ildaura Murrillo-Rohde, Virginia Ohlson, Hildegard Peplau, Rozella Schlotfeldt, Jessie Scott, and Harriet Werley. In the next decade, 41 additional leaders

350

were awarded that distinction. For a complete listing, refer to the AAN Web site (http://www.aannet.org/fellowship/ll/history.asp).

The AAN has made use of these living legends in various ways. A leadership conference is held annually as part of the "Building Academic Geriatric Nursing Capacity" Program, which the AAN manages in partnership with the John A. Hartford Foundation (Conn, 2006). One popular feature has been an interview with living legends, for example, Mary Starke Harper, Florence Wald, Luther Christman, and Claire Fagin, during which the individual reminisces about her or his career trajectory. At its 2004 annual meeting, the AAN instituted "An Emerging Leader" Program. One aspect of that programming has been breakfast discussions with living legends. The commitment to fostering leadership is particularly important if we are to develop future legends in nursing.

ANGELA BARRON MCBRIDE

See Also
American Academy of Nursing

REFERENCE

Conn, V. S. (2006). Innovative model for building academic nursing. *Western Journal of Nursing Research, 28,* 367–368.

M

Magnet Hospitals

IN THE EARLY 1980s, the United States was experiencing a serious nursing shortage. In an effort to assist in solving the problems involved, the American Academy of Nursing appointed a Task Force on Hospital Nursing Practice. The members were: Margaret L. McClure (chair), Muriel A. Poulin, Margaret D. Sovie, and Mable Wandelt.

During the course of their early deliberations, the task force observed that there were a small number of hospitals that, unlike others, were not having difficulty recruiting and retaining professional nurses. Moreover, it was clear that although there was a substantial body of literature related to turnover, virtually no studies had been done regarding the retention of nurses. As a result, the task force undertook a national study, specifically focused on identifying the critical factors that made selected hospitals highly attractive to registered nurses, even in a time of severe shortage. And, because of their ability to attract and retain their staff, the institutions were labeled "Magnet Hospitals." Forty-one institutions comprised the sample and the data were collected through interviews conducted with the nurse executives and staff nurses from each of the institutions. The results of the study were published in 1983 in a monograph, entitled

Magnet Hospitals: Attraction and Retention of Professional Nurses (McClure, Poulin, Sovie, & Wandelt, 1983).

After publication of the study, several nurse scholars, most notably Marlene Kramer and Linda Aiken, continued to conduct research involving the Magnet Hospitals. Their findings not only validated those of the original research but also demonstrated a link between the Magnet organizations and high-quality patient outcomes.

In the early 1990s, the American Nurses Credentialing Center (ANCC) began a new program, designed to allow hospitals to apply to be designated as Magnet Hospitals. Using the 14 characteristics identified in the original study and expanding them further to include findings from other studies as well as the American Nurses Association's *Standards for Organized Nursing Services*, the ANCC developed a rigorous methodology by which the applicant hospitals could be judged; this process involves the submission of extensive written materials, as well as site visits conducted by specially trained appraisers. Hospitals that receive the Magnet designation must repeat the application process every 4 years in order to maintain their standing.

Much of the work that has been done to date, including the research findings and the ANCC Magnet Hospital designation process, is summarized in a volume entitled *Magnet Hospitals Revisited: Attraction and Retention of Professional Nurses* (McClure & Hinshaw, 2002). In addition, information regarding the ANCC Magnet Hospital program can be found on the Web at http://www.nursecredentialing.org.

MARGARET L. MCCLURE

See Also
American Academy of Nursing
American Nurses Association
American Nurses Credentialing Center

REFERENCES

McClure, M. L., Poulin, M. A., Sovie, M. D., & Wandelt, M. (1983). *Magnet hospitals: Attraction and retention of professional nurses.* Washington, DC: American Nurses Publishing.

McClure, M. L., & Hinshaw, A. S. (2002). *Magnet hospitals revisited: Attraction and retention of professional nurses.* Washington, DC: American Nurses Publishing.

Mahoney, Mary Eliza

MARY ELIZA MAHONEY was born in Massachusetts in 1845; she died in 1926 at the age of 81. Mahoney graduated from the New England Hospital for Women and Children Training School for Nurses in 1879 and has the distinction of being the first black nurse trained in the United States. Mahoney was recognized for the quality of her nursing care, which was described as quietly efficient with untiring compassion (American Nurses Association, 2006). Mahoney was active in community affairs and in professional organizations at both local and national levels. She presented the welcome address at the first conference of the National Association of Colored Graduate Nurses (NACGN) in 1909 (Carnegie, 1995). In recognition of her attributes as a trained nurse and as a model for all nurses, the NACGN initiated the Mary Mahoney Award, to be presented to a person(s) exhibiting outstanding contributions to intergroup relations. When the NACGN was merged with the ANA in 1951, ANA kept up the practice of issuing the Mary Mahoney Medal for outstanding contributions to intergroup relations. Mary Mahoney was inducted posthumously into the American Nurses Association Hall of Fame in 1976.

M. JANICE NELSON

See Also
American Nurses Association
ANA Hall of Fame

REFERENCES

American Nurses Association. (2006). *1976 inductee: Mary Eliza Mahoney, 1845–1926*. Retrieved March 22, 2006, from http://www.nursingworld.org/hof/mahome.htm

Carnegie, M. E. (1995). *The path we tread: Blacks in nursing worldwide* (3rd ed.). New York: National League for Nursing Press.

Malcolm Baldrige National Quality Award

MALCOLM BALDRIGE WAS the U.S. Secretary of Commerce from 1981 until his accidental death in 1987. Baldrige was a firm believer and supporter of quality management as a primary focus to enhance the strength and financial success of our country. He was extensively involved in the creation of the quality improvement act that was named after him. To recognize and honor his efforts, Congress named this award after him (National Institute of Standards and Technology, 2006).

The Malcolm Baldrige National Quality Award (MBNQA) (http://www.quality.nist.gov/) is given by the President of the United States to businesses as well as education and health care organizations based on performance excellence as evaluated by independent board members. The seven areas that are judged are: leadership; strategic planning; customer and market focus; measurement, analysis, and knowledge management; human resource focus; process management; and results (American Society for Quality, 2006). The award represents a successful partnership between government and the private sector. The government commits approximately $5 million, which is then enhanced by $100 million in donations from the private sector and state and local organizations. The

Board of Examiners is a collection of 300 industry, educational, government, and nonprofit organization volunteers who are responsible for reading the applications, visiting the nominated businesses, and issuing feedback regarding strengths and weaknesses (National Institute of Standards and Technology, 2006). The education and health care categories were established in 1999.

The following are a few of the recent health care organizations that have won this prestigious award: Bronson Methodist Hospital, Kalamazoo, Michigan 2005; Robert Wood Johnson University Hospital, Hamilton, New Jersey 2004; Baptist Hospital Inc., Pensacola, Florida and Saint Luke's Hospital of Kansas City, Missouri, 2003; SSM Health Care, 2002. Criteria and the application process are available through the National Institute of Standards and Technology Web site located at http://www.quality.nist.gov/Criteria.htm.

RONDA MINTZ-BINDER

REFERENCES

American Society for Quality. (2006). *Malcolm Baldrige National Quality Award*. Retrieved August 19, 2006, from http://www.asq.org/learn-about-quality/malcolm-baldrige-award/overview/overview.html

National Institute of Standards and Technology. (2006). *Frequently asked questions about the Malcolm Baldrige National Quality Award*. Retrieved August 19, 2006, from http://www.nist.gov/public affairs/factsheet/baldfaqs.htm

The Baldrige Program. (n.d.). *Self-assessment for continuous improvement*. Retrieved October 22, 2006, from http://www.quality.nist.gov/Principal_Article.htm

Malpractice

MALPRACTICE WAS DEFINED many years ago as "... a limited class of negligent activities committed within the scope of performance by those pursuing a particular profession involving highly skilled and technical services" (Lesnick & Anderson, 1962). More recently, malpractice has been defined as "... negligence, misconduct, or breach of duty by a professional person that results in injury or damage to a patient" (Reising & Allen, 2007). Negligence, by contrast, is defined as "conduct which falls below the standard established by law for the protection of others against unreasonable risk of harm" (Brent, 2001, p. 54). For negligence to exist, there must be a *duty* between the client and the professional practitioner whose actions, or lack thereof, caused the injury (Brent, 2001). For purposes here, "duty" is constituted by virtue of the fact that the nursing professional has entered into a contract, either written or tacit, with the client to provide reasonable and safe nursing care.

In prior decades, many not-for-profit organizations, such as orphanages, churches, and hospitals were considered to be charitable institutions, which were literally exempt from litigation. Professional practitioners in these facilities—including physicians and nurses—were commonly considered as dedicated and committed "Good Samaritans," who were, by virtue of their "vocational calling," also not subject to lawsuits. Thus, across the years, the incidence of litigation involving malpractice/negligence issues among health care organizations and professions was exceedingly low. This situation remained so until *Darling v. Charleston Memorial Hospital,* in the state of Illinois in 1965. Outcomes of this particular lawsuit dispelled the notion of charitable immunity and paved the way, as it were, for litigation of heath care organizations and health care professionals. From a negative vantage point, since that time, the number of litigations involving hospitals and health care providers has escalated to the point that many physicians and nurses, particularly those engaged in highly vulnerable clinical specialties such as obstetrics or anesthesiology, have opted for other areas of clinical practice, if for no other reason than to seek a reprieve from exorbitantly high malpractice insurance premiums. On the plus side, continuous and escalating health care litigation has led to the development and implementation of standards of practice and standards of care specific to the various categories of health care practitioners and specific to given communities. In addition, personnel manuals, policy manuals, written job descriptions, quality improvement programs, and adherence to standards of accreditation are all part of the *modus operandi* of health care organizations and dictate the conditions of third-party reimbursement, as well as participation in federal Medicare and Medicaid programs.

Reising and Allen (2007) have identified seven of the most common malpractice claims against professional nurses: (1) failure to follow standards of care; (2) failure to use equipment in a responsible manner; (3) failure to communicate; (4) failure to document; (5) failure to access and monitor; (6) failure to act as patient advocate; and (7) inappropriate delegation practices (2007, pp. 40–41). These seven areas provide a framework for the development of competencies intended for patient safety, patient satisfaction, and prevention of litigation for nursing students, nurse educators, and nursing practitioners.

M. JANICE NELSON

REFERENCES

Brent, N. J. (2001). *Nurses and the law* (2nd ed.). Philadelphia: Saunders.
Darling v. Charleston Memorial Hospital, 211 NE2d253 (IL 1965).
Lesnick, M. J., & Anderson, B. E. (1962). *Nursing practice and the law.* Philadelphia: Lippincott.
Reising, D. L., & Allen, P. N. (2007). Protecting yourself from malpractice claims. *American Nurse Today, 2*(2), 39–44.

Management by Objectives

N 1954, **PETER DRUCKER** first published his management concept entitled Management by Objectives (MBO) in his book *The Practice of Management*. Drucker, who died in November 2005 at the age of 95, was known as the father of modern corporate management as well as one of the world's most influential business theorists (Sullivan, 2005). During his life, Drucker published over 36 books and in 30 languages. He believed that strong workers need to be empowered and that the goal of a manager was to prepare and then free their employees to perform at optimal levels (Sullivan, 2005). MBO is an objective-driven approach to performance evaluation that involves five major principles: (1) defined organization based goals and objectives; (2) member driven individualized objectives; (3) shared decision making; (4) a specified time frame for evaluation; and (5) employee work-based evaluation and mutual feedback (12 Manage Rigor and Relevance, 2006). This premise encourages a shared commitment and understanding between the employee and the employer and elicits employee acceptance of individualized objectives to be met in the time frame ahead. In assessing the quality of the objectives, the SMART technique was also introduced by Drucker (1992). Objectives need to be: Specific, Measurable, Achievable, Realistic and Time-related.

Objectives are best met when they are clearly written, easily understood, and appropriate to the situation. The principles of MBO were extrapolated into the more current Value Based Management techniques. In the 1990s, Drucker did state that MBO works well if the objectives are known; however, 90% of the time, employees do not know them (12 Manage Rigor and Relevance, 2006).

RONDA MINTZ-BINDER
JOYCE J. FITZPATRICK

REFERENCES

Drucker, P. (1954). *The practice of management.* New York: Harper and Roy.

Drucker, P. (1992, September-October). The new society of organizations. *Harvard Business Review,* 95–105.

Sullivan, P. (2005). *Management visionary Peter Drucker dies.* Retrieved July 7, 2006, from http://www.washingtonpost.com/wp-dyn/content/article/2005/11/11/AR2005111101038.html

12 Manage Rigor and Relevance. (2006). *Management by objectives (Drucker) SMART.* Retrieved July 7, 2006, from http://www.12manage.com/methods_smart_management_by_objectives.html

McManus, R. Louise

RACHEL LOUISE MCMANUS was born on March 4, 1896; she died on May 29, 1993. A graduate of the Pratt Institute in Brooklyn, New York, McManus later earned her nursing diploma at the Massachusetts General Hospital School of Nursing. She then earned her baccalaureate, Master's, and doctoral degrees at Teachers College (TC), Columbia University. McManus served on the faculty at TC from 1925 until her retirement in 1961; she assumed the department chair position in 1947. In collaboration with the Committee on Measurements and Educational Guidance of the National League for Nursing Education (NLNE), McManus was instrumental in the development of prenursing tests, pretests for clinical nursing courses, achievement tests in the sciences, and tests in clinical nursing. She eventually developed what promised to be one of the most valuable contributions to the profession—the establishment of a state board test pool. The application of these batteries of tests brought about national standardization of nurse licensing exams (Christy, 1969). McManus was recipient of numerous awards including the Columbia University Bicentennial Award, the Mary Adelaide Nutting Award, and the Florence Nightingale Red Cross Society Citation and Medal (Rothwell, 2006). In recognition of her contributions, the National

Council of State Boards of Nursing (NCSBN) established the R. Louise McManus Award and the Meritorious Service Award (Rothwell, 2006). The *R. Louise McManus Medal* was established by the Teachers College Nursing Education Alumni Association to recognize long-standing contributions of a distinguished nature to the nursing profession (NEAA, 2006). Based on her professional achievements, her commitment to advancing the nursing profession, and the fact that she was the first professional nurse to earn the PhD, R. Louise McManus was inducted into the National Women's Hall of Fame (Seneca Falls, New York) in 1994 (Columbia University Record, 1994).

M. JANICE NELSON

See Also
The National Council of State Boards of Nursing, Inc. (NCSBN)

REFERENCES

Christy, T. E. (1969). *Cornerstone for nursing education: A history of the division of nursing education of teachers college, Columbia University, 1899–1947.* New York: Teachers College Press.

Columbia University Record. (1994). *Three alumnae join women's hall of fame.* Retrieved March 30, 2006, from http://www.columbia.edu/cu/record/archives/vol20/vol20_iss12/record1012.27.html

National Council of State Boards of Nursing (NCSBN). (2005). *Award ceremony honors outstanding nurse regulators.* Retrieved March 20, 2006, from http://www.marketwire.com/mw/release_html_bl?release_id=92526

Nursing Education Alumni Association (NEAA). (2006). *Achievement awards: Criteria for specific NEAA achievement awards.* Retrieved April 8, 2006, from http://www.tcneaa.org/pages/9/index.htm

Rothwell, K. (2006). *National women's history month: Honoring nurses' courage and vision.* Retrieved March 20, 2006, from http://www.nursezone.com/spotlightonnurses

Mentoring

FORMAL EDUCATION IS essential in learning the fundamentals so necessary to exerting leadership, but socialization experiences are important, too. The mentoring relationship, whereby the expert provides guidance to the novice in responding to new role expectations and understanding contextual cues, is essential to the development of excellence. Mentoring is crucial to learning what is typically not taught in class, for example, managing time, networking, developing communication skills, deciding where to publish, leading teams, and understanding proprietary issues. The mentor provides the mentee or protégé with perspectives that can only be gained from experience, for example, thinking strategically and responding to criticism.

The mentoring relationship contributes to the mentor's leadership abilities, too. It is personally and professionally gratifying to share what one has learned and to advance future generations of leaders. The mentor is likely to be energized by the mentee's enthusiasm, and the person being mentored may bring special skills to the mentor's projects. Mentees expect their mentors to be role models and to have the demeanor and expertise needed to provide guidance and support; mentors seek mentees who are motivated for success and leadership.

Effective mentoring has assumed even greater importance as professionals endeavor to function effectively in ever-changing environments, and it requires an array of learned competencies (Johnson & Ridley, 2004). For example, mentoring is essential in the development of research competence (Byrne & Keefe, 2002). Gone are the days when institutions can assume experts will "be helpful" to novices without organizational supports in place to expedite mentoring, including expectations for best practices (Pfund, Pribbenow, Branchaw, Lauffer, & Handelsman, 2006). The more complicated new role expectations are, the more necessary mentoring becomes.

ANGELA BARRON MCBRIDE

REFERENCES

Byrne, M. W., & Keefe, M. R. (2002). Building research competence in nursing through mentoring. *Journal of Nursing Scholarship, 34,* 391–396.

Johnson, W. B., & Ridley, C. R. (2004). *The elements of mentoring.* New York: Palgrave Macmillan.

Pfund, C., Pribbenow, C. M., Branchaw, J., Lauffer, S. M., & Handelsman, J. (2006). The merits of training mentors. *Science, 311,* 473–473.

Military Nursing

THE DEMANDS OF war provided the opportunity for Florence Nightingale to develop the skills and knowledge that were the origins of nursing as a profession. Nightingale's military experience provided the impetus for changes in the civilian health care system. Military nursing in America has an equally distinguishing heritage that is evident in the advancement of nursing as a profession in addition to providing women emancipating work outside of the home environment.

Military nursing in America began when General Washington established a hospital organization in the Continental Army. Through the 18th and 19th centuries, women continued to be employed intermittently and in small numbers as military nurses. The Civil War required an increase in the number of nurses to care for soldiers. Women with minimum formal nursing education and training applied to serve as Army contract nurses in addition to other women volunteers. A detailed chronology of the early decades of military nursing is described in *A History of the Army Nurse Corps* (Sarnecky, 1999).

Military nursing languished until 1898 when Dr. Anita Newcomb McGee, representing the Daughters of the American Revolution, volunteered to assist the Army Surgeon General to select the best candidates

369

to become Army nurses in preparation for the Spanish-American War (1898). The skilled and compassionate care provided by contract nurses in the Spanish American War was the impetus for Dr. McGee and a committee from the Red Cross to draft legislation for Congress to create the Army Nurse Corps (female) as part of The Army Reorganization Act. On February 2, 1901, the Army Nurse Corps (female) was founded and was followed by the Navy Nurse Corps in 1908. The Air Force Nurse Corps was created following World War II in 1949.

In between World War I and World War II, the several hundred nurses that were serving in the Army and Navy were not sufficient for a military that waxed and waned in response to national and world events. The Red Cross provided ongoing support to military nursing in terms of training and recruitment of qualified women. The survival of military nursing between wars can be attributed to the professionalism of military nurses and the organizational structure that fostered the education and training of nurses to function in the midst of battlefield hazards, extremes in the environment, and the unique demands of military life.

Even though the need for nurses in the military was validated at the beginning of the 20th century with the creation of the Army Nurse Corps and the Navy Nurse Corps, the status of nurses in the military was ambiguous. Nurses had no military rank, equal pay or other benefits, including retirement or veteran's benefits. In 1944 and later in 1948, Congress passed legislation to give women (mostly nurses) in the armed services full pay and privileges equivalent to what men were receiving; however, the treatment and management of women in the military services was not equal or fair when compared to their male colleagues. There were, for example, limitations on the number of women who could achieve rank and there was no opportunity for a woman to be selected to promotion to general/admiral. At the outset, the military nursing corps was limited to female nurses. Allowing male nurses to serve as officers did not occur until 1955 when male nurses were authorized reserve commissions in the Army Nurse Corps. In 1967, President Lyndon B. Johnson signed Public Law 90-130 "to amend titles 10, 32, and 27, United States Code, to remove restrictions on the careers of female officers in the Army, Navy, Air Force, and Marines, and for other purposes." Additional legislation was needed to remove restrictions on marital status and having children under the age of 16. In the 1970s, the segregation of women in separate corps was eliminated and in 1976 women were allowed admission into the service academies and discussion began to allow women to serve on ships and military airplanes. It is clear that military nurses were on the leading edge for implementing change for the women's rights movement in the United States.

Legacies of military nursing include leadership and innovations in nursing practice. Military nurses are leaders at all levels of unit and hospital management, including the command of major medical units. Many prototypes for nursing practices had their origins in military nursing. These include ward management, team nursing, and advanced nursing practices roles, with the most prominent being the nurse anesthetist and the flight nurse. Military nurses were among the first to use penicillin, renal dialysis, and Stryker frames. A new dimension was provided to nursing research when military nurses in Vietnam conducted research on malaria, shock, and body temperature. In the early 1970s, military nurses were in the vanguard of professional nursing when the services mandated the baccalaureate degree as the entry level requirement for career status as a military nurse.

Current information regarding the military nurse corps can be accessed through several Web sites. The Army Nurse Corps has its own Web site: http://armynursecorps.amedd.army.mil/. The Navy Nurse Corps and Air Force Nurse Corps can be accessed through http://defenselink. mil/ and clicking on links. Select the service and search for nurse corps.

NANCY R. ADAMS

See Also
Florence Nightingale

REFERENCES

Nightingale, F. (1992). *Notes on nursing: What it is, and what it is not.* Philadelphia: J. B. Lippincott Company.

Sarnecky, M. T. (1999). *A history of the U.S. Army Nurse Corps.* Philadelphia: University of Pennsylvania Press.

Montag, Mildred L.

MILDRED LOUISE MONTAG was born August 10, 1908, in Struble, Iowa; she died on January 21, 2004, at the age of 95 (Teachers College, 2004). Montag earned a baccalaureate degree in history from Hamline University, St. Paul, Minnesota, in 1930, a baccalaureate in nursing from the University of Minnesota, and a Master's and doctorate in Nursing Education (EdD) at Teachers College (TC), Columbia University. Montag held a number of professional positions throughout her career, which include a faculty position at the University of Minnesota School of Nursing, instructor at St. Luke's Hospital School of Nursing (New York), and founding director of the School of Nursing at Adelphi University in Garden City, New York. Her doctoral dissertation, *The Education of Nursing Technicians*, completed at TC, ignited the associate degree movement in nursing and helped it evolve from an idea into hundreds of programs held at community and junior colleges across the nation. Montag was instrumental in increasing the number of nurses in this country and changing the nursing population by providing greater access for minorities, males, adult learners, married students, and other diverse populations of students who were interested in becoming nurses

(Teachers College, 2004). Additional information about Mildred Montag can be accessed at http://nursing.adelphi.edu/about/history.php.

M. JANICE NELSON

REFERENCES

Klainberg, M. (n.d.). *About the school of nursing: History of the school: Dr. Mildred Montag.* Retrieved March 22, 2006, from http://www.nursing.adelphi. edu/about/history.php

Teachers College–Columbia University News. (2004). *Mildred Montag, 95, dies.* Retrieved April 20, 2006, from http://www.tc.columbia.edu/news/ article.htm?id-4717

N

National Black Nurses Association, Inc.

T HE **NATIONAL BLACK NURSES ASSOCIATION (NBNA)** was organized in 1971 under the leadership of Dr. Lauranne Sams, former
Dean and Professor of Nursing, School of Nursing, Tuskegee University, Tuskegee, Alabama. The NBNA is a nonprofit organization representing 150,000 African-American registered nurses, licensed voca-
tional/practical nurses, nursing students and retired nurses from the
United States, Eastern Caribbean, and Africa, with 79 chartered chapters
in 34 states.

The NBNA mission "is to provide a forum for collective action by
African American nurses to investigate, define and determine what the
health care needs of African Americans are and to implement change to
make available to African Americans and other minorities health care
commensurate with that of the larger society." The NBNA has had nine
presidents in its 35-year history: Dr. Lauranne Sams, 1973–1977; Dr. Carrie
Rogers Brown, 1977–1979; E. Lorraine Baugh, 1979–1983; Ophelia Long,
1983–1987; Dr. C. Alicia Georges, 1987–1991; Dr. Linda Burnes Bolton, 1991–
1995; Dr. Betty Smith Williams, 1995–1999; Dr. Hilda Richards, 1999–2003;
and Dr. Bettye Davis Lewis, 2003–2007.

COLLABORATIVE COMMUNITY HEALTH MODEL

SINCE its inception, improving the health of African Americans through the provision of culturally competent health care services in community-based health programs has been the cornerstone of the National Black Nurses Association. The NBNA is proud of its Collaborative Community Health Model developed by past presidents Bolton and Georges. This model is the basis for the collaborative partnerships and health programs that are the hallmark of the NBNA. The chapters are the primary mechanism through which the national, state, and local community-based programs are successfully implemented. African-American nurses who are direct members (in cities where no chapters are established) also assume leadership roles in mounting community-based programs.

Working in partnership with community-based organizations, corporations, and other organizations, NBNA has sponsored health fairs and health education and outreach for national organizations, such as the National Urban League, International Black Professional Firefighters, One Hundred Black Men of America, and the National Council of Negro Women. The NBNA has collaborated with the Black Congress on Health, Law, and Economics, a 17-member, multiprofessional organization, Oncology Nursing Society, American Cancer Society, American Heart Association, American Diabetes Association, American Association of Nurses in AIDS Care, National Coalition for Health Professional Education in Genetics, and the International Society for Hypertension in Blacks, among others.

NBNA SIGNATURE PROGRAMS

THE NBNA has signature programs and services, for example, its annual Institute and Conference where nurses and nursing students obtain state of the art clinical instruction on such subjects as cardiovascular disease, cancer, children's health, diabetes, end of life, HIV/AIDS, kidney disease, research, and women's health. Outstanding keynote speakers have included Dr. Risa Lavizzo-Mourey, President and CEO, The Robert Wood Johnson Foundation; Congressman Charles Rangel; Marie Smith, President, AARP; U.S. Surgeon General David Satcher; Ron Williams, President and CEO, Aetna; and Kevin Lofton, President and CEO, Catholic Healthcare Initiatives and Chairman-elect, American Hospital Association. The NBNA presents nursing awards in nine categories and Life Time Achievement and Trailblazer Awards. Scholarships are offered to nursing students at all levels and chapter awards are presented for community service, service to youth, and chapter recruitment and retention.

The National Black Nurses Day on Capitol Hill serves to educate the U.S. Congress on timely topics related to the nursing profession as well as health care disparities. Following the day on Capitol Hill, the National Black Nurses Foundation hosts continuing education unit (CEU) sessions and an awards ceremony honoring public health advocates.

Published twice annually, the *Journal of the National Black Nurses Association* contains peer refereed health research based articles. The quarterly *NBNA Newsletter* includes information on membership and articles written by NBNA members, partners and sponsors on a variety of nursing and health issues. Themes have included public policy, aging, and research. In 2005, NBNA published a special issue on "Surviving the Storms: Katrina, Wilma and Rita." The articles were written by NBNA members as survivors and caregivers. Based on an article that she wrote for the Newsletter, a member of the Fort Bend County Texas Black Nurses Association and St. Luke's Episcopal Hospital, Houston, Texas, received a $50,000 leadership award from Johnson & Johnson.

In September 2005, NBNA and five other organizations were awarded a $300,000 grant from the U.S. Office of Minority Health to provide services to Katrina survivors. In 2006, NBNA published a manual on surviving disasters that was distributed to 1,000 entities in Houston and along the Gulf states. Moreover, for many years, NBNA has had a Memorandum of Understanding with the American Red Cross to help provide nursing services in times of natural and man-made disasters. In 2006, NBNA representatives participated in several American Red Cross workshops on diversity. The purpose of the workshops was to craft curriculum that would help Red Cross volunteers to provide services in a culturally competent manner. At the 2006 Annual Conference, NBNA launched the Institute of Excellence, which is to honor African-American nurses for their contributions in the areas of clinical skills, research, academia, and policy. Twenty-five nurses were inducted in the first class.

In collaboration with other organizations, in 2007, NBNA held three certification programs on HIV/AIDS, end-of-life-care, and corrections. In 2004 and 2005, NBNA received a grant from the John Hartford Geriatric Institute to publish two newsletters that focused on aging. In 2006, the existing articles and new articles were published on the NBNA website as the "Special Report on Aging." The NBNA Web site is www.nbna.org.

In 2003–2004, the National Black Nurses Association and the National Black Nurses Foundation collaborated on a series of workshops on recruitment and retention of African-American nurses into the profession. Funding was provided by the W. K. Kellogg Foundation. The NBNA Women's Health Research Program was established in 1999 for nurse researchers to enhance existing research or develop new research around women's health issues. In 2003, the National Black Nurses Association became one of the five founding organizations of the National Coalition of Ethnic Minority Nurse Associations. This collaboration gives voice to 350,000 minority nurses. Its goals include support for the development of a cadre of ethnic nurses reflecting the nation's diversity; advocacy for culturally competent, accessible and affordable health care; promotion of the professional and educational advancement of ethnic nurses; education of consumers, health care professionals and policy makers on health issues of ethnic minority populations; development of ethnic minority nurse leaders in areas of health policy, practice, education, and research; endorsement of best practice models of nursing practice, education, and research for minority populations.

The NBNA holds membership on various national and federal advisory committees including the National Advisory Committee for the Office of Minority Health; National Advisory Council on Nursing Education and Practice; FDA Nominating Group; National African American Drug Policy Coalition, Inc., Joint Commission of Healthcare Organizations Nursing Advisory Committee, National Council of Negro Women, Balm in Gilead Cervical Cancer Advisory Board, Healthy Mothers, Healthy Babies Coalition, and *Nursing Spectrum Magazine.*

MILICENT GORHAM
BETTYE DAVIS LEWIS

See Also
The National Coalition of Ethnic Minority Nurses Associations

The National Coalition of Ethnic Minority Nurses Associations

S EISMIC SHIFTS in the demographics of the populations in the United States have been well documented and so have the gaps in unequal health care outcomes for people of color. Increasing diversity in the nursing workforce by increasing the nursing pipeline at all levels is thought to be of the utmost importance if the existing gaps are to be closed. In May 1997, the U.S. Department of Health and Human Services, Bureau of Health Professions, and the Division of Nursing held a conference on minority health issues, which brought together distinguished nursing leaders of color representing their respective organizations. The results were the development of a coalition that represents 350,000 ethnic minority nurses and a forum to address the lived health experience of a constituency marginalized from mainstream health delivery systems. The four founding member associations were the National Black Nurses Association (NBNA), the National Association of Hispanic Nurses (NAHN), the National Alaska Native American Indian Nurses Association (NANAINA), and the Asian American/Pacific Islander Nurses Association (AAPINA). A fifth member, the Philippine Nurses

382

THE NATIONAL
COALITION OF
ETHNIC
MINORITY
NURSES
ASSOCIATIONS

Association of America (PNAA), joined the coalition shortly after the formation of the coalition. Individual nurses cannot join the coalition.

From its inception, the coalition has been a collaborative national force and powerful advocate for both the concerns of minority nurses and for the health care needs of ethnic minority populations, which continue to suffer disproportionately high rates of disease and mortality compared to the majority population. In the past seven years, the National Coalition of Ethnic Minority Nurses Associations (NCEMNA) has conducted workshops, prepared white papers on the health status and needs of particular ethnic communities, as well as made recommendations for nursing research to improve the health of these populations. Through a partnership with Aetna and a grant from the Aetna Foundation, a scholars program was initiated to support 10 minority nursing students—two from each NCEMNA member association. A primary focus for NCEMNA is creating programs to increase the number of ethnic minority nurse scientists and researchers who can investigate the causes of minority health disparities and find solutions for eliminating them. The award of a $2.4 million grant from the National Institute of General Medical Sciences (NIGMS) funded a 5-year landmark project designed to engage and cultivate the next generation of nurses scientists from racial and ethnic minority populations known as "NCEMNA: Nurse Stimulation Program." This initiative will create a database of minority nurse researchers and students and provide mentoring development. More information about NCEMNA and the founding members and their various approaches to decrease the gap of unequal health outcomes through the encouragement of minority nurse researchers can be obtained from their Web sites: NCEMNA, http://www.ncemna.org; NBNA, http://www.nbna.org/; NAHN, http://www.thehispanicnurses.org/; NANAINA, http://www.nanaina.com/; AAPINA, http://www.aapina.org/; and PNAA, http://www.pnaa03.org/.

G. RUMAY ALEXANDER

See Also
Mentoring
National Black Nurses Association, Inc.

The National Council of State Boards of Nursing, Inc. (NCSBN)

THE NATIONAL COUNCIL OF STATE BOARDS OF NURSING, INC. (NCSBN) is a not-for-profit organization whose members consist of nursing regulators from boards of nursing in the 50 states, the District of Columbia, and five United States territories—American Samoa, Guam, Northern Mariana Islands, Puerto Rico, and the Virgin Islands. Established in 1978, the purpose of NCSBN is to provide an organization through which state boards of nursing collaborate on matters related to regulation of the profession. A major function of the organization is to develop the National Council Licensing Examination for Registered Nurses (NCLEX-RN®) and National Council Licensing Examination for Practical Nurses (NCLEX-PN®), which are used by all member boards as a requirement for licensure. Additionally, NCSBN maintains a national data bank on disciplinary action taken against nurses' licenses, conducts regulatory research, promotes uniformity in the regulation of nursing practice, provides nurse licensure data, and serves as a venue for dialogue and information exchange for its members. The National Council of State Boards of Nursing provides a Web site (http://www.ncsbn.org), which includes information about its mission, programs, and services.

BARBARA ZITTEL

National Institute of Nursing Research

THE NATIONAL INSTITUTE OF NURSING RESEARCH (NINR) is one
of the institutes at the National Institutes of Health (NIH), which
is the major funding source for health science in the United
States. The NINR was initially mandated as the National Center of
Nursing Research (NCNR) by Public Law 99-156, the Health Research
Extension Act of 1985 and was established at the NIH on April 16,
1986, by U.S. Department of Health and Human Services (HHS) Secretary Otis Bowen, M.D. The Center was redesignated as a National
Institute of Nursing Research in Public Law 103-43 (The NIH Revi-
talization Act of 1993) and federally established by HHS Secretary,
Donna Shalala, on June 14, 1993. The legislative process also established the National Advisory Council for Nursing Research (NACNR)
(http://ninr.nih.gov/ninr/research/diversity/mission.html). The NINR
supports basic and clinical research and research training to establish
a scientific basis for the practice of nursing and health care with individuals, families, and communities. The NINR has provided leadership
for nursing and nursing research through a series of funding priorities and strategic plans initiated and developed with the nursing scientific community and interdisciplinary colleagues, as well as the National

Advisory Council for Nursing Research (NACNR). In the latest plan, the NINR has provided funding opportunities for research in areas central to nursing practice and health care. Those areas include "chronic illness experiences, cultural and ethnic considerations, end of life/palliative care, health promotion and disease prevention, implications for genetic advances, quality of life/quality of care, symptom management of illness and treatment, and tele-health interventions and monitoring" (http://ninr.nih.gov/ninr/research/diversity/mission.html).

The NINR is a major source of funding for nursing research and research training. A number of different grant award mechanisms are available for such funding (http://grants.nih.gov/grants/funding/funding_program.htm).

ADA SUE HINSHAW

REFERENCES

National Institute of Nursing Research (NINR). (2003). Retrieved August 14, 2006, from http://ninr.nih.gov/ninr/research/diversity/mission.html
National Institutes of Health (NIH). (2006). Retrieved August 14, 2006, from http://grants.nih.gov/grants/funding/funding_program.htm

National League for Nursing

S**INCE** its creation in 1893 as a society formed for "the establishment and maintenance of a universal standard of training" for nursing, the National League for Nursing (NLN) has continued to be a leading professional association for nursing education. The mission of the NLN is to advance excellence in nursing education that prepares the nursing workforce to meet the needs of diverse populations in an ever-changing health care environment. This mission is evidenced through the NLN's faculty development programs, Certification in Nursing Education hallmarks of excellence, extensive testing products, position statements on significant issues in nursing education, research, and other efforts designed to advance the science of nursing education and the Centers of Excellence in Nursing Education™ program. The hallmarks of excellence consist of "characteristics or traits that serve to define a level of outstanding performance or service" (http://www.nln.org/excellence/hallmarks_indicators.htm). Hallmarks pertain to: students, faculty, continuous quality improvement, curriculum, resources, innovation, teaching/learning/evaluation strategies, educational research, environment, and leadership.

NLN's membership is threefold: (1) all of nursing education programs, except doctoral; (2) schools of nursing and allied agencies as well as individuals; and (3) any individual (nurse or non-nurse, faculty member or not) who is concerned about and wishes to influence the future of nursing education. At present, NLN members include more than 1,200 schools of nursing and in excess of 18,000 faculty teaching in nursing programs across the country. Each fall, the NLN hosts an Education Summit, a national conference that draws approximately 1,500 educators who come together as a community to discuss innovations in nursing education and how together we can transform the educational enterprise to best prepare graduates who can successfully implement their roles in today's complex, uncertain, ever-changing health care, educational and social environments, and create a preferred future for nursing.

THERESA M. VALIGA

WEB REFERENCE

National League for Nursing, www.nln.org

National League for Nursing Accrediting Commission (NLNAC)

ESTABLISHED in 1893 as the American Society of Superintendents of Training Schools for Nurses (the "Society"), later to become the National League for Nursing, was the first nursing organization in the United States, the purpose of which was to establish and maintain a universal standard for the training of nurses. Throughout the early years following the turn of the 20th century, the Society issued numerous publications addressing the standardization of curricula for schools of nursing and, eventually through the collaborative efforts of faculty at Teachers College, Columbia University, issued the well-known *Goldmark Report*, which was the first survey of nursing and nursing education in the United States (Christy, 1969). In 1912, the Society became the League for Nursing Education. Ever concerned about standardization and quality of the education of nurses, by 1938, the "League" initiated accrediting activities for schools of nursing. It wasn't until 1952, however, that the process of accreditation of nursing schools was brought under the aegis of the National League for Nursing (NLN).

In 1996, the NLN Board of Governors approved the recommendation for the establishment of an independent organization to be known as the National League for Nursing Accrediting Commission (NLNAC).

The 15 Commissioners consist of: nine nurse educators, three executives, and three public members. These commissioners assume full responsibility for the management, financial decisions, policy making, and general administration of the NLNAC. The NLNAC is recognized by the U.S. Department of Education as the national accrediting body for all types of programs in nursing education. NLNAC is also recognized by the National Council of State Boards of Nursing, State Boards of Nurse Examiners, the U.S. Department of Health and Human Services, Bureau of Health Professions, Nursing, and the U.S. Uniformed Nursing Services, to name a few. As of December 2006, NLNAC has been responsible for the accreditation of nursing programs ranging from licensed practical nursing (LPN) through the Master's level. NLNAC accreditation offers to schools of nursing the following:

1. National recognition that the program or school has been evaluated by a competent and respected independent group, which decides that the program meets or exceeds predetermined criteria as set forth by the NLNAC for nursing programs within a certain category (e.g., practical nursing, diploma granting, or degree granting);
2. The opportunity to demonstrate that the program or school fosters ongoing self-examination and reevaluation of nursing education programs for purposes of quality improvement; and
3. The assurance that the program or school demonstrates a quality education and that students and graduates of the program are eligible for educational mobility.

M. JANICE NELSON

See Also
The National Council of State Boards of Nursing, Inc. (NCSBN)
National League for Nursing

REFERENCES

Christy, T. E. (1969). *Cornerstone for nursing education.* New York: Teachers College Press, Teachers College, Columbia University.
National League for Nursing Accrediting Commission. (n.d.). Retrieved on May 26, 2007, from http://nlnac.org

National Organization of Nurse Practitioner Faculties

THE **NATIONAL** Organization of Nurse Practitioner Faculties (NONPF) was established in 1974 to promote national and international quality nurse practitioner education. "...the NONPF domains and core competencies for nurse practitioner (NP) practice have provided guidance to curriculum development across NP programs. NONPF also has led the development of entry-level competencies for NP specialty practice and of national guidelines for NP educational programs. These seminal documents support the preparation of highly qualified health professionals" (http://www.nonpf.com/). NONPF is a resource to faculty and practitioners. In addition to the core competencies in primary and acute care, NONPF has published a number of statements on seminal topics in nursing education, including a response to the National Council of State Boards for Nursing *Vision Paper: The Future Regulation of Advanced Practice Nursing*, recommendations on the practice doctorate in nursing, and a monograph on mentoring. Listed on the NONPF Web site are resource centers of the organization, namely, Practice Doctorate Resource Center, Community Health Resource Center, and Faculty

390

391

*National
Organization of
Nurse
Practitioner
Faculties*

Practice Resource Center. These are designed, in part, to convey the perspective of NONPF, the latest updates on committee work, and available resources for members, so that members are educated about the latest issues that may affect their practice in clinical and academic areas.

HARRIET R. FELDMAN

See Also
Advanced Practice Registered Nurses
National Council of State Boards of Nursing
Regulatory Bodies

WEB REFERENCE

National Organization of Nurse Practitioner Faculties, http://www.nonpf.com/

National Quality Forum

NURSING LEADERS need to understand the mission and goals of the National Quality Forum (NQF), and the incredible force they are in the health care performance improvement arena in the United States. As noted in the Continuous Quality Improvement entry of this *Encyclopedia*, improving care and the outcomes of patients is strategically important for health care organizations (Gosfield & Reinertsen, 2005) and the forces of the "pay for performance" movement will soon "up the performance bar" in ways never before experienced. Performance improvement will be an "imperative," not just a "strategic goal." Pay for Performance (P4P) is an emergent issue on health care executives' radar screen, and it is here to stay for the foreseeable future. Therefore, nursing leaders must fully comprehend P4P and its tie to the role of the NQF mission.

"P4P has arisen in response to concerns that traditional payment schemes reward the volume of services provided, while placing too little emphasis on the quality and efficiency of health care. By paying differentially based on quality and efficiency, public and private purchasers seek to encourage and reward performance improvement efforts" (National Quality Forum Executive Institute, 2006). Nurses are best served when performance improvement initiatives are aligned with the broad set of NQF endorsed measures.

WHO IS THE NQF?

THE NATIONAL Quality Forum is a private, not-for-profit membership organization created to develop and implement a national strategy for health care quality measurement and reporting. The mission of the NQF is to improve American health care through endorsement of consensus-based national standards for measurement and public reporting of health care performance data that provide meaningful information about whether care is safe, timely, beneficial, patient-centered, equitable, and efficient.

ORGANIZATIONAL GOALS

THE SPECIFIC goals of the NQF (http://www.qualityforum.org) are to:

1. Promote collaborative efforts to improve the quality of the nation's health care through performance measurement and public reporting;
2. Develop a national strategy for measuring and reporting health care quality;
3. Standardize health care performance measures so that comparable data are available across the nation (i.e., establish national voluntary consensus standards);
4. Promote consumer understanding and use of health care performance measures and other quality information; and
5. Promote and encourage the enhancement of system capacity to evaluate and report on health care quality.

The four strategic goals of NQF (http://www.qualityforum.org) are:

1. NQF-endorsed standards will become the primary standards used to measure the quality of health care in the United States;
2. The NQF will be the principal body that endorses national health care performance measures, quality indicators, or quality of care standards;
3. The NQF will increase the demand for high quality health care;
4. The NQF will be recognized as a major driving force for and facilitator of continuous quality improvement of American health care quality.

All NQF activities involve the active participation of representatives from across the spectrum of health care stakeholders. Projects are guided by a Steering Committee and many are assisted by a Technical Advisory Panel. Agreement around recommendations is developed through the NQF formal consensus development process.

NURSING CARE QUALITY AT THE NQF

N URSING is the largest health care profession in the United States, with nurses serving as principal caregivers in hospitals and other settings, thereby constituting the single largest operating expense of any health care delivery system. Considering this reality, however, it is surprising how before the NQF Nursing Performance Measures project little attention had been directed toward developing a comprehensive set of nursing care performance measures. Recognizing nurses' contributions to patient safety and quality outcomes, NQF embarked on the "Nursing Care Performance Measures" project in February 2003 to:

* Identify a framework for how to measure nursing care performance, with particular attention to the performance of nurses as teams and their contributions to the overall health care team;
* Endorse a set of voluntary consensus standards for evaluating the quality of nursing care (including designating consensus standards that are appropriate for public reporting); and
* Identify and prioritize unresolved issues regarding nursing care performance measurement and research needs.

This resulted in 15 NQF-endorsed[TM] consensus standards[1] for nursing-sensitive care (U.S. Office of Management and Budget, 1998) (See Figure N.1). These standards must be considered as a "fabric" defining nursing's impact on care, rather then "individual threads" of stand-alone measures. Viewed together, they provide consumers with a way to assess the quality of the nurse's contribution to inpatient hospital care, and they enable providers to identify critical outcomes and process of care for continuous improvement. As "nursing-sensitive," these consensus standards include measures of processes and outcomes—and structural proxies for

---

[1] Voluntary consensus standards are defined as "common and repeated use of rules, conditions, guidelines or characteristics for products or related processes and production methods and related management systems practices; the definition of terms; materials, performance, designs, or operations; measurement of quality and quantity in describing materials, processes, products, systems, services or practices; test methods and sampling procedures; or descriptions of fit and measurement of size or strength."

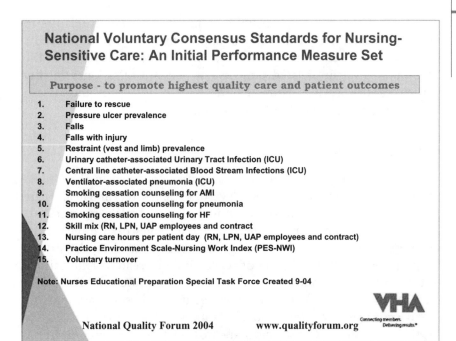

National Voluntary Consensus Standards for Nursing-Sensitive Care: An Initial Performance Measure Set

Purpose - to promote highest quality care and patient outcomes

1. Failure to rescue
2. Pressure ulcer prevalence
3. Falls
4. Falls with injury
5. Restraint (vest and limb) prevalence
6. Urinary catheter-associated Urinary Tract Infection (ICU)
7. Central line catheter-associated Blood Stream Infections (ICU)
8. Ventilator-associated pneumonia (ICU)
9. Smoking cessation counseling for AMI
10. Smoking cessation counseling for pneumonia
11. Smoking cessation counseling for HF
12. Skill mix (RN, LPN, UAP employees and contract
13. Nursing care hours per patient day (RN, LPN, UAP employees and contract)
14. Practice Environment Scale-Nursing Work Index (PES-NWI)
15. Voluntary turnover

Note: Nurses Educational Preparation Special Task Force Created 9-04

VHA
Connecting members.
Delivering results.*

National Quality Forum 2004   www.qualityforum.org

FIGURE N.1   National Quality Forum consensus standards for nursing-sensitive care.

these processes and outcomes (e.g., skill mix, nurse staffing hours)—that are affected, provided, or influenced by nursing personnel, but for which nursing is not exclusively responsible (National Quality Forum, 2006). Funded through a grant by The Robert Wood Johnson Foundation, the final work was published in 2004 in a document known as the first "National Voluntary Consensus Standards for Nursing-Sensitive Care: An Initial Performance Measure Set" (National Quality Forum, 2004).

In addition, a key factor for the Steering Committee responsible for guiding the project was the issue that without a standardized approach for measuring the nursing practice environment and nursing's contribution to patient care delivery, it is impossible to consistently evaluate the extent to which the nursing shortage affects the quality of health care in the United States or to understand how to actually improve nursing performance. Therefore, this standardized set of nursing—sensitive voluntary consensus standards was also developed in order to help address future initiatives in the areas of:

* Quality improvement
* Public accountability and pay for performance initiatives
* Patient safety
* Nursing performance measurement.

During the period 2003 to 2006, so much information relating to nursing measurement had begun to appear that the NQF developed a Web site to serve as a "one-stop" comprehensive resource for all of the NQF nursing quality related projects and measures (National Quality Forum, 2004). Known as "Nursing Care Quality at the NQF," the site can be accessed at http://216.122.138.39/nursing/.

CONCLUSION

THE PRIMARY purpose of measuring care delivered in the United States is to promote the highest level of patient safety and health care outcomes. The NQF nursing project initially focused solely on acute care, but a set of research recommendations and a framework for measuring nursing performance in other settings also was developed. The NQF nursing project has fueled a number of academic and research organizations to further study the practice of nursing in a scientific way. The entire scope of the NQF work relevant to the quality of hospital and nursing care deserves the keen attention of all nursing leaders. For example, the "National Voluntary Consensus Standards for Hospital Care: An Initial Performance Measure Set" (National Quality Forum, 2003) identifies 39 hospital care performance measures that should be publicly reported by all acute care hospitals. The nursing project links to this work, because seven of the endorsed hospital measures, which have quantifiable links to nursing, also have been endorsed as voluntary consensus standards for nursing sensitive care.

The National Quality Forum (NQF) has made a huge impact on the industry since it was incorporated in 1999. In a short period of time, a shared sense of urgency about the impact of health care quality on patient outcomes, workforce productivity, and health care costs have prompted leaders in the public and private sectors to support the NQF as a mechanism to bring about national change. Broad participation from all parts of the health care system (including national, state, regional, and local groups representing consumers, public and private purchasers, employers, health care professionals, provider organizations, health plans, accrediting bodies, labor unions, supporting industries, and organizations involved in health care research or quality improvement) have united in a common cause. Together, they are working to promote a common approach to measuring health care quality and fostering a national, system wide capacity for quality improvement. And importantly, nursing has a visible, credible key role in it all.

LILLEE SMITH GELINAS

See Also
Continuous Quality Improvement

REFERENCES

American Nurses Association. (1999). *Nursing sensitive quality indicators for acute care settings and ANA's safety & quality initiatives.* Retrieved August 18, 2007, from http://www.nursingworld.org/MainMenuCategories/The PracticeofProfessionalNursing/PatientSafetyQuality/NDNQI/Research/QIforAcuteCareSettings.aspx

Gosfield, A. G., & Reinertsen, J. L. (2005). The 100,000 Lives Campaign: Crystallizing standards of care for hospitals. *Health Affairs, 24*(6), 1560–1570.

National Quality Forum. (2003). *National voluntary consensus standards for hospital care: An initial performance measure set.* Retrieved August 24, 2007, from http://216.122.138.39/publications/reports/

National Quality Forum. (2004). *National voluntary consensus standards for nursing sensitive care: An initial performance measure set.* Retrieved August 24, 2007, from http://216.122.138.39/publications/reports/

National Quality Forum. (2006). *National quality forum: Nursing care quality at NQF.* Retrieved August 18, 2006, from http://www.qualityforum.org/nursing/default.htm

National Quality Forum Executive Institute. (2006). *Navigating quality—Current topics: Pay for performance.* Retrieved September 26, 2006, from http://www.nqfexecutiveinstitute.org/currenttopics/pfp.cfm

U.S. Office of Management and Budget, Office of Information and Regulatory Affairs. (1998). *Circular A-119. Revised. Federal participation in the development and use of voluntary consensus standards and in conformity assessment activities.* Retrieved September 4, 2007, from http://www.whitehouse.gov/omb/circulars/a119/a119.html

National Student Nurses' Association

FOUNDED in 1952, the National Student Nurses' Association (NSNA) is a nonprofit organization for students enrolled in associate, baccalaureate, diploma, and generic graduate nursing programs. It is dedicated to fostering the professional development of nursing students. Over the years, hundreds of thousands of nursing students have carried the NSNA membership card as a tangible symbol of their early commitment to the nursing profession. As the only independent organization for nursing students, NSNA:

* Brings together and mentors students preparing for initial licensure as registered nurses, as well as those enrolled in baccalaureate completion programs;
* Conveys the standards and ethics of the nursing profession;
* Promotes development of the skills that students need as responsible and accountable members of the nursing profession;
* Advocates for high quality, evidence-based, affordable and accessible health care;
* Advocates for and contributes to advances in nursing education;
* Develops nursing students who are prepared to lead the profession in the future.

NSNA members participate in community health projects, legislation education, and activities to recruit students into the profession. Special activities include:

* Breakthrough to Nursing Project, designed to increase the number of underrepresented populations into the nursing profession;
* Community health projects offering opportunities to address the health needs of the public;
* Implementation of the Bill of Rights and Responsibilities for Students of Nursing and model Code of Ethics for students to adopt;
* Legislation Education program to encourage involvement in understanding the legislative process, voter registration, and get-out-the-vote activities;
* NSNA Leadership University (http://www.nsnaleadershipu.org) encouraging students to earn academic credit for participating in NSNA's many shared governance and leadership activities;
* Opportunity to build and maintain an electronic, Web-based professional portfolio.

Success in nursing school is an important focus for NSNA. Education programs at the Annual Convention and Annual MidYear Conference cover a wide range of topics that broaden a student's perspective as well as to help them pass the licensure examination and launch a successful nursing career. Approximately 5,000 nursing students attend educational programs and participate in leadership and professional development activities. Faculty who attend NSNA meetings are awarded continuing education credit for several programs designed to enhance their teaching skills.

NSNA is governed by a Board of Directors and House of Delegates. Ten nursing students who are elected to serve for 1 year comprise the Board of Directors. Two consultants appointed by the American Nurses Association and the National League for Nursing provide guidance to the Board (without vote). Four students are also elected to serve on the Nominating and Elections Committee. A House of Delegates meets annually to elect officers and to debate resolutions that focus on issues relevant to nursing education and practice. Delegates come from 700 school and state NSNA chapters. National staff provides administrative support. Scholarships, ranging from $1,000 to $5,000, are offered through the Foundation of the National Student Nurses' Association (FNSNA). In addition to the general scholarship program, the Promise of Nursing Regional Scholarship Program, administered by the FNSNA, provides undergraduate and graduate nursing scholarships, fellowships, and school grants. Funds for Promise of Nursing program are raised by regional events sponsored by Johnson & Johnson.

All NSNA members receive *Imprint* magazine, published five times during the academic year. Other publications include: *NSNA News, NSNA e-News, Dean's Notes,* and several *Guidelines for Planning* booklets. A variety of programs produced by NSNA include DVDs and videos on the following: mentoring; recruitment into the nursing profession; convention keynote address by the U.S. Surgeon General, Dr. Richard Carmona; history of NSNA; history of the American Nurses Association; and NSNA membership recruitment. Membership and involvement in NSNA has grown over time. Nursing students with a desire to share their experiences and passion for nursing and to have a voice in the future of the profession comprise over 45,000 members nationwide. Involvement in leadership activities as a student has inspired many NSNA alumni to become leaders of the nursing profession.

National Student Nurses' Association, Inc.
45 Main Street, Suite 606
Brooklyn, New York 11201
(718) 210-0705
FAX (718) 210-0710
E-mail: nsna@nsna.org
http://www.nsna.org
http://www.nsnaleadershipu.org

DIANE MANCINO

See Also
American Nurses Association
Mentoring
National League for Nursing

Nightingale, Florence

FLORENCE NIGHTINGALE was born of wealthy parents in Florence, Italy, on May 12, 1820. She died in her sleep, blind and infirm, on August 13, 1910, at the age of 90.

Nightingale was a study in contrasts. She has been described as a "... woman of brilliance and contradiction—stubborn and inspiring, witty and impatient, dedicated and meddling...." (Vicinus & Nergaard, 1989). What is for sure, certain, and inarguable is that Nightingale was a force to be reckoned with. She was a staunch hospital reformer and a brilliant statistician, yet was affectionately referred to as "the lady with the lamp."

She was schooled primarily by her father and later, at the age of 32, studied nursing at the Institute of Protestant Deaconesses in Kaiserwerth, Germany. Nightingale's accomplishments during the Crimean war are legend. Her ingenious application of soap, water, and clean bandages reduced the death rate from nearly 50% to 2.5% among the casualties who were dying of disease rather than of war wounds. Nightingale pioneered the use of graphics in statistical analysis; she originated the use of pie graphs and line diagrams to illustrate her points—a tactic that was previously unknown. Nightingale's organizational skills revolutionized hospital environments when she introduced ventilation and sanitation.

Many of her strategies introduced in the Crimea (1854–1856) predated concepts of germ theory, clean and sterile technique, and pasteurization—all introduced in the 1870s (Bellis, 2006), and the introduction of penicillin in 1928 (Singletary, 2000). When she established the *Nightingale Training School for Nurses* in London (1860), the day was declared as the birthday of modern nursing. Fifteen years later (1875), Nightingale founded the *Metropolitan and National Nursing Association* to provide home care, the first of visiting nurse associations the world over (Gillie, 1984). Despite her incapacitation in later years, Nightingale published books and pamphlets, and she wrote more than 10,000 letters—most of which are housed in the Library of the British Museum and the Greater London Record Office (Vicinus & Nergaard, 1989).

M. JANICE NELSON

REFERENCES

Bellis, M. (2006). *Inventors. Louis Pasteur*. Retrieved May 14, 2006, from http://www.inventors.about.com/library/inventors/blpasteur.htm

Dolan, J. A., Fitzpatrick, M. L., & Herrmann, E. K. (1983). *Nursing in society: A historical perspective* (15th ed.). Philadelphia: W. B. Saunders Company.

Gillie, R. B. (1984). *Florence Nightingale's cap: Saga & symbolism*. Unpublished pamphlet, Westerly Hospital, Westerly, RI.

National Archives Learning Curve. (2006). *Florence Nightingale*. Retrieved March 20, 2006, from http://www.spartacus.schoolnet.co.uk/REnightingal.htm

Singletary, M. (2000). *Penicillin. The wonder drug*. Retrieved May 14, 2006, from http://www.web1,caryacademy.org/chemistry/rushin/Student/Projects/CompoundWebSites/2000/

Vicinus, M., & Nergaard, B. (Eds.). (1989). *Ever yours, Florence Nightingale: Selected letters*. London: Billings & Sons, Ltd.

Nurse Residency

R ESIDENCY PROGRAMS, first reported in the literature in the 1980s, are of documented value in the successful transition of the graduate nurse into professional practice (Altier & Krsek, 2006). It has become increasingly more difficult for new graduates in acute care hospitals to transition to the staff nurse role. To meet the needs of hospitalized patients, today's graduates must have the knowledge and skills necessary to care for acutely ill patients presenting with complex needs (Goode & Williams, 2004). A well-designed residency program enables the nurse resident to progress from the comprehension of evidence-based practice to the actual application of learned knowledge and skill in the work setting (Krugman et al., 2006). Various descriptions of nurse residency programs exist in the literature (Goode & Williams, 2004; Rosenfeld, Smith, Iervolino, & Bowar-Ferres, 2004). A residency program is a unique educational opportunity that allows the expansion of skills in a nurturing, supportive environment. Effort is acknowledged, the individual's importance is validated, and positive outcomes result. Collegial relationships established during the program continue to grow after residency completion (Altier & Krsek, 2006). Residency programs generally include extended orientation time, relationship with a mentor, and structured educational/didactic sessions (Goode & Williams, 2004; Herdrich & Lindsay, 2006; Rosenfeld et al., 2004). Nurse residency programs have been acknowledged as a key strategy in the recruitment and retention of graduate nurses (Herdrich & Lindsay, 2006; Joint Commission on Accreditation of Healthcare Organizations, 2002; Nursing Executive Watch, 2002; The Robert Wood Johnson Foundation, 2002).

In 2002, The University HealthSystem Consortium and The American Association of Colleges of Nursing (UHC/AACN) jointly developed The National Post-Baccalaureate Residency Program curriculum. This standardized curriculum is based on a series of learning and practice experiences involving cohort relationships and clinical narratives. Core content is divided into three topic areas: leadership, patient outcomes, and professional role development. Critical thinking and communication threads are woven throughout the yearlong program (Krugman et al., 2006). A unique feature of the UHC/AACN residency model is the partnership between the academic hospital and the paired college of nursing. This collaboration affords an opportunity to share resources, strengthen the relationship between service and academe, and incorporate the cross-fertilization of knowledge between the clinical enterprise and the university (Goode & Williams, 2004). Desired outcomes of this project are the reduction of new graduate turnover, enhanced job satisfaction and autonomy, increased critical thinking skills, increased support for the new graduate, and attainment of the additional competencies needed to function as a staff nurse in a manner that promotes patient safety (Goode & Williams, 2004). Further evaluation of nurse residency programs is needed but evidence is available that supports their impact in increasing nurse retention (Altier & Krsek, 2006; Goode & Williams, 2004; Krugman et al., 2006; Rosenfeld et al., 2004), improving critical thinking skills (Herdrich & Lindsay, 2006), improving organizing and prioritizing abilities, and reducing graduate nurse stress (Krugman et al., 2006).

MARY ANN MCGINLEY

See Also
Accreditation in Nursing Practice
American Association of Colleges of Nursing
Mentoring
Staff Recruitment
Staff Retention

REFERENCES

Altier, M. E., & Krsek, C. A. (2006). Effects of a 1-year residency program on job satisfaction and retention of new graduate nurses. *Journal for Nurses in Staff Development, 22*(2), 70–77.

Goode, C. J., & Williams, C. A. (2004). Post-baccalaureate nurse residency program. *Journal of Nursing Administration, 34*(2), 71–77.

Herdrich, B., & Lindsay, A. (2006). Nurse residency programs: Redesigning the transition into practice. *Journal for Nurses in Staff Development, 22*(2), 55–62.

Joint Commission on Accreditation of Healthcare Organizations. (2002). *Health care at the crossroads: Strategies for addressing the evolving nursing crisis.* White paper. Retrieved from www.jointcommission.org/NR/rdonlyres/ 5C138711-ED76-4D6F-909F-B06E0309F36D/0/health_care_at_the_ crossroads.pdf

Krugman, M., Bretschneider, J., Horn, P. B., Krsek, C. A., Moutafis, R. A., & Smith, M. O. (2006). The national post-baccalaureate graduate nurse residency program: A model for excellence in transition to practice. *Journal for Nurses in Staff Development, 22*(4), 196–205.

Nursing Executive Watch. (2002). *Hospitals exploring nurse residencies to improve retention.* Washington, DC: Healthcare Advisory Board.

Robert Wood Johnson Foundation, The. (2002). *Health care's human crisis: The American nursing shortage.* Princeton, NJ: The Robert Wood Johnson Foundation.

Rosenfeld, P., Smith, M. O., Iervolino, L., & Bowar-Ferres, S. (2004). Nurse residency program: A 5-year evaluation from the participants' perspective. *Journal of Nursing Administration, 34*(4), 188–194.

Nurse Satisfaction in the Professional Practice Environment

OVER THE YEARS, renewed emphasis has been placed on the reorganization and redesign of the professional practice environment of nurses and other health care providers (Champy, 1996). The latest nursing shortage along with the recruitment and retention of nurses, particularly within the acute care environment, has focused increased attention on nurses' practice environments (Lake, 2007). It is essential to create nurse practice environments that foster cost-effective, quality, safe and efficient patient care, and practice settings that cultivate growth, development, professional autonomy, and multidisciplinary collaboration. Today, the consumer as well as the clinician seeks to work/be cared for in a setting that promotes patient/family centered care and supports professional practice. As restructuring of health care environments continues, the evaluation of the patient's satisfaction with care keeps advancing. Equally important is the impact of the work setting for the clinician. The organizational culture that creates the environment in which the care is delivered plays a very important role in impacting clinical practice and patient outcomes (Aiken, Sochalski, & Lake, 1997). Thus, measuring the effectiveness of the professional practice environment continues to be a big challenge.

In the early 1980s, the work of McClure and colleagues (1983) in collecting data to identify successful work environments was initiated in the United States by the American Academy of Nursing's Task Force on Nursing Practice in Hospitals (McClure, Poulin, Sovie, & Wandelt, 2002). Data from this work indicated characteristics such as autonomy, control over practice, and collaborative nurse-physician relationships increased retention, were places where nurses liked to work and were characterized as Magnet Hospitals where staff turnover was low. This research was followed by a series of studies conducted by Kramer (1990) and Kramer and Schmalenberg (1993) that supported the findings from the original Magnet Study. The elements of autonomy, control over practice, and effective communication among nurses and physicians continued to yield a positive work experience and supported a positive work environment for clinicians. Data from the work of Kramer and colleagues resulted in the first multidimensional measure of satisfaction with the professional practice environment. The Nursing Work Index (NWI), developed by Kramer and Hafner (1989), consisted of 65 items designed to measure those organizational elements first identified by the Magnet Hospitals. Nurses were asked to evaluate their level of agreement with items measured on a 4-point Likert scale, indicating what elements were important for them to experience job satisfaction and be able to offer patients high quality care. In 2000, Aiken and Patrician evaluated the NWI and reduced it to 55 items. The NWI-Revised (NWI-R) measured three conceptually derived elements that support an effective professional practice environment: nurse autonomy; control over practice, and relationships with physicians. For both the NWI and NWI-R, specific scoring procedures have been developed.

In 2002, Lake revised the NWI and created the Practice Environment Scale (PES), which contained 45 items from the original 65 items. Through research, she established the psychometric properties of the PES and defined five factors: nurse participation in hospital affairs, nursing foundations for quality care, nurse manager ability, support for nurses, and staffing and resource adequacy. In 1998, the Professional Practice Environment (PPE) scale was developed by a team from the Massachusetts General Hospital (MGH) to expand on the elements included in both the NWI-R and the PES. In addition to measuring the original Magnet constructs, this new instrument addressed the challenges of the current health care environments, including: cultural diversity; responsiveness potential for workplace conflicts emerging in a fast-paced work setting; and motivation of the workforce in the face of limited resources and demands for cost effectiveness. The original PPE scale consisted of 35 items anchored on a 4-point Likert scale that measured eight professional practice environment characteristics, namely: leadership and autonomy over practice; clinician-physician relationships; control over

408

NURSE
SATISFACTION
IN THE
PROFESSIONAL
PRACTICE
ENVIRONMENT

practice; communications about patients; teamwork; conflict management; internal work motivation; and cultural sensitivity. The 35-item PPE scale was used between 1999 and 2001 with satisfactory internal consistency reliability estimates for the subscales (above .75). In 2004, a revised 40-item PPE scale was developed to clarify problem items identified by respondents. The scale was psychometrically evaluated with a sample of 849 respondents from within the professional practice staff (across disciplines) at the MGH. In the data analysis, all items, with two exceptions, met the minimum item-total correlation criterion of .30. The resulting 38-item scale, with a Cronbach's alpha of .93, produced an eight-component solution with Cronbach's alphas ranging from .78 to .88. These results established the instrument as a valid and reliable measure of staff perception of the professional practice work environment (Ives Erickson et al., 2004).

In 2006, MGH staff undertook more editorial revision on the PPE Scale that included making each item a complete declarative statement and adding two items to the Handling Disagreement/Conflict subscale. In addition, the now 40-item scale was developed for use online and called the Revised Professional Practice Environment Scale–Online (RPPE–Online) (Jones, Duffy, Ditomassi, & Ives Erickson, unpublished). The RPPE–Online, distributed electronically to the professional practice staff across the MGH environment, yielded a 61% response rate (n = 1,837). Psychometric evaluation of the RPPE–Online was then undertaken on all nurses in the 2006 sample who had no missing data on the scale (n = 1,550). A random sample cross-validation procedure (Cudeck & Brown, 1983) was used to test whether the eight factors in the calibration sample (n = 775) could also be derived in a second, comparable validation sample (n = 775) drawn from the same population of MGH nurses. The two samples were comparable with no significant differences on demographic characteristics. Sample size for both samples was more than adequate to undertake principal components analyses with each sample having an approximate 20:1 case-to-variable ratio (Comrey, 1988; Tabachnick & Fidell, 2007).

Internal consistency for the 40-item RPPE–Online was .93 for the calibration sample and .92 for the validation sample. Principal components analysis was next undertaken on the calibration and validation samples with the original eight PPE scale components being demonstrated. In the calibration sample, 59.0% of total variance was explained by the eight components; in the validation sample, 59.5% was accounted for by the same eight components. Cronbach's alpha internal consistency reliabilities ranged from .76 to .87 in the calibration sample and from .76 to .88 in the validation sample. In both samples, the same three items were dropped because of low item-total correlations. Thus, findings from this cross-validation psychometric evaluation indicated that the 37-item RPPE-Online is reliable and valid for use in health outcomes research examining eight characteristics of the professional practice environment of RN staff working in acute care settings.

DOROTHY A. JONES
JEANETTE IVES ERICKSON
MARIANNE DITOMASSI

See Also
American Academy of Nursing
Consumer Satisfaction
Magnet Hospitals
Staff Recruitment
Staff Retention

REFERENCES

Aiken, L. H., & Patrician, P. A. (2000). Measuring organizational traits of hospitals. The Revised Nursing Work Index. *Nursing Research, 49*(3), 146–153.

Aiken, L., Sochalski, J., & Lake, E. (1997). Studying outcomes of organizational change in health services. *Medical Care, 35*(11 Suppl), NS6–NS18.

Champy, J. (1996). *Reengineering management: The mandate for new leadership.* New York: HarperBusiness.

Comrey, A. (1988). Factor analytic methods of scale development in personality and clinical psychology. *Journal of Consulting and Clinical Psychology, 56,* 754–761.

Cudeck, R., & Brown, M. (1983). Cross validation of covariance structures. *Multivariate Behavioral Research, 18,* 147–167.

Ives Erickson, J., Duffy, M., Gibbons, P., Fitzmaurice, J., Ditomassi, M., & Jones, D. (2004). Development and psychometric evaluation of the professional practice environment (PPE) scale. *Journal of Nursing Scholarship, 36*(3), 279–284.

Jones, D., Duffy, M., Ditomassi, M., & Ives Erickson, J. M. (unpublished) Development and psychometric evaluation of the Revised Professional Practice Environment Scale – Online Version.

Kramer, M. (1990). The magnet hospitals: Excellence revisited. *Journal of Nursing Administration, 20*(9), 35–44.

Kramer, M., & Hafner, L. P. (1989). Shared values: Impact on staff nurse job satisfaction and perceived productivity. *Nursing Research, 38,* 172–177.

Kramer, M., & Schmalenberg, C. (1993). Learning from success: Autonomy and empowerment. *Nursing Management, 24*(5), 58–64.

Lake, E. (2002). Development of the practice environment scale of the nursing work index. *Research in Nursing & Health, 25,* 176–188.

410

Nurse
Satisfaction
in the
Professional
Practice
Environment

Lake, E. (2007). The nursing practice environment: Measurement and evidence. *Medical Care Research and Review, 64*(2), 104S–122S.

McClure, M., Poulin, M., Sovie, M., & Wandelt, M. (1983). *Magnet hospitals: Attraction and retention of professional nurses.* Kansas City, MO: American Nurses Association.

McClure, M., Poulin, M., Sovie, M., & Wandelt, M. (2002). *Magnet hospitals: Attraction and retention of professional nurses (original study).* In M. McClure & A. Hinshaw (Eds.), *Magnet hospitals revisited: Attraction and retention of professional nurses* (pp. 1–24), Washington, DC: American Nurses Publishing.

Tabachnick, B., & Fidell, L. (2007). *Using multivariate statistics* (5th ed.). Needham, MA: Allyn & Bacon.

Nurses Educational Funds, Inc.

NURSES EDUCATIONAL FUNDS, INC. (NEF) is solely dedicated to providing scholarships for registered nurses to advance their education at the gradate level. Established in 1910, NEF has endowed 14 named scholarships as well as a general scholarship fund. Applicants must be registered nurses enrolled full time in an accredited Master's degree or full- or part-time in a doctoral degree program in nursing or a nursing-related field. Other eligibility requirements include membership in a professional nursing association and U.S. citizenship (or declaration of official intention of becoming a U.S. citizen). The criteria that are given the greatest consideration when selecting candidates include academic excellence and the potential for contributing to the nursing profession. NEF is a not-for-profit organization. Contributions to NEF are tax deductible.

Nurses Educational Funds, Inc.
304 Park Avenue South, 11th Floor
New York, NY 10010
Phone: (212) 590-2443
Fax: (212) 590-2446
Email: info@n-e-f.org
www.n-e-f.org

DIANE MANCINO

411

Nurses Improving Care for Health System Elders (NICHE)

NURSES IMPROVING CARE FOR HEALTH SYSTEM ELDERS (NICHE) is the only national nursing program designed to address the specialized needs of the older adult patient. A program of the John A. Hartford Foundation Institute for Geriatric Nursing at New York University College of Nursing (NYUCN), NICHE was founded by Drs. Terry Fulmer and Mathy Mezey in 1992, and comprises a national network of hospitals and their affiliate health care organizations. The program provides initial and ongoing resources to assist hospitals to develop and strengthen both the individual nurse's geriatric expertise, as well as a hospital's capacity to develop, use, and evaluate best-practice nursing care for older adults (Fulmer et al., 2002).

NICHE hospitals are linked though a listserv, ongoing conferences, and task forces that inform policy and resource development at the Hartford Institute for Geriatric Nursing at NYUCN. The core components of NICHE include self-evaluation tools for the hospital, evidence-based clinical protocols, access to an information sharing listserv, a resource-laden Web site, a geriatric curriculum for nurses, and other educational

413

*Nurses
Improving Care
for Health
System Elders
(NICHE)*

materials. The Geriatric Institutional Assessment Profile (GIAP) is an instrument that helps NICHE-participating hospitals identify organizational attributes of the hospital relevant to geriatric care, including gaps in knowledge about geriatric care, attitudes and perceptions that influence how staff work with older patients, and specific practice issues and concerns (Abraham et al., 2002). Results are benchmarked against other NICHE hospitals and utilized to measure organizational readiness to provide quality care to older adults prior to implementing NICHE (NYU Hartford Institute NICHE Benchmarking Service, 2006). Additionally NICHE provides nursing practice models of care with consultation and guidelines provided for start-up and maintenance of the selected model (Mezey et al., 2004).

Recognizing the contribution of NICHE to improved outcomes for hospitalized older adults, the American Organization of Nurse Executives (AONE) Institute for Patient Care Research and Education collaborated with the Hartford Institute to establish an award for a hospital that embodies best practices in nursing care for older adults. AONE has also spearheaded an initiative to develop guiding principles for an "elder friendly" hospital.

PRACTICE MODELS

NICHE hospitals implement one or more geriatric practice models. The *Geriatric Resource Nurse (GRN) Model* is based on the belief that primary nurses know the most about the daily patterns and needs of the older adults on their units, and is associated with the institutional values of nurse autonomy and professional development (Fulmer, 2001). After receiving specialized education in nursing care of the older adult, the geriatric resource nurse (GRN) receives ongoing mentorship and clinical support from an advance practice nurse. The GRN in turn provides consultation to nurse colleagues at the unit level.

The *ACE unit model* provides a self-contained, specially prepared environment, nurse/geriatrician comanagement, and interdisciplinary collaboration. The program components include interdisciplinary team management, patient-centered nursing care, early discharge planning, and review of medical care for older adult patients (Mezey et al., 2004). ACE units provide elder-friendly furniture, sitting areas, low beds, sensory aids, such as hearing amplifiers, equipment to support ADL performance, and environmental design that is specialized to the needs of older adults (Siegler, Glick, & Lee, 2002).

The *Chicago Syndrome-specific model* focuses on hospital-wide dissemination of a clinical protocol aimed at the prevention, early detection, and management of delirium. An advance practice nurse provides

414

NURSES
IMPROVING
CARE FOR
HEALTH
SYSTEM
ELDERS
(NICHE)

consultation and education to improve nurses' accuracy and efficiency in detecting and managing delirium in hospitalized older adults (NICHE Web site: www.hartfordign.org/programs/niche).

NICHE OUTCOMES

HOSPITALS have reported improved clinical outcomes, enhanced nurse knowledge, increased compliance with protocol application, and decreased length of stay upon implementing the NICHE program (Guthrie, Edinger, & Schumacher, 2002; Lee & Fletcher, 2002; Lopez et al., 2002; Pfaff, 2002; Swauger & Tomlin, 2002). Also, NICHE programs are associated with improved Joint Commission performance and Magnet initiatives. The following key factors are instrumental in successfully implementing NICHE: a clear vision of geriatric care, interdisciplinary collaboration, a process of including staff in relevant decision making, and mechanisms to address staff needs for education, equipment, and other geriatric specific resources (Boltz, 2007). Thus, NICHE requires the commitment of nursing leadership to meet the requirement of ongoing NICHE designation, that is, implementation of a geriatric model and ongoing evaluation of its effectiveness.

MARIE BOLTZ
ELIZABETH CAPEZUTI

See Also
American Organization of Nurse Executives
Evidence-Based Practice

REFERENCES

Abraham, I. L., Bottrell, M. M., Dash, K. R., Fulmer, T., Mezey, M., O'Donnell, L., et al. (2002). Profiling care and benchmarking best practice in care of hospitalized elderly: The Geriatric Institutional Assessment Profile. *Nursing Clinics of North America, 34*(1), 237–255.

Boltz, M. (2007). *Hospital nurses' perceptions of the geriatric care environment.* PhD dissertation, New York University (UMI Number: TBD).

Fulmer, T. (2001). The geriatric resource nurse: A model of caring for older patients. *American Journal of Nursing, 102,* 62.

Fulmer, T., Mezey, M., Bottrell, M., Abraham, I., Sazant, J., Grossman, C., et al. (2002). Nurses Improving Care for Health System Elders (NICHE): Nursing outcomes and benchmarks for evidence-based practice. *Geriatric Nursing, 23*(3), 121–127.

415

*Nurses
Improving Care
for Health
System Elders
(NICHE)*

Guthrie, P. F., Edinger, G., & Schumacher, S. (2002). TWICE: A NICHE program at North Memorial Health Center (CE). *Geriatric Nursing, 23*(2), 133–139.

Lee, V. K., & Fletcher, K. R. (2002). Sustaining the geriatric resource model at the University of Virginia. *Geriatric Nursing, 23*(3), 128–132.

Lopez, M., Delmore, B., Young, K., Golden, P., Bier, J., & Fulmer, Y. (2002). Implementing a geriatric resource model. *Journal of Nursing Administration, 32*(11), 577–585.

Mezey, M., Kobayashi, M., Grossman, S., Firpo, A., Fulmer, T., & Mitty, E. (2004). Nurses Improving Care to Health System Elders: (NICHE): Implementation of best practice models. *Journal of Nursing Administration, 34*(10), 451–457. Retrieved May 1, 2007, from www.hartfordign.org/programs/niche

NYU Hartford Institute NICHE Benchmarking Service. (2006). *NICHE.* Retrieved May 1, 2007, from http://www.hartfordign.org/programs/niche/index.html

Pfaff, J. (2002). The Geriatric Resource Nurse Model: A culture change. *Geriatric Nursing, 23*(3), 140.

Siegler, E. L., Glick, D., & Lee, J. (2002) Optimal staffing for Acute Care of the Elderly (ACE) units. *Geriatric Nursing, 23,* 152.

Swauger, K., & Tomlin, K. (2002). Best care for the elderly at Forsyth Medical Center. *Geriatric Nursing, 23*(3), 145–150.

Nursing Informatics

THE PHRASE NURSING INFORMATICS (NI) brings to mind nurses using computers to access patient information and document care in an electronic health record (EHR); however, NI is far more than nurses using computers. NI focuses on how nurses structure knowledge and organize data to support nursing management, practice, and research. Recognized as a nursing subspecialty in 1992, NI uses information technology and processes to support patient and nurse decision making across the care continuum through the integration of data, information, and knowledge (American Nurses Association [ANA], 2001). NI supports nurse leaders' daily decision making by providing accurate, accessible, usable information and by developing cost-effective systems to enhance patient safety and quality care. NI specialists address federal goals to create a "consumer centric and information rich" health care system with widespread adoption of interoperable EHRs by 2014 (Thompson & Brailer, 2004). NI specialists help clinicians and leaders develop required informatics competencies for today's health care environment. Key areas of interest in NI are defining and representing nursing knowledge to optimize storage, retrieval, and clinical use; developing clinical intervention and management applications across care settings; and discovering new nursing knowledge through analyzing large datasets.

Defining, representing, and storing nursing knowledge: Data alone are meaningless. When combined with other data in an understandable manner, data become information. When placed in a clinical context, data become knowledge that nurse leaders can use to make decisions. The quality of these decisions depends on the initial data standardization and data specificity about nursing phenomena and clear communication to increase data quality. Health information technology (HIT) systems require robust processes for retrieval, storage, presentation, sharing, and use of data. The enormous amount of data generated in the daily processes of care must be coded and stored in ways that can be used by health care practitioners and institutions. Standardized vocabularies translate clinical observations into discrete, unambiguous terms understandable to both people and computers. Nursing has eight standardized vocabularies (e.g., NANDA, Omaha), which describe nursing processes and classify nursing-specific phenomena into recognizable forms. Health care systems use standardized vocabularies (e.g., SNOMED) and need a translator for data communication. Reference terminology models act as translators by mapping terms among standardized languages and provide a framework for combining terms with concepts to create meaningful information (Hardiker, Bakken, & Coenen, 2005). To exchange data, HIT systems must be able to communicate and interpret exchanged messages. System interoperability standards allow communication, while messaging structures (e.g., the HL7 reference information model, http://hl7.org) apply "grammar rules" to information facilitating exchange across multiple software/hardware platforms. Stringent security and privacy protection is vital.

Effective HIT systems support nurse leaders by collecting and analyzing data pertinent to nursing practice, quality, and outcomes. This fosters benchmarking and best practices identification. Financial and administrative databases offer useful information but are not sufficient for nursing decisions. The Nursing Minimal Data Set (NMDS) and Nursing Management Minimal Data Set (NMMDS) identify essential data necessary to characterize nursing practice. The NMDS collects demographic, service, and nursing care data (Werley, Devine, Zorn, Ryan, & Westra, 1991). The NMMDS includes 18 environmental, nursing care, and financial elements (Huber, Schumacher, & Delaney, 1997). At a broader level, ANA's National Database of Nursing Quality Indicators (NDNQI) collects unit-specific nurse-sensitive data from hospitals in the United States; member institutions use the database for benchmarking and quality improvement (ANA, 1999).

Nursing informatics applications: NI specialists integrate knowledge into practice through technology-enhanced practice and patient-centered applications that promote effective health care across the care continuum. The federal HIT Strategic Framework (Thompson & Brailer,

2004) presents a vision of consumer-centered, information-rich, electronically enhanced health care. In this vision, a comprehensive EHR follows the consumer across care settings, offering point-of-care accessibility and decision support to individuals and providers. EHR systems in multiple care settings and consumers' personal health records (PHRs) link across the National Health Information Infrastructure (NHII) through interoperability standards. EHRs support improved health care quality through clear and accessible documentation, diagnostic findings, clinical decision support, and computerized provider order entry (CPOE). Many issues need resolution as the EHR and NHII initiatives progress. Nurse leaders must be actively involved in the process by clearly identifying nursing needs to ensure EHR functionality supports and streamline nurses' work, critical thinking, and communication with health care team members. Active involvement in EHR system selection, deployment, and evaluation enhances stewardship of human and capital resources. Public–private efforts to identify EHR core functionality and to develop vendor product certification based on a minimum set of functionality, interoperability, and security elements provide decision support.

PHRs offer opportunities for engaging consumers in health self-management and active participation in seamless, nongeographically limited care. PHRs are defined as "an Internet based set of tools that allows people to access and coordinate their life-long health information and make appropriate parts of it available to those who need it" (Markle Foundation, 2003). The debate about PHRs centers on issues of core functions and applications, information storage, system complexity and independence, and safeguards governing access, privacy, confidentiality and security of personal health information (Tang, Ash, Bates, Overhage, & Sands, 2006). Hurricane Katrina highlighted the need for interoperable PHR and EHR systems to preserve health information fundamental to coordinated health care disaster response.

Consumer health informatics (CHI) encompasses a variety of applications of computer technology employed to meet lay people's needs for information, self-care, and health service participation, including tailored health information, peer-support groups, communication resources, risk assessment, and monitoring tools and patient portals (Kaplan & Brennan, 2001). CHI initiatives reflect a patient- rather than provider-centered perspective. They may be designed for consumer use alone or in collaboration with health care providers. Nurse leaders can capitalize on CHI applications as outreach methods for provision of seamless care across health care settings.

Knowledge discovery in databases: NI specialists build nursing science through knowledge discovery in databases (KDD), a method of searching large datasets using statistical and machine learning techniques to discover patterns and relationships that may lead to new nursing knowledge (Abbott & Lee, 2005). Data mining procedures identify associations and create predictive models to test the relationships or patterns; nurse experts interpret output that may lead to theory development and knowledge dissemination. The process leverages information in existing massive datasets to form new nursing knowledge relevant to nursing practice, care delivery, outcomes, and health policy.

SUSAN P. KOSSMAN
PATRICIA FLATLEY BRENNAN

REFERENCES

Abbott, P. A., & Lee, S.-M. (2005). Data mining and knowledge discovery. In V. K. Saba & K. A. McCormick (Eds.), *Essentials of nursing informatics* (4th ed., pp. 469–478). New York: McGraw-Hill.

American Nurses Association. (1999). Nursing-sensitive quality indicators for acute care settings and ANA's safety & quality initiative. Retrieved January 20, 2006, from http://www.nursingworld.org/readroom/fssafe99.htm

American Nurses Association. (2001). *Scope and standards of nursing informatics practice*. Washington, DC: American Nurses Publishing.

Hardiker, N. R., Bakken, S., & Coenen, A. (2005). Advanced terminology systems. In V. K. Saba & K. A. McCormick (Eds.), *Essentials of nursing informatics* (4th ed., pp. 279–289). New York: McGraw-Hill.

Huber, D., Schumacher, L., & Delaney, C. (1997). Nursing management minimum data set (NMMDS). *Journal of Nursing Administration, 27*(4), 42–48.

Kaplan, B., & Brennan, P. F. (2001). Consumer informatics supporting patients as co-producers of quality. *Journal of the American Medical Informatics Association, 8*(4), 309–316.

Markle Foundation. (2003). *The personal health working group final report: Connecting for health: A public-private collaborative*. Retrieved March 2, 2006, from http://www.connectingforhealth.org/resources/final_phwg_report1.pdf

Tang, P. C., Ash, J. S., Bates, D. W., Overhage, J. M., & Sands, D. Z. (2006). Personal health records: Definitions, benefits, and strategies for overcoming barriers to adoption. *Journal of the American Medical Informatics Association, 13*(2), 121–126.

Thompson, T. G., & Brailer, D. J. (2004). *The decade of health information technology: Delivering consumer-centric and information-rich health care. Framework for strategic action*. Washington, DC: Office for the National Coordinator for Health Information Technology, U.S. Department of Health and Human Services. Retrieved from http://www.hhs.gov/healthit/documents/hitframework.pdf

Werley, H. H., Devine, E. C., Zorn, C. R., Ryan, P., & Westra, B. L. (1991). The nursing minimum data set: Abstraction tool for standardized, comparable, essential data. *American Journal of Public Health, 81*(4), 421–426.

WEB REFERENCES

American Medical Informatics Association (AMIA), http://www.AMIA.org/
  • AMIA Nursing Informatics working group:
    http://www.amia.org/mbrcenter/wg/ni/
American Nurses Association (ANA) Nursing Practice Information Infrastructure, http://www.nursingworld.org/npii/
  • Nursing-sensitive quality indicators for acute care:
    http://www.nursingworld.org/readroom/fssafe99.htm
Office of the National Coordinator for Health Information Technology, http://www.hhs.gov/healthit/

Nursing Organizations Alliance

T
HE NURSING ORGANIZATIONS ALLIANCE, also known as The Alliance, was created on November 17, 2001, when two organizations elected to merge into one. The prior two organizations were the National Federation for Specialty Nursing Organizations (NFSNO) and the Nursing Organizations Liaison Forum (NOLF). The decision to join forces was based on the desire of the members to provide a more unified and stronger solidarity for nurses (Nursing Organizations Alliance, 2005). Any nursing organization with a strong national focus on current issues related to nursing and health care may become a member of The Alliance. The headquarters of The Alliance is located in Lexington, Kentucky, and in 2006 there were 70 member organizations, including the American Nurses Association, Sigma Theta Tau International, the National League for Nursing, the National Student Nurses Association, and a variety of specialty associations. Every November, a summit is held at a rotating location around the United States. The purpose of the summit is to provide opportunities for networking and sharing of new knowledge across all areas of education, research, advocacy, practice, and profession advancement among the top management of the membership.

The Annual Nursing Alliance Leadership Academy is also offered to present and future board members and leaders and their support staff (Nursing Organizations Alliance, 2006). Additionally, The Alliance offers an annual 4-day Nurse in Washington Internship (NIWI) Program, which teaches nurses or nursing students how to impact health care policy decision making through networking and participating within the legislative structure.

RONDA MINTZ-BINDER

See Also
American Nurses Association
National League for Nursing
National Student Nurses' Association
Sigma Theta Tau International

REFERENCES

Nurses Organizations Alliance. (2005). *About us*. Retrieved July 6, 2006, from http://www.nursing-alliance.org/about.cfm
Nurses Organizations Alliance. (2006). *NALA: 3rd Annual Nursing Alliance Leadership Academy*. Retrieved July 6, 2006, from http://www.amrinc.net/alliance/2006nala.cfm

Nursing Shortage in the United States

N EVERY DECADE since the Medicare and Medicaid programs were established in 1965, the nation has experienced a shortage of registered nurses (RNs). Each of these shortages generally lasted 1 to 2 years before they resolved. From an economic perspective, these shortages were classic "dynamic" shortages: (1) the demand for RNs increased; (2) the supply of RNs remained constant or did not rise to the level to meet demand at the going market rate; (3) eventually, organizations raised wages after trying nonwage strategies to increase supply (e.g., by developing internal float pools, employing nurses from temporary employment agencies and traveling nurses, and importing RNs from other countries); (4) the increase in wages stimulated short- and long-run increases in nurse labor supply (in the short run, existing RNs increased their participation in the labor market by reentering the market if they were not employed, increasing their hours from part- to full-time, working overtime hours, taking on second jobs; and, in the long run, the wage increases stimulated increased enrollment into nursing education programs, thereby increasing the *future* supply of RNs); and (5) the shortage resolved.

The current nursing shortage began in 1998, is now in its 9th year of duration, and is the longest lasting nursing shortage in over half a century. The shortage resulted from the interplay of economic forces but with some notable differences: (1) the current shortage has lasted four times longer than its predecessors—it is static versus dynamic in the classical economic sense; (2) its impact is more apparent as a growing number of studies have established that patients cared for in low-staffed hospitals are at increased risk of in-hospital complications, including mortality (Aiken, Clarke, Sloane, Sochalski, & Silber, 2002; Needleman & Buerhaus, 2003); and (3) the shortage has a significant demographic component reflected by a decreasing number of younger age RNs (under 35 years) and strong growth of RNs in the workforce over the age of 50 (Buerhaus, Staiger & Auerbach, 2000, 2004).

As of 2006, the current shortage has been addressed largely by the private sector: hospitals raised wages; organizations have made significant efforts to improve noneconomic factors (working conditions); schools of nursing, hospitals, and other health care organizations have formed partnerships aimed at increasing the supply of RNs; the importation of foreign-born RNs rose to the highest known levels in decades; and corporations such as Johnson & Johnson, CIGNA, and others have developed national campaigns to resolve the shortage. On the public sector side, many states have developed commissions, implemented initiatives to help hospitals and nursing education programs, and some states have passed significant appropriations. At the congressional level, there has been very little if any material response.

Looking ahead, what can we expect in the future? The large baby boom cohorts (born 1945–1965) entered nursing in the 1970s and early 1980s at a time when there were few career options available to women; hence, the bulk of the current RN workforce is composed of baby-boom RNs who are now in their 40s and 50s. After the baby-boom generation, the size of cohorts born in the 1970s and 1980s was smaller, and when individuals born in these cohorts graduated from high school, there were more career opportunities available for women; hence, the propensity of young women entering nursing programs decreased significantly from the mid-1980s forward. Because the size of cohorts was also much smaller than those of the baby-boom generation, the result was a drop-off in enrollments in nursing education program in the mid 1990s, a 20-year decline in percentage of RNs in the workforce under the age of 35, a substantial increase in the average age of the RN workforce, and a 15% annual growth in the number of RNs over 50 in the workforce from 2001 to 2004. The implications of these trends are that the RN workforce is getting older, will eventually shrink in size as baby-boom RNs retire during the next decade, and, because we have thus far been unable to replace these aging RNs with a younger workforce, shortages of RNs ranging from 400,000 to 800,000 are projected to develop in the next decade.

PETER I. BUERHAUS

REFERENCES

Aiken, L. H., Clarke, S. P., Sloane, D. M., Sochalski, J., & Silber, J. H. (2002). Hospital nurse staffing and patient mortality, nurse burnout, and job dissatisfaction. *The Journal of the American Medical Association, 288*, 1987–1993.

Auerbach, D., Buerhaus, P., & Staiger, D. (2000). Associate degree graduates and the rapidly aging registered nurse workforce. *Nursing Economic$, 18*(4), 178–184.

Buerhaus, P., Donelan, K., Norman, L., & Dittus, R. (2005). Nursing students' perceptions of a career in nursing and impact of a national campaign designed to attract people into the nursing profession. *Journal of Professional Nursing, 21*(2), 75–83.

Buerhaus, P., Donelan, K., Ulrich, B., Norman, L., & Dittus, R. (2005). Is the shortage of hospital registered nurses getting better or worse? Findings from two recent national surveys of RNs. *Nursing Economic$, 23*(2), 61–72.

Buerhaus, P., Needleman, J., Mattke, S., & Stewart, M. (2002). Strengthening hospital nursing, *Health Affairs, 21*(5), 123–132.

Buerhaus, P., Staiger, D., & Auerbach, D. (2000). Implications of a rapidly aging registered nurse workforce. *Journal of the American Medical Association, 283*, 2948–2954.

Buerhaus, P., Staiger, D., & Auerbach, D. (2003). Is the current shortage of hospital nurses ending? Emerging trends in employment and earnings of registered nurses. *Health Affairs, 22*(6), 191–198.

Buerhaus, P., Staiger, D., & Auerbach, D. (2004). New signs of a strengthening nurse labor market? *Health Affairs Web Exclusive*, W4-526–W4-533. Retrieved August 24, 2007, from http://www.medscape.com/viewarticle/556417_4

Needleman, J., & Buerhaus, P. (2003). Nurse staffing and patient safety: Current knowledge and implications for action. *International Journal of Quality Health Care, 15*(4), 275–277.

Needleman, J., Buerhaus, P., Mattke, S., Stewart, M., & Zelevinsky, K. (2002). Nurse staffing and quality of care in hospitals in the United States. *New England Journal of Medicine, 346*(22), 1715–1722.

Norman, L., Buerhaus, P., Donelan, K., McCloskey, K., & Dittus, R. (2005). Nursing students' assess nursing education. *Journal Professional Nursing, 21*(3), 150–158.

Staiger, D., Auerbach, D., & Buerhaus, P. (2000). Expanding career opportunities for women and the declining interest in nursing as a career. *Nursing Economic$, 8*(5), 230–236.

Nutting, M. Adelaide

MARY **ADELAIDE NUTTING** was born in Quebec, Canada, on November 1, 1858. She died in New York City in 1948. Nutting graduated from the Johns Hopkins Hospital Training School for Nurses (1889–1891). Within 2 years of graduation, Nutting became the assistant Superintendent of Nurses and Principal of the Training School. She held the position of Superintendent of Nurses until 1907 when she was persuaded by Dean James Earl Russell to assume charge of the course in Hospital Economics at Teachers College (TC), Columbia University (Christy, 1969b). Nutting was the director of the first university-connected department of nursing, and the first nurse ever to be appointed to a professorship in a university (Christy, 1969b). Eventually, the nursing program at TC became a hub for international nursing education. Nutting laid the foundation for graduate education in nursing when she insisted that only those nurses with a high school diploma who had completed a 2- or 3-year nurses training program would be eligible for admission to nursing courses at TC. Additionally, Nutting laid the groundwork to create an accelerated nursing curriculum for college graduates. Through her work with the American Society of Superintendents of Training Schools for Nurses (later to become the National

League for Nursing Education), Nutting worked ardently to establish a universal standardized nursing curriculum. Nutting also was influential in securing funding from the Rockefeller Foundation to conduct a national survey on nursing education, later published in 1923 as the *Goldmark Report*. Although this report did not enjoy the same impact as the 1910 *Flexner Report for Medicine*, it did pave the way to establish a Rockefeller-endowed experiment in university education for nurses at Yale University. When Nutting died, it was commonly thought that she was second only to Nightingale in standardizing nursing education and in advancing the profession (Christy, 1969a). Nutting was posthumously inducted into the American Nurses Association Hall of Fame in 1976. Further information about Nutting can be accessed on the Web at www.teacherscollege.edu/nursing/history.

M. JANICE NELSON

See Also
ANA Hall of Fame
National League for Nursing

REFERENCES

Christy, T. E. (1969a). *Cornerstone for nursing education: A history of the division of nursing education of Teachers College, Columbia University, 1899–1947.* New York: Teachers College Press.

Christy, T. E. (1969b). Portrait of a leader: M. Adelaide Nutting. *Nursing Outlook, 7,* 71–75.

O

Orientation and Staff Development: The Way We Learn

REDEFINING ORIENTATION and staff development to promote professional development and create a meaningful path for nursing practice to excel in the 21st century of health care is critical to the profession's contribution to discipline specific education. The academic model of Orientation and Staff Development has shifted in the workplace just as the health care industry has changed dramatically in the 21st century. The term "in-service" has become an outdated approach to postgraduate learning for nurses. Mindful learning best captures the transition from the "stage" of learning from the classroom to the bedside. Nurse educators need to focus their clinical teaching to the process of clinical reasoning as opposed to limited to the tasks of learning sequential and isolated knowledge and skills in a linear manner, as in a classroom. Case-based learning combines the knowledge and skills with the practice of nursing and the patient's story—wherever that may be. Most nurses have grown up with a traditional learning model that is teaching-centric. Today—a learning centric model is critical. According to Benner (1984) nurses move along the developmental framework from novice to competent and finally to proficient and to expert. This process is the way nurses grow professionally, and they learn by talking about their experiences, what Benner refers to as "the patient story." This is accomplished educationally by having educators and nurses engage in a discussion rather than sitting passively listening to a lecture.

Orientation can accomplish this aspect of learning through the acknowledgment of one's experience and developing levels of orientation to meet individual needs. For example, using Benner's model as an academic framework for orientation, new graduates can be supported through more teaching and coaching while experienced nurses are assessed for their competency. Meeting together in a group learning environment interspersed within the orientation framework can provide rich and diverse learning exercises when time is allotted for facilitation about patient cases and dialogue about application of new skills and knowledge. Meaningful connections can be made with this teaching methodology, and collaboration in setting priorities and developing a plan of care can be initiated. There is no longer a "right" or "wrong," but rather a respect for responses and answers and the recognition of strengths of the learners.

Team teaching is another valuable asset to any academic exercise in the workplace because it allows for real time interdisciplinary collaboration and role-modeling of how an effective health care team works. Furthermore, staff development should take on the aspect of rounding and bedside teaching. Nurses must move beyond the collection of data and move to the development of clinical reasoning abilities. According to Benner, astute clinical judgment and expert caring practices are more important than ever for quality health care outcomes. Clinical reasoning gives nurses the ability to make a difference in their roles. Nurses who feel influential can look at the outcomes for their patients. This view goes beyond the practice of nursing to completing tasks but thinking with the end in mind. According to Pesut and Herman (1999), education in the workplace must focus on getting nurses to helicopter above the forest and look down at it, rather than through it. When nurses can effectively do this, they can develop a reflective and creative approach to patient care. Consequently, staff development today has to move beyond the pre-test, lecture/workshop/post-test techniques and complement with probing questions such as: "Tell me about your plan"; "What is the outcome you are looking for"; in addition to "What are you doing now for this patient." Framing situations, according to Pesut and Herman, also guides perceptions and behaviors, not just develops tasks and skills. Education in the workplace can be very instrumental in promoting these higher levels of practice

MARIA L. VEZINA

REFERENCES

Benner, P. (1984). *From novice to expert: Excellence and power in clinical nursing practice*. Menlo Park, CA: Addison Wesley Publishing.

Enhancing nursing excellence in a time of change and cost-containment: Benner Associates Brochure Statement. (n.d.). Retrieved July 9, 2006, from http://home.earthlink.net/~bennerassoc/brochure.html

Haag-Heitman, B. (1999). *The clinical practice development using novice to expert theory*. Baltimore, MD: Aspen Publishers.

Kelly-Thomas, K. (1998). *Clinical and nursing staff development: Current competence, future focus* (2nd ed.). Philadelphia: Lippincott.

Pesut, D., & Herman, J. (1999). *Clinical reasoning: The art and science of critical and creative thinking*. Albany, NY: Delmar Publishers.

Outcomes Management

OUTCOMES MANAGEMENT (OM) is the enhancement of physiologic, psychological or socioeconomical results through implementation of exemplary health practices and services driven by ongoing quantitative performance analyses (Wojner, 2001). The term Outcomes Management was first coined by Ellwood (1988), and defined as a "technology of patient experience designed to help patients, payers, and providers make rational medical care-related choices based on better insight into the effect of these choices on patient life." Ellwood suggested four essential principles for inclusion in an OM program:

1. An emphasis on standards that providers can use to select appropriate interventions;
2. The measurement of patient functional status and well-being, along with disease-specific clinical outcomes;
3. Pooling of outcome data on a massive scale; and
4. Analysis and dissemination of the database to appropriate decision makers.

Ellwood's theoretical vision of OM extends from earlier work proposed first by Codman in 1917, and later by Donabedian (1976). Codman pioneered the concept of OM by advocating for the measurement and publication of what he called physiologic and psychosocial "end-results," as well as determination of the cause of all untoward outcomes. He radically suggested that hospitals use this information to improve the practice of their medical staff. Ironically, Codman's "End-Result Idea" was scoffed by his peers, who viewed measurement and possible public knowledge of health outcomes as detrimental to the advancement of medical practice. In fact, he was labeled as an eccentric for recommending publicly that hospitals should know their results, compare their results with those of other hospitals, promote medical staff on the basis of their results, and commit to continuous improvement (Wojner, 2001).

In 1976, Donabedian proposed measurement and evaluation of the quality of health care services at three levels: structure, process, and outcome. Donabedian further proposed that foundational contributors such as manpower, technology, and other resources (structure), methods used to provide or access health care services (processes), as well as proximal and distal results (outcomes) must be assessed in a systematic manner given their interrelatedness, to provide an understanding of quality and opportunities for improvement. Interestingly, despite Donabedian's well-crafted definitions and widespread adoption of his quality framework, it was not until Ellwood's vision for OM emerged that measurement of outcomes became apparent within most health care settings (Wojner, 2001). Even today, process measurement is common among health care providers, whereas outcomes measurement remains somewhat evasive, and many providers still are unable to differentiate processes from outcomes.

In 1997, Wojner published an OM Model that applied Ellwood's work to clinical measurement and management of patient outcomes. The model provided guidance to clinical application of OM techniques using a four-phase approach:

1. Phase One: Establishment of outcome targets; development of definitions and measurement systems; and capture of baseline performance.
2. Phase Two: Comparison of baseline performance to results achieved from implementation of evidence-based structures/processes through review of related literature, networking, and dialogue with experts in the field; negotiation with practice stakeholders for adoption of best practices; and, construction of structured care methods (SCMs) (e.g., pathways, algorithms, protocols, order sets) that

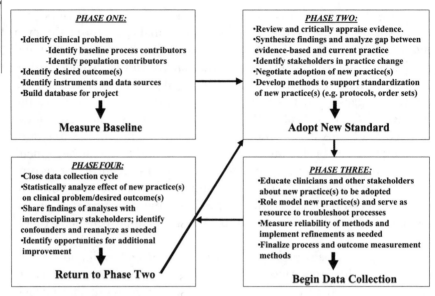

FIGURE O.1   Outcomes Management Model.

standardize interdisciplinary care according to adopted evidence-based practices (EBPs).

3. Phase Three: Implementation of SCMs and practice change(s), including role modeling new practices and educating interdisciplinary team members, measurement of performance reliability, and collection of structure, process, and outcome data.

4. Phase Four: Analysis of post-test data to determine if outcome target(s) have been achieved; widespread dissemination of results among interdisciplinary stakeholders and dialogue about additional opportunities for improvement; and return to Phase Two as needed to identify further methods that may impact outcomes positively.

The OM Model uniquely illustrates a cyclical approach to measurement and methodical management strategies based on Ellwood's (1988) work. A guiding premise for the OM Model is the need to fully define at the start the goals/outcome targets that are desired, with emphasis on the need to capture and understand baseline performance contributors to substandard results before initiating changes in clinical practice. Additionally, the model places an emphasis on the need to review the published literature for evidence of what was previously referred to as "best practices" but currently are referred to as evidence-based practices (EBPs). Figure O.1 illustrates an updated version of the OM Model using EBP terminology.

Today, many health care settings are embarking on a journey of implementing EBPs to support outcomes enhancement. It is important that this work be guided by a methodical approach to measurement of the impact of EBP on system, provider, and patient outcomes. Similar to the approach used when critical pathways came on the scene in health care in the early 1990s, many institutions are immediately climbing aboard the EBP bandwagon without establishing a clear understanding of baseline opportunities for improvement against which they can measure impact. OM provides a mechanism that in concert with EBP enables quantification of the effect of implementing evidence in practice. Using a wide lens for analyses of outcomes, providers that blend OM with EBP are capable of measuring a variety of results including: reduction in complications and case severity; improved perception of the care experience, functional status, post-illness return to productivity, quality of life and resource utilization; staff retention, workload and satisfaction with the work environment; and cost and length of stay.

OM is not an easy process to establish, but its rewards are vast. It requires administrative and clinical support personnel with a background in research methods and statistics, an engaged interdisciplinary team, and technology to capture, manipulate, and analyze variables of interest. Many automated health care systems can be integrated in the process to reduce the workload associated with widespread OM, from electronic medical record systems to accounting and billing systems. Last, experience with the OM process is the best teacher of its widespread application. Experimentation with implementation should be encouraged, lessons learned from the process, and continual refinements made to ensure optimal OM.

ANNE W. WOJNER-ALEXANDROV

See Also
Consumer Satisfaction
Evidence-Based Practice
Staff Retention

REFERENCES

Codman, E. A. (1917). The value of case records in hospitals. *Modern Hospitals, 9,* 426–428.

Donabedian, A. (1976). Measuring and evaluating hospital and medical care. *Bulletin of New York Academic Medicine, 52*(1), 51–59.

Ellwood, P. M. (1988). Outcomes management: A technology of patient experience. *New England Journal of Medicine, 318,* 1549–1556.

Wojner, A. W. (1997). Outcomes management: From theory to practice. *Critical Care Nursing Quarterly, 19*(4), 1–15.

Wojner, A. W. (2001). *Outcomes management: Application to clinical practice.* St. Louis, MO: Mosby.

P

Palmer, Sophia

SOPHIA FRENCH PALMER was born in 1853 in Milton, Massachusetts, and died in 1920. Palmer graduated from the Boston Training School for Nurses and spent a period of time in private duty nursing before returning to New Bedford, Massachusetts, as Nursing Superintendent at St. Luke's Hospital, where she also established a school of nursing. Early in her career, Palmer was charge nurse at Massachusetts General Hospital, Superintendent of Nurses at Garfield General Hospital in Washington, DC, where she again established a training school, and later was Superintendent of Nurses at Rochester (NY) General Hospital. Sophia Palmer was one of the early nursing leaders involved in establishing the Associated Alumnae of United States & Canada (later to be renamed the American Nurses Association), and the Society for Superintendents of Training Schools for Nurses (later to become the National League for Nursing Education). Her greatest achievements, however, involved her influence in the establishment of the New York State Nurses Association (NYSNA) and the Genesee Valley Nurses Association in Rochester, New York. Palmer also expended great effort to obtain legislation requiring licensure for nurses. Palmer was the first president of the New York Board of Examiners. She was the first editor of the *American*

Journal of Nursing, a position that she held until her death. More information about Sophia Palmer can be obtained by accessing the following Web site: http://viahealth.org/body_rochester.cfm?id=516.

M. JANICE NELSON

See Also
American Nurses Association
National League for Nursing

REFERENCES

American Nurses Association. (2006). *Sophia French Palmer (1853–1920). 1976 inductee*. Retrieved August 31, 2007, from http://www.nursingworld.org/FunctionalMenuCategories/AboutANA/WhereWeComeFrom_1/HallofFame/19761982/palmsf5561.aspx

Pavri, J. M. (2000). *Honoring our past: Building our future, a history of the New York State Nurses Association, NYSNA*. Franklin, VA: Q Publishing.

Rochester General Hospital. (n.d.). *Sophia French Palmer*. Retrieved March 29, 2006, from http://www.viahealth.org/body_rochester.cfm?id=642

Santa Fe Community College. (n.d.). *Nursing leaders: Sophia Palmer*. Retrieved March 29, 2006, from http://inst.sfcc.edu/~health/nursing/Nursing_old/old%20stuff/Leaders.htm

Patient Care Delivery Models

IT COULD BE STATED without argument that the first nursing care delivery model was initiated by Florence Nightingale (c. 1859) during the Crimean War. It was Nightingale who differentiated between the "head" nurse (she who did the thinking, planning, and directing of patient care), and the "floor" nurse, who in essence was the provider of that care (Nightingale, 1859). Thus was born a hierarchical model for the delivery of patient care that prevailed for nearly a century in English and American health care facilities.

In the early years following the turn of the 20th century, professional nursing was dominated by private-duty nurses who were employed through a "registry." These nurses cared for a single patient in the home or in the hospital (before the introduction of intensive care units). Oftentimes, the director of the nursing school also was the director of nursing in the hospital; nursing "pupils" provided the care of patients "on the wards," and nursing faculty provided the supervision of these students in their clinical rotations. Graduate nurses were not usually hired in hospitals until after the stock market crash of 1929, when families could no longer afford private duty nurses. It was then that hospitals began to staff the wards with graduate nurses (new graduates not yet licensed) utilizing the original Nightingale hierarchical model.

Although by the mid-20th century, registered nurses (RNs) were still primarily hospital diploma graduates, the influence of those with college degrees slowly became evident. The nurse as college graduate was much more inclined to seek out opportunities, which would grant greater autonomy and control over clinical practice and greater opportunities for clinical decision making. Thus, the professional freedom offered by community health agencies, that is, district nursing, whereby the professional nurse was responsible for clients within a specified regional locality or district, was an attraction to the collegiate nursing population. The nurse was responsible for client assessment and for appropriate delegation of client-oriented tasks to nonlicensed personnel. College graduates were attracted to this model because it fit with the values of freedom and autonomy promulgated within the academic classroom.

In an effort to recruit and retain professional nurses, little by little, models such as *team* and *primary* nursing, as well as *all RN staffs* began to evolve in health care settings, as did *clinical ladders* and *advanced practice roles* such as the clinical nurse specialist and the nurse practitioner— which had an impact on the effective delivery of clinical nursing services, regardless of the setting. These models were popular in the second half of the 20th century.

Team Nursing is undoubtedly one of the earliest models designed to replace the hierarchical structure of the Nightingale model. Within this context, each team is comprised of a mix of RNs, licensed practical nurses (LPNs), and certified nursing assistants (aides) responsible for a single group of patients. The number of teams on a given patient unit is obviously determined by the size of the unit. The onset of the *advanced practice nurse*, such as the *clinical nurse specialist* and/or the *nurse practitioner*, has had a major impact on professional practice in the organizational setting, while giving new meaning to the concept of team nursing. Although the nurse practitioner is generally thought of as providing primary care to a group of clients outside the hospital setting, many are employed within hospital-operated ambulatory care setting, or within the hospital itself, many times providing the initial physical assessments of patients required by regulating agencies such as the State Health Department and the Centers for Medicare and Medicaid Services (CMS). Primarily prepared at the Master's level, these nurses in advanced practice roles serve as consultants to the nursing staff; they fill roles such as staff educator, researcher, administrator/manager, and, in many instances, as master clinician.

Primary nursing in its truest form assigns a "caseload" to the professional nurse, who is then responsible for each of his or her patients "around the clock," as it were. It is the responsibility of the primary nurse to make clinical rounds and to prescribe appropriate nursing interventions depending on client diagnosis. In the case of a hospital admission, the primary nurse maintains responsibility for the client(s) from admission to discharge; in a community health or long-term care, or home care setting, it is possible that the primary nurse maintains responsibility for the client over an extended period of time.

Like most of these other professional practice models, the *clinical ladder* concept was initiated as a retention mechanism for registered nurses. The concept was intended to provide an avenue for clinical advancement within the organization by way of achieving certain preset criteria intended for each level of performance. Each advanced step denotes a new level of clinical expertise and therefore also carries additional financial reimbursement.

An *all RN staff* is expensive but self-explanatory. Within this model, professional nurses provide all dimensions of direct patient care whereas ancillary personnel are responsible for those tasks not involved in direct patient care. With the tightening of fiscal belts, cutbacks in Medicare and Medicaid reimbursement, organizational mergers, changes in organizational philosophy, and the like, except for limited instances one might conclude that the all RN staff has largely become a phenomenon of the past. Medicare regulations, in particular, however, mandate that clients in home care and in hospice are continuously assessed by registered nurses, thus limiting the use of ancillary nursing personnel in these circumstances (Kaiser Family Foundation, 2005).

M. JANICE NELSON

See Also
Advanced Practice Registered Nurses
Clinical Ladder
Florence Nightingale

REFERENCES

Bocchino, C. A. (1991). An interview with Joyce C. Clifford. *Nursing Economic$, 9*(1), 7–17.

Forchuk, C., Mound, B., & Yamashita, M. (2005). Nurse case management: Negotiating care together with a developing relationship. *Perspectives in Psychiatric Care, 41*(2), 62.

Hall, L. E. (1969). The Loeb Center for Nursing and Rehabilitation. *International Journal of Nursing Studies, 6,* 81–95.

Kaiser Family Foundation. (2005). *Navigating Medicare and Medicaid.* Retrieved March 27, 2007, from http://www.kff.org/medicare/7240.cfm

Nightingale, F. (1859). *Notes on nursing: What it is, and what it is not.* Philadelphia: J. B. Lippincott Company.

Patient Classification
Systems

PATIENT CLASSIFICATION SYSTEMS or taxonomies (PCS) date back to the 1960s in the United States and were developed as *workload management* or *patient acuity* tools for staffing. Contemporaneously, PCS are required for Medicare reimbursement and accreditation by the Joint Commission on Accreditation of Health Care Organizations. These tools are used to determine the number and mix of staff needed to care for a group of patients, medical diagnosis, medical billing, and epidemiological study. Types of Patient Classification Systems are the *critical indicator,* also referred to as a prototype evaluation, and *summative* types, also referred to as a factor evaluation (Seago, 2002; Yoder-Wise, 2007). A critical indicator type categorizes patient activities using general factors of patient care activities, such as hygienic care, positioning, feeding, and medication administration. A relative intensity measure (RIM) is one example based upon the patient's diagnosis related group (DRG). A summative type uses nursing care time per activity, for example, amount of time for teaching. The Nursing Intervention Classification (NIC) system is a factor system. These systems may help leaders determine staffing mix on a daily basis; however, they are not a panacea. Reliability and validity issues related to nurses' self-reporting and legal issues related to inability to meet predicated staffing levels determined by the measures have caused some organizations to use other mechanisms to determine staffing needs. Other examples are the Physician's Current Procedural Terminology (CPT), the International Classification of Disease, Ninth Edition (ICD-9), and the Diagnostic and Statistical Manual of Mental Disorders (DSM-IV). Some of these taxonomies, such as the DSM-IV, can be stored on PDA's (personal digital assistants) for easy and accessible use for clinicians and students.

MARTHA J. GREENBERG

See Also
Accreditation in Nursing Practice

REFERENCES

Marquis, B. L., & Huston, C. J. (2006). *Leadership roles and management functions in nursing: Theory and application* (5th ed.). Philadelphia: Lippincott Williams & Wilkins.

Seago, J. (2002). A comparison of two patient classification instruments in an acute care hospital. *Journal of Nursing Administration, 32*(5), 243–249.

Yoder-Wise, P. S. (2007). *Leading and managing in nursing* (4th ed.). St. Louis, MO: Mosby/Elsevier.

Young, K. M. (2000). *Informatics for healthcare professionals*. Philadelphia: F. A. Davis.

Patient Safety

CCORDING TO THE INSTITUTE OF MEDICINE (IOM; 2000), tens of thousands of Americans die each year from errors in medical care and hundreds of thousands are injured, or almost injured, during their care. In *Crossing the Quality Chasm: A New Health System for the 21st Century* (IOM, 2001), the IOM identified six dimensions in which health care systems were failing and where major gains would lead to improvement. According to the IOM, health care should be safe, effective, patient-centered, timely, efficient, and equitable. Although health care organizations have a long history of devoting resources to measuring contributing factors and outcomes related to quality of care, the IOM reports served as a wakeup call that more was needed to prevent harm to patients, and improve quality.

LOOKING TO OTHER INDUSTRIES FOR SOLUTIONS

AN IMPORTANT and paradigm-changing reaction to the IOM reports was the search for solutions from industries other than health care for effective approaches to improving and sustaining safety.

Patient safety health care leaders (e.g., Leape et al., 2000) called for adoption of strategies used by other industries, such as the airline industry, to prevent high stakes failures and reduce the harm surrounding error. As a result of turning to expert resources outside health care, a major change in thinking occurred as to why errors happen, the role of the individual in error generation, and the roles that health care providers and leaders play in increasing and sustaining patient safety.

Health care leaders learned that to make sustainable improvements in patient safety, their focus had to switch from individual health care providers and workers to the complex systems in which they work and to the complexity as well as limitations within individuals themselves. The new focus for understanding error turned from the traditional approach to patient safety that demanded perfect individual performance in imperfect situations, to understanding the imperfect situations in which imperfect performers work. Reason's (1990) framework explained that the usual route to failure, or error, is the contribution of multiple latent failures and gaps across multiple systems in an organization. Thus, although an individual makes a decision that may result in death, harm, or near harm to a patient, the complexity surrounding the event is what leads the individual to thinking it was the right decision given the circumstances (Cook & Woods, 1994).

A CHANGE IN ORGANIZATIONAL CULTURE REGARDING ERROR

T HE SWITCH of health care to a focus on systems that contribute to error and away from the individual continues to be a challenge. Changing from a traditional health care culture of blaming individuals to a culture of nonblame surrounding error has been difficult at best. The tendency for those not associated with an error event to simplify the event after the fact, called hindsight bias, is a formidable hindrance in the search for details that explain how flawed systems are involved. And yet learning about the details of a situation and how systems as well as human factors contribute to error will provide the knowledge necessary to make improvements in and sustain patient safety.

The traditional accountability for health care providers involved performing perfectly without error. The expectation in this new approach to patient safety is for health care providers to be open about their own errors and near misses, and to share and discuss the stories that surround error events. Furthermore, the new accountability is that providers be open about the system barriers that make it difficult to provide safe care, speak up about those barriers, and participate in planning to reduce or eliminate them.

Likewise, the new expectation for health care leaders is to facilitate a culture in which providers feel free to speak up about their errors and the barriers to providing safe and quality care. Rather than the weakest link in an otherwise unrealistic fail-proof system, this new approach positions the health care provider as the resilient component in the health care environment for learning about, making improvements in, and rescuing within the systems in which care is delivered.

TOWARD A SAFER HEALTH CARE DELIVERY SYSTEM

A LTHOUGH ongoing efforts to change the culture surrounding error continue in health care across the Unites States, many other strategies have been developed to improve the safety of care. Design and production of equipment and information technology to support provider work and overcome human limitations has become a major industry as health care organizations search for effective interventions. As new products are implemented, leaders are learning the challenges related to implementing and sustaining any change in a complex system. Seemingly perfect solutions can cause unexpected changes that result in a more complicated environment and thus a higher risk for error.

And, yet, some approaches have galvanized health care providers and educators across the nation in organized efforts that show promise. Berwick's leadership of the Institute for Healthcare Improvement (IHI Web site: http://www.ihi.org/ihi) has resulted in national patient safety improvement efforts to develop best-demonstrated practices in care delivery and adoption of care practices toward saving lives in health care. A new focus for research on understanding the actual work of health care providers and decision making in health care environments is increasing and will contribute to a knowledge base for redesign of health care environments for safe practice and health care provider education (Ebright, Patterson, Chalko, & Render, 2003; Potter et al., 2005). The National Patient Safety Foundation (NPSF Web site: http://www.npsf.org/) and the Agency for Healthcare Research and Quality (AHRQ Web site: http://ahrq.gov/) fund research on patient safety and potential interventions for reaching patient safety outcomes.

Health care leaders are beginning to realize the enormous challenges to achieving major and sustainable improvements in patient safety (Leape & Berwick, 2005). Strategies that incorporate culture change, new mechanisms for reporting and investigation of error and near-miss events, human factors limitations in design of environments, and new patient safety accountabilities for direct care providers and leaders are being used to address these challenges (IOM, 2004; Morath & Turnbull, 2005).

PATRICIA R. EBRIGHT

See Also
Agency for Healthcare Research and Quality
Institute for Healthcare Improvement

REFERENCES

Cook, R. I., & Woods, D. D. (1994). Operating at the "sharp end": The complexity of human error. In M. S. Bogner (Ed.), *Human error in medicine* (pp. 255–310). Hillsdale, NJ: Lawrence Erlbaum.

Ebright, P., Patterson, E., Chalko, B., & Render, M. (2003). Understanding the complexity of registered nurse work in acute care settings. *Journal of Nursing Administration, 33*(12), 630–638.

Institute of Medicine. (2000). *To err is human: Building a safer health system.* Washington, DC: National Academies Press.

Institute of Medicine, Committee on Quality of Healthcare in America. (2001). *Crossing the quality chasm: A new health system for the 21st century.* Washington, DC: National Academies Press.

Institute of Medicine. (2004). *Keeping patients safe: Transforming the work environment of nurses.* Washington, DC: National Academies Press.

Leape, L. L., & Berwick, D. M. (2005). Five years after "To err is human." *Journal of the American Medical Association, 293*(19), 2384–2390.

Leape, L. L., Kabcenell, A. I., Gandhi, T. K., Carver, P., Nolan, T. W., & Berwick, D. M. (2000). Reducing adverse events: Lessons from a breakthrough series collaborative. *Joint Commission Journal of Quality Improvement, 26*(6), 321–331.

Morath, J., & Turnbull, J. (2005). *To do no harm: Ensuring patient safety in health care organizations.* San Francisco: Jossey-Bass.

Potter, P., Wolf, L., Boxerman, S., Grayson, D., Sledge, J., Dunagan, C., et al. (2005). Understanding the cognitive work of nursing in the acute care environment. *Journal of Nursing Administration, 35*(78), 327–335.

Reason, J. (1990). *Human error.* Cambridge: Cambridge University Press.

WEB REFERENCES

Agency for Healthcare Research and Quality (AHRQ), http://ahrq.gov/
Institute for Healthcare Improvement (IHI), http://www.ihi.org/ihi
National Patient Safety Foundation (NPSF), http://www.npsf.org/

Pay-for-Performance

PAY-FOR-PERFORMANCE (**P4P**) is a current movement that is gaining momentum, calling for providers to be rewarded for providing superior care and intended to improve the management of patient outcomes (Goldberg, 2006). Under the standard system, health care providers are paid based on the quantity or type of services they provide to patients, with few quality measures involved. Pay-for-performance in health care refers to the idea that providers should be compensated based on the quality of the care provided. Providers supply data on specified quality measures, and purchasers of health services pay differentially based on the outcomes resulting from those preset measures.

The P4P movement has grown, in part, out of concerns surrounding the adequacy of care received by patients. Despite the rising cost of health care, there is strong evidence to suggest that not all patients receive adequate care in America's hospitals. Reports such as the Institute of Medicine article, "To Err is Human: Building a Safer Health System" (1999), have led to increased public scrutiny of the quality of health care. As a result, the private and public sectors have called for consistent, improved provider quality and performance measurement supported by payment incentives that reward high performance.

452

Although there are several players in the P4P movement, the main influence is the Centers for Medicare and Medicaid Services (CMS; www.cms.hhs.gov), by far the nation's largest purchaser of health care services. CMS and U.S. Department of Health and Human Services (HHS; www.hhs.gov) have worked together to initiate several P4P initiatives. In 2001, the HHS announced the *Quality Initiative* (CMS, 2005), which has led to several P4P projects across hospitals, nursing homes, home health care providers, and kidney dialysis centers. Next, CMS, working with Premier (an alliance of not-for-profit hospitals) began a demonstration project titled the Hospital Quality Incentive Demonstration (HQID). Under HQID, hospitals that achieve superior performance in a variety of clinical areas, such as heart failure and hip or knee replacements, would receive financial incentives and public recognition as top performing hospitals. Hospitals that did not improve their outcomes above a predefined quality threshold would be subject to financial penalties.

Physician Group Practice (PGP) Demonstration (http://www.parknicollet.com/patientsCommunity/PGPdemo.cfm), the first physician-aimed P4P program, gives physician groups in 10 communities across the nation the opportunity to receive financial bonuses by demonstrating proactive patient care and innovative disease management strategies that save health care dollars in the long term. The Physician Voluntary Reporting Program, initiated in 2006, asks physicians to submit data for certain expensive, high-volume procedures for chronic diseases. The purpose of the additional data collection is to give CMS more insight into practices that allow avoidance of unnecessary hospital admissions and reduction in emergency department readmissions. Using this information, CMS can develop future quality metrics and initiatives. Finally, the Hospital Consumer Assessment of Health Plans Survey (HCAHPS; https://www.cahps.ahrq.gov/default.asp) is a voluntary program designed to measure patient satisfaction. Although most hospitals already measure consumer satisfaction, HCAHPS seeks to standardize patient satisfaction data across all providers to make more valid comparisons among hospitals.

In the private realm, there are three primary P4P catalysts. First, there are several Institute of Medicine reports, such as "To Err is Human" and "Crossing the Quality Chasm" (2001) which call the quality of American health care into question. Also, the National Committee for Quality Assurance (NCQA) set up the Health Plan Employer and Data Information Set (HEDIS) in the 1990s. This program compares health plans and other entities across a variety of performance measures. Although HEDIS does not have payment incentives tied to its quality measures, it has been a strong supporter of CMS pay-for-performance initiatives. Finally, the Integrated Healthcare Association of America, a nonprofit collection of California health systems and plans, has set up the largest pool of private funds for incentive payments for medical groups based on quality.

Current movement within the public and private sectors suggests that the health care industry is headed toward an increased P4P focus; however, P4P has received some criticism (Safavi, 2005). For example, P4P is inherently provider focused and assumes that providers and payers (rather than the patients) know best if a care experience was valuable, and P4P rewards clinical competence and outcomes, yet patients are increasingly interested in compassion, respect, and aesthetics. The patients' perceptions of quality and what they are willing to pay for must factor into the future P4P equation.

NANCY HOLLINGSWORTH

REFERENCES

Centers for Medicare and Medicaid Services. (2005). *Hospital quality initiative overview*. Baltimore, MD: Author. Retrieved from http://www.cms.hhs.gov/HospitalQualityInits/downloads/HospitalOverview200512.pdf

Goldberg, L. (2006, March). *Paying for performance: A call for quality healthcare*. Washington, DC: Deloitte Center for Health Solutions.

Safavi, K. (2005). Moving pay-for-performance to pay-for-value. *Healthcare Technology, 3*. Retrieved from www.hctproject.com

Peplau, Hildegard

HILDEGARD **P**EPLAU was born on September 1, 1909, in Reading, Pennsylvania, and died at the age of 89, on March 17, 1999, in Sherman Oaks, California. Peplau graduated from Pottstown, Pennsylvania, Hospital School of Nursing in 1931. She received a Bachelor of Arts degree in Interpersonal Psychology from Bennington College in Vermont in 1943. She earned a Master's degree in Psychiatric Nursing at Teachers College (TC), Columbia University, in 1947, and a Doctor of Education degree (EdD) in Curriculum Development from TC in 1953 (McCalla, 1998). Peplau was awarded honorary doctoral degrees from universities around the world including Ohio State and Rutgers Universities, and the University of Ulster in Ireland (McCalla, 1998). Peplau is considered a legend in the field of nursing and universally regarded as the mother of psychiatric nursing. Peplau was the only nurse to serve as the Executive Director and then President of the American Nurses Association. She served on the International Council of Nurses, received the Christiane Reimann Prize from that organization. Peplau contributed revolutionary and pivotal ideas to the field of nursing and health care, such as patient-nurse relationship, mental health nursing constructs, inciting patients to more actively participate in their health care, and interpersonal relationships between health care providers and their clients. Peplau was a committed figurehead in nursing education and an advocate of higher education in nursing. She fought for the mentally ill, founded and continuously remodeled psychiatric nursing, and brought about a change of thought regarding therapeutic health care relationships. Peplau was posthumously inducted into the American Nurses Association Nursing Hall of Fame in 1998. Additional information about Hildegard Peplau can be accessed at http://rutgersuniversity.org/nursing/peplau.htm

M. JANICE NELSON

See Also
American Nurses Association
ANA Hall of Fame

REFERENCES

American Nurses Association. (2006). *Hildegard Peplau (1909–1999) 1998 inductee*. Retrieved August 31, 2007, from http://www.nursingworld.org/FunctionalMenuCategories/AboutANA/WhereWeComeFrom_1/HallofFame/19962000Inductees/peplauh5563.aspx

Callaway, B. (2002). *Hildegard Peplau: Psychiatric nurse of the century*. New York: Springer Publishing.

McCalla, C. (1998). *Welcome to the Hildegard Peplau nursing theorist homepage*. Retrieved March 22, 2006, from http://publish.uwo.ca/-cforchuk/peplau/hpcb.html

Philanthropy/ Fund-Raising

PHILANTHROPY—WHETHER it takes the form of fund-raising, service learning, mobilizing volunteers, or board work—is likely to gain in importance as a component of nursing leadership. Too often, however, the only overlap recognized between leadership and philanthropy is that successful leaders are expected to raise money for their organizations. That viewpoint grossly underestimates the profound relationship between the two (McBride, 2000). Both leadership and philanthropy require clarity regarding mission, values, and goals; ongoing strategic planning; making the "case" for why stakeholders should invest in the future; friend raising; image building; resource development; and fund-raising, leveraging assets, and stewardship.

At the end of the 1980s, Sigma Theta Tau International revamped its strategic plan—which had previously emphasized knowledge development, dissemination, and utilization—to add a fourth goal, resource development, in order to accomplish the other three. Having mounted the first major fund-raising campaign in nursing in order to build the International Center for Nursing Scholarship in Indianapolis, this organization recognized the importance of philanthropy in achieving nursing's preferred future. Faced with mounting financial pressures, nonprofit organizations and those employed by them would have to be more creative in expanding the resource base through greater emphasis on gifts as investments (DeLellis, Kardos, & Langston, 1999). Scholarships are an investment in workforce development; endowed lectureships are a guaranteed means of bringing professionals together to discuss the issues of the day. Endowed chairs and professorships have grown significantly in the last two decades as a strategy for addressing the faculty shortage by attracting senior faculty capable of providing program leadership (Fitzpatrick, Fitzpatrick, & Dressler, 2005).

Rarely do health care professionals assume leadership positions with an interest in or knowledge about fund-raising. To address this need, Fitzpatrick and Deller (2000) wrote a book on fund-raising skills for health care executives in which they confronted myths (no special skills are required; the primary responsibility for fund-raising belongs to the development officer; gifts will naturally follow if programs are strong), articulated basic principles (people give to people; people give to vision not just need; if you don't ask you're not likely to receive), and provided information regarding strategies and available resources. More and more leadership-development programs are covering fund-raising fundamentals because of the demand for that material. For example, Sigma Theta Tau International's Omada Board Leadership Institute includes that topic in its curriculum. Universities are developing centers to teach philanthropic principles and to expand the knowledge base of participants. One of the largest of these in the world is the Center for Philanthropy at Indiana University, which can be accessed at: http://www.philanthropy.iupui.edu.

Philanthropy is also important to leadership because the dollars available stimulate creativity. Foundations are organizations that exist, typically, to leverage dollars into programs of a model-developing nature that can, once proven, be widely adopted and supported by other means (Maraldo, Fagin & Keenan, 1988). The W. K. Kellogg Foundation has had a long-standing relationship with the nursing profession, particularly in support of healthy communities. Their historic investment in nursing exceeds that of all other foundations combined. Two nurses who shaped that legacy, Helen Grace and Gloria Smith, have contributed to a book that describes the Foundation's shaping of American nursing between 1930 and 1980 (Lynaugh et al., 2007).

Nurses are increasingly playing a role in providing leadership to foundations. For example, at the time of this writing, Sheila Burke chaired the Henry J. Kaiser Family Foundation; Rebecca Rimel was president and CEO of The Pew Charitable Trusts; and Susan Sherman headed the Independence Foundation. Also, nursing has long been represented on The Robert Wood Johnson Foundation board in the persons of Rheba de Tornyay and Marla Salmon. In the last 7 years, the John A. Hartford

Foundation has invested heavily in nursing in order to meet the challenges created by an aging patient population (go to http://www.hgni.org for information about this initiative).

ANGELA BARRON MCBRIDE

See Also
Sigma Theta Tau International

REFERENCES

DeLellis, A. J., Kardos, E. G., & Langston, N. F. (1999). Development in schools of nursing: Fund-raising to further long-range strategic plans. *Nurse Educator, 24*(3), 29–34.

Fitzpatrick, J. J., & Deller, S. S. (2000). *Fundraising skills for health care executives.* New York: Springer Publishing.

Fitzpatrick, J. J., Fitzpatrick, M. L., & Dressler, M. B. (2005). Endowed chairs and professorships in schools of nursing: A 2004 update. *Journal of Professional Nursing, 21,* 244–252.

Lynaugh, J. E., Grace, H. K., Smith, G. R., Sena, R. R., de Villalobos, M. M. D., & Hlale, M. M. (2007). *The W. K. Kellogg Foundation and the nursing profession: Shared values, shared legacy.* Indianapolis, IN: Sigma Theta Tau International.

Maraldo, P. J., Fagin, C., & Keenan, T. (1988). Nursing and private philanthropy. *Health Affairs, 7*(1), 130–136.

McBride, A. B. (Compiled) (2000). *Nursing & philanthropy. An energizing metaphor for the 21st century.* Indianapolis, IN: Center Nursing Press.

Power and Leadership

THE RELATIONSHIP OF POWER to leadership is unmistakable. Power is a key component of leadership. It fuels it. But just what do we mean by power? There are many different kinds of power: The power of position, the power of beauty, the power of truth, personal power. What is power, really? It is energy of emotion that either arises from within or is triggered from without. Its surge is ignited by one's own thoughts and feelings about things that matter to them. Power can emanate from symbols like a cross or a flag or even a slogan. Anything that generates meaning generates power.

As it relates to leadership, it has been said that power that arises from within is true power, whereas externally imposed power is more appropriately called "force" (Hawken, 2002). Arising from within, the power of leaders emerges from the depths of the soul, so to speak. In fact, as leadership expert Warren Bennis put it, "If you don't see any need to change the world or improve the quality of our lives, you will not be motivated to become a leader" (Bennis & Goldsmith, 1997).

Great leaders inspire us. They move us. Daniel Goleman, founder of the idea of emotional intelligence, calls these leaders, "limbic attractors," signifying their influence on the limbic system, the emotional seat of the

460

brain. They move us emotionally. If you think about some of the leaders that are most outstanding in our minds, for each there was an inner conviction, a defining moment that brought forth an eruption of power from within; a power so compelling that it transformed the culture of a nation.

Several legendary examples are Mahatma Gandhi, a 90-pound Indian man who managed to bring the British Empire to its knees; Rosa Parks, a tired African-American woman who refused to give up her seat on the bus on which only whites were permitted to sit and made gigantic strides toward racial equality; Margaret Sanger, who watched countless women suffer from repeated pregnancies and die in childbirth and revolutionized family planning; and Lillian Wald, who watched poor public health conditions ravage immigrant families throughout New York City and founded the Visiting Nurse Service of New York.

In each of these cases, the power of their leadership derived its potency from the depth of meaning and principle their situations had for them, as distinguished from power for one's personal aggrandizement. This is the crux of the power of leadership: it shapes a new reality by giving new meaning and altering power relationships. Power arises from principles (Hawken, 2002).

New paradigms and new realities are shaped by the power of principles exercised by leaders. In the process of leadership, the world we once knew changes. We see things very differently. Indeed, the context proffered by the leader is very powerful; as it is context that renders meaning. Stephen Covey gives a good example of the power of context. He is on a subway where several children are behaving wildly. Running into others on the train and causing quite a disturbance, Covey tells how he approached their father and points out that he should make an effort to prevent them from disturbing so many people on the train (Covey, 1989). "Oh I suppose I should do something . . . but I'm in the state of shock myself. We just came from the hospital where my wife just died. And they lost their mother. I'm just not sure how to handle the situation myself. I'm sorry." Such is the power of context; it dramatically shifts the meaning of everything.

Another aspect of the power of leadership is the crucial distinction to be made between the exercise of power to advance a collective purpose, and the power of self-advancement. When true power is exercised, it is shared and given freely. In fact, our most memorable leaders are empowering; in the sense that their power is about influence, confluence, and synergy versus domination, control, or willfulness. To be empowering is to attract and allow things (people, process, technology, and opportunity) to *self-organize* versus imposing order and "making things happen."

Empowerment is the foundation of "Transformational Leadership," which has been referred to as "Leadership of the 21st Century." It is the kind of leadership that we want most for ourselves. As old models of wielding power through fear and coercive, controlling tactics have been found to be lacking, new leadership models based on a sense of shared power have emerged (Porter-O'Grady, 1992). Transformational leadership represents leadership in the new paradigm, leaving old models of leading behind. Earlier models were based on the premise that prediction and control are possible, and that interactions occur in straightforward ways (in a linear fashion). We know now, thanks to years of experience and discoveries in science, that this is not so. New leadership models in the transformational vein reflect the latest progress in science revealing that mechanistic concepts fall short when dealing with human beings. The new science takes into account that the power inherent in leadership occurs in interaction; and power is generated in complex and self-organizing ways. Leadership is seen as an opportunity for change and learning, not for control (Wheatley, 2004).

Transformational leadership begins with self-awareness, as it creates energy exchanges in power relationships that transform followers as well as situations and leaders themselves. Leaders create an atmosphere that encourages change to emerge; allowing for unforeseeable consequences. Increasingly, the best lead not by virtue of position, but by excelling in the art of relationship. Leadership excellence is being redefined in interpersonal terms. These leaders generate power by virtue of striking chords of response among followers; surfacing simmering issues and creating synergies among groups (Goleman, 2002). Therein lies their power.

PAM MARALDO

See Also
Emotional Intelligence
Leadership Development
Lillian Wald

REFERENCES

Bennis, W., & Goldsmith, J. (1997). *Learning to lead.* Cambridge, MA: Perseus Books.

Covey, S. (1989). *The seven habits of highly effective people.* New York: Simon and Schuster.

Goleman, D. (2002). *Primal leadership.* Boston: Harvard Business School Press.

Hawken, D. (2002). *Power vs force.* Los Angeles, CA: Hay House.

Porter-O'Grady, T. (1992). *Implementing shared governance.* Baltimore: Mosby Publishers.

Wheatley, M. (2004). *Leadership and the new science.* Palo Alto, CA: Berrett-Koehler Publishers, Inc.

Preceptorship: The Gatekeepers for Professional Nursing Development

PRECEPTORSHIP IS A STRATEGY for the acculturation of new nurses into the practice setting. The preceptor serves as coach and mentor as the new nurse endeavors to understand the practice environment and adapt to the responsibilities associated with being a nurse. Throughout their professional careers, nurses vividly remember their first preceptor as well as their first work experience as a nurse. This fact alone tells us that the preceptor role is a critical variable in the development of a nurse's perception of the profession. A positive experience with a preceptor validates one's choice to take a particular job and perhaps to choose a particular career path. It often progresses to a decision to "stay or to leave." Thus, the concept of the gatekeeper is born—someone who holds the key to another's new nursing career (Vezina, 2004). Development of a preceptor program in a health care institution today is considered to be a "best practice strategy" for nursing recruitment and retention. Understanding the nurse's role in and influence on professional development of other nurses and nursing students is paramount.

Most nurses are not inherently successful preceptors. Unique knowledge and skills need to be introduced, role-modeled, assessed, and supported for success to be achieved in this role. Consequently, a fully developed nurse preceptor training program is instrumental in achieving successful recruitment and retention outcomes.

Successful recruitment and retention outcomes may result from a variety of initiatives, including the development of a preceptor program enriched with a pool of trained preceptors and the creation of a culture to support recruitment and retention. Because nursing is a practice discipline, acquiring knowledge and attitudes as well as skills is the foundation to developing competence. Preceptors act as role models and clinical experts, socializers, and educators, to accomplish the attainment of these competencies.

The first step to a successful Preceptor Program is developing criteria for the selection and assignment of preceptors. The preceptor role must be operationally defined, a financial benefit assigned if possible, selection criteria specified, and distinct responsibilities outlined. This first step establishes productive communication among all interested parties. Some basic prerequisites for the assignment of preceptor include: (1) completion of a predetermined amount of time as a registered nurse (RN) within an institution, for example, of 6–9 months if an experienced nurse, 1 year or more if a new graduate; (2) ability to communicate effectively with colleagues and patients; (3) ability to teach colleagues and patients; (4) ability to apply the nursing process and practice in a competent manner; and (5) attributes as a professional role model. With expectations clear, a curriculum must be devised. The teaching methodology needs include an active workshop format with role-playing, case-based learning exercises, and strategies for resolving conflicts and giving feedback to enhance growth and development of the new nurse.

The next crucial step in curriculum development is to identify a conceptual model. This framework directs how professional development and teaching can best be understood and applied. One example is to combine a nursing and educational approach to development—such as Benner's *From Novice to Expert* (1984) and Knowles and others' *The Adult Learner* (1998). As such, the curriculum provides a frame of reference from which to approach new nurses, recognize their stage of professional development, and support expected behaviors. In addition, by using adult principles of learning rather than traditional pedagogical approaches, a more facilitative, independent strategy replaces the "sage on stage" approach to teaching. The content outline for a model preceptor program is shown in Table P.1.

Newly hired staff can feel more supported in their orientation because a framework and process has been established within the institution.

TABLE P.1 Content Outline for a Model Preceptor Program

1) Orientation Description	✴ Process of orientation ✴ Model(s) of professional development ✴ Experiential learning methods
2) Role of the Preceptor	✴ Preparing for preceptorship ✴ Principles including communication, adult learning, and evaluation ✴ Purpose of orientation ✴ Goal of the preceptor-orientee relationship ✴ Preceptor selection criteria ✴ Desirable preceptor characteristics ✴ Rewards perceived by preceptors ✴ Coordination of unit orientation by preceptor, educator and clinical nurse manager
3) Making an Assignment Plan for an Orientee 4) Assessment of Skills in Problem Management 5) Assessment of Skills in Communication and Conflict Resolution 6) Assessment of Priority-Setting Skills	
7) Evaluation Process	✴ Principles of evaluation ✴ Methods of feedback such as giving examples that are: specific rather than general; factual rather than opinionated; descriptive rather than judgmental. ✴ Action plans/performance improvement plans ✴ Evaluation conference

This provides security and opens the door to learning and growing rather than a fear-based introduction to the work world. Facilitating others to perform on their own is incredibly rewarding and a confidence builder in the end.

MARIA L. VEZINA

See Also
Mentoring
Staff Recruitment
Staff Retention

REFERENCES

Benner, P. (1984). *From novice to expert: Excellence and practice power in clinical nursing*. Menlo Park, CA: Addison Wesley.

Billings, D., & Halstead, J. (1998). *Teaching in nursing: A guide for faculty*. Philadelphia: Saunders.

Flynn, J. P., & Stack, M. C. (Eds.). (2006). *The role of the preceptor: A guide for nurse educators and clinicians* (2nd ed.). New York: Springer Publishing.

Knowles, M., Holton, E., & Swanson, R. (1998). *The adult learner: The definitive classic in adult education and human resource development*. Houston, TX: Gulf Professional Publishing.

Merriam, S., & Caffarella, R. (1999). *Learning in adulthood, a comprehensive guide* (2nd ed.). San Francisco: Jossey-Bass.

Vezina, M. (2004). The gatekeepers. *ADVANCE for Nurses, Serving RNs in the Greater NY/NJ Metro Area, 4*(21), 29–30.

Professional Practice Model

THE IMPORTANCE OF WORKING in a professional practice environment has been well known since the first Magnet Hospital Study (McClure, Poulin, Sovie, & Wandelt, 1983). From this landmark study, essential components of professional practice were identified including: autonomy, control over practice, and collaborative relationships with physicians. Professional practice models are generally based on theory, are not stagnant, are designed to evolve over time and are a basis for guiding ways nurses can clearly articulate belief systems (Ives Erickson, 1996; McEwen & Willis, 2002). Professional practice models describe the relationships of important organizational concepts and can support organizational activities designed to advance nursing practice. One of the most effective strategies for aligning nurses and clinicians across the disciplines is the articulation of a professional practice model. When a team becomes aligned, a commonality of direction emerges, and individual energies harmonize. There is a shared purpose and understanding of how to complement one another's efforts (Senge, 1995). In the white paper *Hallmarks of the Professional Nurse Practice Environment* (2002), the American

Association of Colleges of Nursing cites the following as characteristics of the practice setting that best support professional nursing practice:

* Manifest a philosophy of clinical care emphasizing quality, safety, interdisciplinary collaboration, continuity of care, and professional accountability;
* Recognize contributions of nurses' knowledge and expertise to clinical care quality and patient outcomes;
* Promote executive level nursing leadership;
* Empower nurses' participating in clinical decision making and organization of clinical care systems;
* Maintain clinical advancement programs based on education, certification, and advanced preparation;
* Demonstrate professional development support for nurses;
* Create collaborative relationships among members of the health care provider team; and
* Utilize technological advances in clinical care and information systems.

The operational challenge in articulating a professional practice model is in defining concepts in such a way that brings significance to daily practice. Each component is critical to practice and care delivery. If a model is to work, each clinician needs to understand, embrace, and master the skills involved and be willing to learn—continuously learn—because the environment in which care is delivered is rapidly changing. This is a journey that the health care team takes together.

An example of a professional practice model is the interdisciplinary model utilized at Massachusetts General Hospital, which provides a comprehensive view of professional practice (Picard & Jones, 2005). This Professional Practice Model consists of nine essential elements including vision and values, standards of practice, narrative culture, professional development, patient-centeredness, clinical recognition and advancement, collaborative decision making, research and innovation, and entrepreneurial teamwork. The Professional Practice Model is a framework for achieving clinical outcomes, assuring the identity, integrity, and development of each discipline and for working collaboratively in the care of patients and families. Because each component is inherently related to all others, an "interlocking" puzzle was chosen to represent the model. Each is connected to the need to truly understand the patient experience and ways to improve the patient care process (Figure P.1).

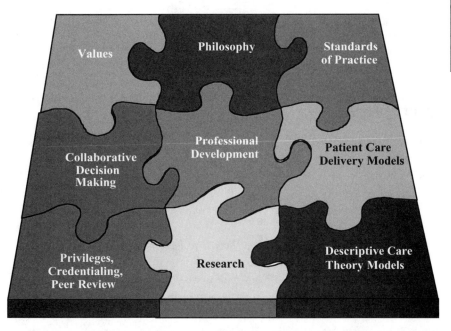

FIGURE P.1 Massachusetts General Hospital Professional Practice Model.

The creation of a professional practice model serves many purposes, including:

* Articulates the work of clinicians across a variety of settings;
* Provides a framework to guide clinical practice, education, administration, and research;
* Promotes communication among disciplines and between clinicians and the organization;
* Provides a framework for setting a strategic direction and achieving goals and clinical outcomes;
* Guides the allocation of resources;
* Serves as a framework for the evaluation of practice; and
* Functions as a marketing tool to visually describe clinical practice both internally and externally.

The model gathers the components of nurses' contributions and fits them together to reveal the whole or essence of nursing practice. In addition, it takes the often-invisible work of nurses and other members of the health care team and makes it visible.

JEANNETTE IVES ERICKSON
MARIANNE DITOMASSI

See Also
American Association of Colleges of Nursing
Magnet Hospitals

REFERENCES

American Association of Colleges of Nursing. (2002). *Hallmarks of the professional nurse practice environment*. White paper. Washington, DC: Author.

Ives Erickson, J. (1996). *Caring headlines*. Boston: Massachusetts General Hospital.

McClure, M. L., Poulin, M. A., Sovie, M. D., & Wandelt, M. (1983). *Magnet hospitals: Attraction and retention of professional nurses*. Washington, DC: American Nurses Publishing.

McEwen, M., & Willis, E. M. (2002). *Theoretical basis for nursing*, Philadelphia: Lippincott Williams & Wilkins.

Picard, C., & Jones, D. (2005). *Giving voice to what we know: Margaret Neuman's theory of health as expanding consciousness in practice, research and education*. Sudbury, MA: Jones and Bartlett Publishers.

Senge, P. (1995). *The fifth discipline*. New York: Doubleday/Currency.

R

Rapid Response
Teams

RAPID RESPONSE TEAMS (RRT), also known as Medical Emergency Teams (MET) have been utilized in a number of facilities both in the United States and internationally. They were first developed as a result of the Robert Wood Johnson Foundation grant, "Transforming Care at the Bedside," conducted by the Institute for Healthcare Improvement (IHI). These teams function by bringing consultation from critical care experts directly to the bedside no matter the location. Their development results in better support to patients and the staff caring for them, improved patient outcomes, and decreased untoward events that may require a higher level of care, improved survival rates, and altered patterns of transfers into critical care areas. These teams can also function in an educational role, assisting their colleagues in gaining knowledge and experience in the care of complex patients.

Although protocols and membership of RRTs are structured differently in each setting, most have some combination of the following: the process is initiated by the nurse caring for the patient and the RRT is comprised of a critical care nurse, a respiratory therapist, a senior resident and/or a hospitalist. Criteria established for initiating the RRT varies but generally includes acute changes in the following: respiratory status, blood pressure and heart rate, level of consciousness, and decreased urine output without a history of renal dysfunction. In the evolution of RRTs, the level of discomfort of the nurse caring for the patient has been added to the criteria for calling the RRT. The RRT is expected to arrive at the patient's bedside within 10 minutes of a call initiating the team response. Communication is critical in this process and use of SBAR (Situation, Background, Assessment, and Recommendation) techniques have assisted in the effective use of the RRTs.

Studies of the effectiveness of RRTs are varied with and while the RRT provides a systems approach to dealing with critically ill patients the benefits are not yet well defined in measuring outcomes, such as mortality and cardiac arrest rates (Cretikos & Hillman, 2003). Recent studies (Hillman et al., 2005) suggest that the use of the RRT has increased but that the negative outcomes such as unplanned admission to critical care, unexpected deaths, or the incidence of cardiac arrest has not occurred.

INGRID E. BRODIN

See Also
Institute for Healthcare Improvement

REFERENCES

Cretikos, M., & Hillman, K. (2003). The medical emergency team: Does it really make a difference? *Journal of Internal Medicine, 33*(11), 511–514.

Hillman, K., Chen, J., Cretikos, M., Bellomo, R., Brown, D., Doig, G., et al. (2005). Introduction of the medical emergency team (MET) system: A cluster-randomised controlled trial. *Lancet, 365*(9477), 2091–2097.

Scholle, C., & Mininni, N. (2006). How a rapid response team saves lives. *Nursing 2006, 36*(1), 36–40.

Simmons, T. C. (2005). Best-practice protocols: Implementing a rapid response system of care. *Nursing Management, 36*(7), 41–59.

Regulatory Bodies

THE 10TH AMENDMENT to the U.S. Constitution reserves to the states, as part of their police powers, the right to regulate professions in order to protect the health, safety, and welfare of the public. Regulatory boards are created when state legislators are convinced that the practice of a profession requires regulation in order to protect the public. The resulting laws that are passed are referred to as *practice acts*. For nursing, the first such practice acts were passed in 1903. Practice acts distinguish the practice of nursing from that of other health care providers and define and differentiate the scope of practice and professional responsibilities for registered professional nurses, licensed practical nurses, and advanced practice nurses. Generally, practice acts are written in broad terms to permit the acquisition of new knowledge, technological advances, and the gradual evolution of the profession. Practice acts designate the creation of a regulatory board and grant authority to the board to enforce the provisions of the law. The regulatory board serves as the administrative body to assure that provisions of the practice act are met. A list of nursing regulatory boards can be found at http://www.ncsbn.org by clicking on the link labeled *Boards of Nursing*. There is at least one nursing regulatory body in each of the 50 states and the District of Columbia; some states have two such bodies, one for Licensed Practical Nurses and one for Registered Professional Nurses. Regulatory boards, based on the authority provided in the practice act, generally function to establish criteria for licensure, including education, experience, examination, age, and citizenship; determine grounds for removal of a license; establish policies to conduct disciplinary proceedings; determine licensure renewal requirements, including continuing competence or continuing education; and arbitrate scope of practice issues, that is, make legal opinions on those activities that can and cannot be provided by the licensed professionals within the board's purview. Requirements for membership on regulatory boards are specified in the nursing practice act. In the early history of nursing, regulatory boards included only registered professional nurses as members. Licensed practical nurses began to be added in the 1940s and in the 1970s jurisdictions began to include public members as board members with full voting rights and privileges. The structure of regulatory boards across states and jurisdictions is marked by considerable diversity. Some boards are essentially independent and operate autonomously on licensure revenues. Such boards have the authority to promulgate regulations, initiate new legislation and make declarative statements regarding scope of practice issues. Other boards function within an umbrella organization in a department, such as health, education or labor, which regulates numerous other disciplines. This hierarchical structure impacts strongly on the authority of the regulatory board and its ability to control its budget, determine the outcome of licensure for applicants, and make decisions on scope of practice issues. Regulatory boards also have gathered to form associations of regulatory boards. Voting membership in such associations is usually limited to the regulatory board or body within each individual state authorized to regulate the specific profession. The National Council of State Boards of Nursing (NCSBN) serves as an example of an association of regulatory nursing boards. Further information about NCSBN can be obtained by accessing their Web site at http://www.ncsbn.org.

BARBARA ZITTEL

See Also
Continuing Professional Education
The National Council of State Boards of Nursing, Inc. (NCSBN)

Reiter, Frances

FRANCES REITER was born 1904 and died in 1977 at the age of 73. Reiter graduated from Teachers College (TC), Columbia University, with a Master of Arts degree in teaching the biological sciences. She was also on the faculty at TC. Reiter assumed the deanship of the Graduate School of Nursing at New York Medical College in 1960, which, in 1966, merged with and became the Pace University Lienhard School of Nursing, where she became dean emerita in 1969. In 1943, she coined the term, "nurse clinician," and advocated for advanced academic preparation for this role. Reiter was Chair of the American Nurses Association (ANA) Committee on Education when the first position paper was published in 1965, calling for the standardization of pre-licensure professional nursing education at the baccalaureate level (ANA, 1965). She was the recipient of numerous awards including the Medal of Excellence from the New York Medical College. She received an Honorary Membership Award from ANA, the International Red Cross Award, the Florence Nightingale Award, and the Distinguished Service Award from the National League for Nursing. Reiter was an early grant recipient of the American Nurses Foundation (ANF, 2005). She was an honorary fellow of the American Academy of Nursing and was inducted into the American Nurses Association Hall of Fame in 1984.

M. JANICE NELSON

See Also
Advanced Practice Registered Nurses
American Academy of Nursing
American Nurses Association
American Nurses Association Hall of Fame
American Nurses Foundation
National League for Nursing
Florence Nightingale

REFERENCES

American Nurses Association, Committee on Education. (1965). *Educational preparation for nurse practitioners and assistants to nurses: A position paper*. New York: Author.

American Nurses Association. (2006). *Frances Reiter (1904–1977) 1984 inductee*. Retrieved August 31, 2007, from http://www.nursingworld.org/FunctionalMenuCategories/AboutANA/WhereWeComeFrom_1/HallofFame/19761984/reitfx5573.aspx

American Nurses Foundation. (2005). The American Nurses Foundation—1955–2005. Special 50th Anniversary Retrospective. *Foundation Focus*, 1–2. Retrieved August 31, 2007, from www.anfonline.org/anf/ffocus0106.pdf

Research Integrity

THE 2006 POSITION STATEMENT on Nursing Research from the American Association of Colleges of Nursing (AACN) articulates nursing's commitment to research integrity: "Nursing's commitment to an egalitarian application of professional standards and ethics has earned the trust of the public. Similarly nursing research is guided by commitment to ethical standards in all phases of scientific discovery and use of knowledge" (AACN, 2006). Integrity requires rigor, systematic care, and accountability in scholarship. The involvement of either humans or animals in research calls for ethical investigator behavior and practices.

According to Lo (2001), three major principles guide research, especially with human subjects. One major principle is respect for people and their rights for choosing to participate in studies based on full disclosure of the opportunities and possible consequences. This principle guides the processes/procedures for informal consent and Institutional Review Boards basic to the protection of human subjects. The principle of beneficence dictates that the benefits of the research outweigh either the physical or psychological risks to subjects. The principle of justice "requires that the benefits and burdens of research be distributed fairly"

(Lo, p. 215). This third principle particularly refers to vulnerable populations and the need to not study such populations when others would be as appropriate. Operationally, these ethical principles require that:

* all research should be approved by an appropriate ethics committee;
* study findings will justify any risk or inconvenience to the subjects;
* researchers must have the qualifications, training, and competence to conduct the study with a high degree of scientific integrity;
* the rights and feelings of subjects must be respected at all times; and
* subjects must be provided with information on the purpose, requirements, and demands of the protocol prior to their giving consent and they must be free to withdraw consent at any time. (Peat, Mellis, Williams, & Xuan, 2001, Table 8.7)

Creating an environment for research integrity that fosters intellectual integrity, open communication and trust is the responsibility of all investigators, institutions, and funding agencies. Research integrity involves, foremost, the protection of subjects, but also includes avoiding research misconduct, that is, fabrication, falsification, or plagiarism during the inquiry process, reporting conflicts of interest of all types and negotiating fairly with colleagues in terms of credit (e.g., presentations, authorship) for the scientific ideas and conduct of the research. In order to protect subjects, major infrastructures have been built at federal and institutional levels. Research misconduct that threatens or harms subjects is not acceptable, and federal as well as institutional policies/procedures have evolved for their protection. The federal policies/procedures must be met by institutions applying for and accepting federal funds for research. In general, the same policies/procedures are used with all investigations. The Office of Research Integrity (ORI) in the U.S. Department of Health and Human Services (HHS) (http://ori.dhhs.gov/) monitors for responsible research conduct in institutions receiving federal financing for investigations through educational, preventive, and regulatory activities. Institutions conducting research with federal funds establish an infrastructure of Offices (e.g., Office of Vice President in Universities) that educate for the conduct of responsible research (CRR), foster an environment for research integrity and above all, adhere to, and operationalize the federal policies/procedures for protecting subjects. Policies and procedures for monitoring, reporting and handling cases of research misconduct are part of the responsibility of these offices. There are two main protections for human subjects: Institutional Review Board approval of all investigations involving people, and Informed Consent policies/procedures. A major aspect of federal and institutional oversight of research is providing educational requirements and opportunities for principal investigators of studies.

The major responsibility for ethical behavior in research lies with the scientists. For example, all investigators in institutions receiving federal funds must complete a National Institutes of Health module on the responsible conduct of research (RCR) (http://cme.cancer.gov/clinicaltrials/learning/humanparticipant-protections.asp), and especially the protection of human subjects/participants. National and institutional conferences and seminars reinforce these basic ethical principles and policies. To generate knowledge regarding research integrity and RCR, the Office of Research Integrity offers grants to study the issues involved, especially strategies for protecting human subjects.

ADA SUE HINSHAW

See Also
American Association of Colleges of Nursing
Informed Consent (Research)

REFERENCES

American Association of Colleges of Nursing (AACN). (2006). *Position statement on nursing research*. Retrieved June 30, 2006, from http://www.aacn.nche.edu/Publications/positions/NsgRes.htm

Lo, B. (2001). Addressing ethical issues. In S. Hulley et al. (Eds.), *Designing clinical research: An epidemiological approach* (pp. 215–225). Philadelphia: Lippincott Williams & Wilkins Company.

Peat, J., Mellis, C., Williams, K., & Xuan, W. (2001). Appraising research protocols. In *Health science research. A handbook of quantitative methods* (pp. 283–286). London: Sage Publications.

WEB REFERENCE

U.S. Department of Health and Human Services (HHS), Office of Research Integrity (ORI), http://ori.dhhs.gov/

Risk Management in the Health Care Setting

THE JOINT COMMISSION (2007) defines Risk Management as "clinical and administrative activities undertaken to identify, evaluate, and reduce the risk of injury to patients, staff, and visitors, and the risk of loss to the organization itself." Risk management was practiced in the insurance industry for many years before becoming a specific competency within health care organizations. The initial function of risk management was to help mitigate the escalating costs of health care premiums, which had been rising as a result of an increasing number of claims and lawsuits. As expenses rose in the 1970s, a need developed to examine the liability concerns that affected patient care and the outcomes of these situations. In addition, the risk manager's role was focused on proactively managing activities within the health care system that could broaden the knowledge and behaviors of providers in response to negative outcomes of care. Risk managers were initially seen as the guardians of the information chest of adverse events and their effect on patients.

In many institutions today, risk managers collect and analyze occurrence reports, participate in the defense of malpractice cases, offer guidance and education dealing with difficult patients and situations, as well as initiate sentinel event case review. It is through the risk manager's assessment and interaction with providers that liability concerns are identified. In addition, the risk manager helps to identify system weaknesses or vulnerabilities within hospital settings that may allow adverse events to occur.

Since the release of the 2001 Institute of Medicine publication *To Err Is Human,* the world of risk management and patient safety has begun to coalesce and move to new prominence in health care. Identification of risk, development of corrective action plans, event disclosure, and providing apology to patients and their families are some of the responsibilities that risk managers undertake.

There are many ways that risk managers can help to analyze concerns. Communication is the number one tool of an effective risk manager. Understanding the causes of errors is crucial to preventing their recurrence as well as litigation in the future. Risk managers look for ways to make improvements in work processes to prevent harm from reaching others. Nurses are key to the process of a case analysis or root cause analysis (RCA); however, it is often challenging to create an environment free from blame that allows people to speak freely about their fears and concerns. Reviewers have moved away from the process of asking, "Who did it?" to asking "What happened and why?"

Creating a *fair and just culture* is one way that nurse leaders can collaborate with risk managers to prevent errors and identify system vulnerabilities. According to Frankel (2004), "A fair and just culture means giving constructive feedback and critical analysis in skillful ways, doing assessments that are based on facts, and having respect for the complexity of the situation. It also means providing fair-minded treatment, having productive conversations, and creating effective structures that help people to reveal their errors and help the organization learn from them."

As nurse leaders work to create transparencies in health care and patient care delivery systems, it is important to involve patients in the prevention and management of risk. At times, the fear of litigation prevents health care providers from acknowledging to the patient that something has gone wrong. The provider often feels unable to offer an apology. Most patients don't sue their providers because of the mistake but, rather, because of a lack of communication and impression of hiding information. "In a survey conducted by the National Patient Safety Foundation (NPSF) as many as 95% of the respondents wanted to know about even the most insignificant error" (Federico, 2003, p. 2). By receiving open and honest communication from their providers, patients have the potential to be knowledgeable about their health care and feel safer. Open and direct communication is crucial for a patient to understand what has happened when there is an error, and it is essential to remaining in control of health care decisions. This in turn will lead to a more satisfied patient relationship and also may lead to a decrease in malpractice litigation.

For too long, health care providers have not been accountable to their patients and society for errors that have occurred. The public now demands more. The core competencies of risk managers are focused on supporting providers with information about risk avoidance as well as the management of adverse events when they occur. Their contributions help to foster and create a patient care culture of transparency, safety and performance improvement and will expect no less from the hands they place their lives in. This is not unlike teaching our children the importance of owning up to a mistake.

DENISE PETERSON

See Also
Accreditation in Nursing Practice
Sentinel Events

REFERENCES

Carroll, R. (2006). *Risk management handbook*. Chicago: American Hospital Publishing.

Federico, F. (2003). Disclosure of medical error. *Forum, 23*(2), 2–3.

Frankel, A. (2004). *Dana-Farber Cancer Institute: Principles of a fair and just culture*. Retrieved August 24, 2007, from http://www.macoalition.org/Initiatives/docs/Dana-Farber_PrinciplesJustCulture.pdf

Institute of Medicine. (2001). *To err is human*. Washington, DC: National Academies Press.

The Joint Commission. (2007). *Sentinel event glossary of terms*. Retrieved August 24, 2007, from http://www.jointcommission.org/SentinelEvents/se_glossary.htm

Robb, Isabel Hampton

ISABEL HAMPTON ROBB was born in Canada, in July 1860; she died in Cleveland, Ohio, in 1910 at the age of 50. Robb was a graduate of the Collegiate Institute of St. Catherine's (Ontario, Canada) and was subsequently admitted to the Bellevue Hospital Training School for Nurses (Christy, 1969b). Robb was largely responsible for gaining access to Teachers College (TC) Columbia University, to establish the course in Hospital Economics, designed for graduate nurses serving in administrative or teaching roles across the country. She was committed to the concept of higher education for nurses and during her tenure at the Johns Hopkins Training School for Nurses, Robb served as mentor to M. Adelaide Nutting in this regard and she played a pivotal role in convincing Nutting to accept the director position at TC (Christy, 1969b). Before serving as Superintendent of Nurses and Principal of the Training School at "the Hopkins," Robb served as Superintendent of the Illinois Training School in Chicago. She was one of the few nurses of the time who was able to manage marriage, family, and a professional career (Christy, 1969a). Robb was active in the formation of the American Society of Superintendents of Training Schools for Nurses (later to be renamed the National League for Nursing Education), and of the Nurses' Associated Alumnae

485

of United States and Canada (later to become the American Nurses Association), and she served as the first president of the Associated Alumnae (1896–1897). She also was among the original members of the committee to establish the *American Journal of Nursing*. She was dubbed the "Architect of Modern Nursing," and was considered responsible for many of the significant advances in nursing which took place during the latter years of the 19th century (Noel, 1979). Robb was posthumously inducted into the ANA Hall of Fame in 1976. Additional information about Robb can be found at www.hopkinsmedicine.org/about/history/history8html.

M. JANICE NELSON

See Also
American Nurses Association
ANA Hall of Fame
National League for Nursing

REFERENCES

Christy, T. E. (1969a). *Cornerstone for nursing education: A history of nursing education of Teachers College, Columbia University, 1899–1947*. New York: Teachers College Press.

Christy, T. E. (1969b). Portrait of a leader: Isabel Hampton Robb. *Nursing Outlook, 17*(3), 26–29.

Noel, N. L. (1979). *Isabel Hampton Robb: Architect of modern nursing*. Unpublished doctoral dissertation. New York: Teachers College, Columbia University.

Rogers, Martha E.

MARTHA ELIZABETH ROGERS was born in Dallas, Texas, on May 12, 1914; she died in Phoenix, Arizona, in 1994. Rogers received her diploma in nursing from Knoxville General Hospital in 1936. She attended a number of colleges and universities including the University of Tennessee at Knoxville, George Peabody College, Teachers College, Columbia University, and the Johns Hopkins University. In the first years of her career, Rogers practiced public health nursing in Michigan, Connecticut, and Arizona. She was appointed professor and head of the Division of Nursing at New York University in 1954 and remained in that position until 1975 (American Association of the History of Nursing, 2006). Rogers's greatest contribution to nursing was the publication of her revolutionary theory on *The Science of Unitary Human Beings,* which spearheaded nursing's search for a scientific base. Rogers received numerous citations and awards throughout her highly productive career. She also received honorary doctorates from institutions of higher education such as Duquesne University, the University of San Diego, Iona College, Fairfield University, and Mercy College (Hornberger, n.d.). Rogers published extensively, and lectured in nearly all of the United States plus in numerous countries around the world including China, Brazil, Holland, Puerto Rico, and Mexico. She is one of nursing's outstanding leaders and considered to be one of nursing's most original thinkers (Hornberger, n.d.). Rogers was active in a number of nursing organizations and remained active until her death. She was posthumously inducted into the American Nurses Association Hall of Fame in 1996. Additional information on Rogers can be accessed at http://www.foundationnysnurses.org/collections/martharogers.htm

M. JANICE NELSON

See Also
ANA Hall of Fame

REFERENCES

American Association of the History of Nursing. (2006). *Gravesites of prominent nurses: Martha E. Rogers, 1914–1994*. Retrieved March 29, 2006, from http://www.aahn.org/gravesites/rogers.html

American Nurses Association. (2006). *Martha Elizabeth Rogers (1914–1994) 1996 inductee*. Retrieved August 31, 2007, from http://www.nursingworld.org/FunctionalMenuCategories/AboutANA/WhereWeComeFrom_1/HallofFame/19962000Inductees/rogeme5577.aspx

Hornberger, C. (n.d.). *M. Rogers and the science of unitary human beings*. Retrieved August 31, 2007, from http://www.washburn.edu/washburn/gen/washburn_generated_pages/School_of_Nursing_Who_is_Martha_Rogers_p186.html

S

Sanger, Margaret

MARGARET HIGGINS SANGER was born in Corning, New York, on September 14, 1879; she died in 1966 at the age of 87 in Tucson, Arizona. An avid advocate of women's rights and women's health, Margaret Sanger is credited with creation of the term "birth control," and was responsible for the establishment of the "American Birth Control League," which later became the "International Planned Parenthood Federation." Shortly after the death of her mother in 1899, Sanger left Claverack College in Hudson, New York, and enrolled in a nursing program at a hospital in White Plains, New York. Tuberculosis, poor health, marriage, and a subsequent pregnancy all prevented Sanger from completing the 3rd year of training and attaining certification as a trained nurse. Nevertheless, her experiences in working with impoverished women in the East Side slums of Manhattan prompted her to defy the Comstock Law of 1873, which prohibited the distribution of contraceptive information and dissemination of contraceptive devices. Sanger continually risked scandal and imprisonment for these activities. In 1916, she opened the first family planning and birth control clinic in the United States in Brooklyn, New York. The clinic was raided by police and Sanger was arrested for violating the post office's obscenity laws by sending birth control information by mail. Undeterred, she fled to Europe to escape prosecution and launched two periodicals there: *The Birth Control Review* and *Birth Control News*. In 1917, Sanger was sent to the workhouse for "creating a public nuisance."

Sanger organized the first World Population Conference in 1927 in Geneva, Switzerland. She lectured on birth control throughout the world, including Asia, Africa, and Japan. She also held a number of offices, including president of the Birth Control International Information Center, chair of the Birth Control Council of America, and president of The International Planned Parenthood Federation. Regardless of the fact that she never completed her program in nurses' training, Margaret Sanger was inducted into the ANA Hall of Fame in 1976.

M. JANICE NELSON

See Also
ANA Hall of Fame

REFERENCES

Chestler, E. (1992). *Woman of valor: Margaret Sanger and the birth control movement in America*. New York: Simon & Schuster.

Lewis, J. J. (2006). *Margaret Sanger*. Retrieved July 20, 2006, from http://www.women'shistory.about.com/library/bio/blbio_margaret_sanger.htm

Steinem, G. (1998). *Margaret Sanger: Her crusade to legalize birth control spurred the movement of women's liberation*. Retrieved July 18, 2006, http://www.time.com/time/time100/leaders/profile/sanger.html

Schlotfeldt, Rozella M.

ROZELLA M. SCHLOTFELDT was born in Dewitt, Iowa, in 1914 and she died in 2005 in Cleveland, Ohio at the age of 91. She earned her BS in Nursing from the University of Iowa and practiced for several years in maternity nursing. She later pursued employment with the U.S. Veterans Hospital in Des Moines and subsequently returned to the University of Iowa Hospitals as an instructor-supervisor in maternity nursing. It was here that Schlotfeldt entertained the idea of combining teaching and practice, which, in later years, became the foundation of her "Unification Model" (Rozella M. Schlotfeldt Papers, 1993). Schlotfeldt entered the Army Nurse Corps in early 1944. On completion of service, she pursued a graduate degree and then a PhD from the University of Chicago. Following employment as associate dean for research and development at Wayne State University, Schlotfeldt became dean and professor at the Frances Payne Bolton School of Nursing at Case Western Reserve University. It was here that she solidified and developed her thoughts on a collaboration model for nursing schools and clinical agencies (Rozella M. Schlotfeldt Papers, 1993). Schlotfeldt held numerous professional positions, including consultant to the Surgeon General's Advisory Group on Nursing and to the Walter Reed Army Institute for Nursing Research.

She served on the American Nurses Association Study Committee on Credentialing in Nursing and on the governing council of the American Academy of Nursing, of which she was a fellow. Schlotfeldt was honored numerous times by her colleagues and was the recipient of several honorary doctorates. Additional information about Rozella Schlotfeldt can be accessed at http://www.fpb.case.edu/AlumDev/schlotfeldt.shtm.

M. JANICE NELSON

See Also
American Academy of Nursing
American Nurses Association

REFERENCES

Case Western Reserve University. (1998). 1960–1982: Rozella M. Schlotfeldt and the nursing revolution. *CWRU Magazine.* Retrieved March 29, 2006, from http://www.cwru.edu./pubs/cwrumag/fall1998/features/nursing/fpb75_7.shtml

Glazer, G. (2005). Overview and summary: The doctor of nursing practice (DNP): Need for more dialogue. *Online Journal of Issues in Nursing, 10*(3). Retrieved March 29, 2006, from http://www.nursingworld.org/ojin/topic28/tpc28ntr.htm

The Rozella M. Schlotfeldt Papers. (1993). Retrieved March 29, 2006, from http://www.nursing.upenn.edu/history/collections/schlotfeldt.htm

Sentinel Events

I N THE MID-1990S, the Joint Commission on Accreditation of Health-care Organization Accreditation (JCAHO) used the term "sentinel events" to describe serious health care errors or complications that should be reviewed and corrected immediately. In those organizations using the JCAHO accreditation process, JCAHO may review a patient care event that: has resulted in an unanticipated death or major permanent loss of function, not related to the natural course of the patient's illness or underlying condition or is one of the following: suicide of any individual receiving care, treatment or services in a staffed around-the-clock care setting or within 72 hours of discharge; unanticipated death of a full-term infant; abduction of any individual receiving care, treatment or services; discharge of an infant to the wrong family; rape; hemolytic transfusion reaction involving administration of blood or blood products having major blood group incompatibilities; surgery on the wrong individual or wrong body part; unintended retention of a foreign object in an individual after surgery or other procedure; or prolonged fluoroscopy with cumulative dose or any delivery of radiotherapy to the wrong body region (JCAHO, 2006).

The Joint Commission for Healthcare Organization Accreditation requires review of sentinel events using the root cause analysis format. The root cause analysis methodology avoids personal blame by analyzing error objectively in the context of the system. JCAHO further requires an action plan for any issues identified as a result of the analysis. Sentinel events may be voluntarily reported to JCAHO, which uses the data to identify trends. Out of these data, the JCAHO has issued "Sentinel Event Alerts" designed to assist organizations in identifying, mitigating, and eliminating health care patient safety issues. Sentinel event statistics that organizations may use as comparative data are available on the JCAHO Web site. JCAHO additionally uses the sentinel event data to formulate the JCAHO National Patient Safety Goals.

Although other industries, such as airlines, have used a similar reporting format with success for many years, the concept of sentinel events was quite controversial when first introduced. Because sentinel events also may be litigated events, many organizations feared that peer review information reported to JCAHO could lose privilege and become admissible in a lawsuit. Over time, however, the sentinel event concept has successfully identified and provided an evidence base and methodology for the prevention and mitigation of health care error. Please refer to the JCAHO Web site for a complete and current description of the Sentinel Event Policy.

KATHRYN GARDNER RAPALA

See Also
Accreditation in Nursing Practice
Risk Management in the Health Care Setting

REFERENCE

Joint Commission on Accreditation of Healthcare Organizations. (2006). *Sentinel event policies and procedures*. Retrieved June 23, 2006, from www.jointcommission.org/SentinelEvents/PolicyandProcedures/se_pp.htm

Shared Governance Is Structure Not Process

S HARED GOVERNANCE is a structure, not a program or process (Porter-O'Grady, 2001). This is an important distinction as it informs both thinking and acting with regard to making it a sustainable reality. Too many leaders have seen shared governance as another contemporary process that reflects the current landscape of health care and therefore something that must be considered and implemented. More organizations say they have shared governance than actually demonstrate that they do.

What is shared governance, exactly? There are any number of definitions, but most converge around the notion that shared governance is an organizational frame for configuring accountable professional decision making that fully engages the stakeholders by placing right decisions made by the right people in the right place at the right time for the right purposes (Prince, 1997). The simplicity of this definition belies the complexity of its construction. The mechanics of shared governance require an organizational construct that makes shared decision making the way of doing business within an accountable, professional work setting.

Shared governance is an accountability-based concept insofar as it builds on the notion of legitimate accountability and ownership for the outcomes of particular work (McDonagh, 1991). The system approaches accountability from its defining elements and constructs the organization frame around the locus-of-control for the exercise of particular accountabilities. Construction depends on the articulation of the definers of accountability, autonomy, authority and competence, and the specific enumeration of just what accountabilities exist in the organization, and where best they are placed to assure their appropriate and sustainable exercise.

Once accountability for decisions has been clearly numerated and role and performance expectations outlined, decisions that relate to the expression of those accountabilities are allocated and distributed throughout the organization. An infrastructure for advancing their legitimacy and its exercise is constructed to define, link, and integrate decisions and activities through an intersecting and seamless dynamic that assures organizational integrity and the achievement of related outcomes. Normally, decision capacity is identified within the context of management or organizational decisions and clinical or professional decisions. Traditionally, shared governance structures build on the delineation of the five management accountabilities of human, fiscal, material, support, and systems processes and the professional alignment of accountability for practice, quality, and competence (Porter-O'Grady, 1992). The general rule of engagement for a shared governance system is the clear (exclusive or reserved) delineation of these functional alignments, demonstrating the partnership necessary to make each demarcation work effectively and intersect safely and productively. In shared governance systems, managers do not make clinical decisions and clinicians do not make management decisions.

This distinction between organizational and management accountability (often called resource accountability or contextual accountability) and professional accountability (also called content accountability) is a critical distinction within a shared governance system (Evans, Hawkins, Curley, & Porter-O'Grady, 1995). Accountability does assume some exclusivity or reserved powers based on the rule and performance expectations related to them. Within this logic, it is essential that the accountability specific or distinct to managers be articulated and allocated, and, just as vital, is the need to clearly state the accountabilities that belong to the professional. In the case of nursing shared governance, the professional accountabilities that are unique to the discipline are practice, quality, and competence, as would be delineated within the context of any professional discipline. Within the shared governance rubric, these would be reserved to the profession, and all decisions, activities, and processes related to them would fall within the performance expectations of the professional. The obligation of the system, managers, and support structures would be evidenced in their responsiveness to these decisions made exclusively by the professional staff. The shared elements in the decisional process are exercised in the strategic integration between organizational goals and professional obligations. The organizational and work infrastructure of shared governance is designed to support and advance these intersecting accountabilities and unique role capacities.

Finally, one of the critical elements related to implementation and exercise of shared governance principles is the notion of partnership. Organizational infrastructure and systems support must be constructed within the context of horizontal linkages between the parties accountable and the partnerships among them necessary to sustain the mutual goals of all stakeholders. In these partnership arrangements, all members have specific and unique obligations to the partnership and roles to play in advancing its purposes. Professionals at the point of service, consultants, experts, and clinical specialists (or advanced practitioners) all play a role and make a unique contribution to the clinical concert that is nursing practice. Managers, too, play a significant role in creating a context and advancing the effective decisions of the organization regardless of their locus of control. Each party to this mosaic of interactions and intersections must fully engage his or her role and play that part that maintains and sustains the collaboration necessary to achieve the outcomes that cannot be obtained without it. This mutuality and collateral set of relationships is pivotal to both the structuring and expression of shared governance in the clinical system.

Shared governance represents the consonance of necessary forces to assure both professional and collaborative practices converge to sustain the positive impact on purpose and patient care. Built on the foundations of accountability, reflecting the fundamental characteristics of professional obligation, constructed on an appropriately conceived organizational infrastructure, representing the characteristics of professional partnership and exhibiting the elements of a clearly articulated locus of control, shared governance reflects the best in supporting organizational architecture (Malloch & Porter-O'Grady, 2006). In an increasingly complex and horizontally linked clinical environment, prerequisites of accountability partnership and discipline-specific integrity are accelerated. The shared governance organizational infrastructure creates a frame for the behaviors and relationships necessary to truly advance an evidence-driven patient centered clinical environment necessary to build the future of professional, quality-based health care.

TIM PORTER-O'GRADY

REFERENCES

Evans, K., Hawkins, M., Curley, T., & Porter-O'Grady, T. (1995). Whole systems shared governance: A model for the integrated health system. *Journal of Nursing Administration, 25*(5), 18–27.

Malloch, K., & Porter-O'Grady, T. (2006). *Introduction to evidence-based practice in nursing and healthcare.* Boston: Jones & Bartlett.

McDonagh, K. (1991). *Nursing shared governance.* Atlanta, GA: KJ McDonagh Associates, Inc.

Porter-O'Grady, T. (1992). *Implementing shared governance.* Baltimore: Mosby Publishers.

Porter-O'Grady, T. (2001). Is shared governance still relevant? *Journal of Nursing Administration, 31*(10), 468–473.

Prince, S. (1997). Shared governance: Sharing power and opportunity. *Journal of Nursing Administration, 27*(3), 28–35.

Sigma Theta Tau International (STTI)

T HE HONOR SOCIETY OF NURSING, Sigma Theta Tau International (STTI) provides leadership and scholarship in practice, education, and research to enhance the health of all people. STTI supports the learning and professional development of members striving to improve nursing care worldwide. Membership is by invitation to baccalaureate and graduate nursing students who demonstrate excellence in scholarship, and to nurse leaders exhibiting exceptional achievements in nursing. Established in 1922 by six nurses, the name is derived from the Greek words *Storgé*, *Tharos*, and *Timé*, meaning "love," "courage," and "honor." The honor society was incorporated in 1985 as Sigma Theta Tau International, Inc., a not-for-profit organization with a 501(c)(3) tax status in the United States. The society's 446 chapters are located at 535 institutions of higher education throughout the United States, as well as in Australia, Botswana, Brazil, Canada, Ghana, Hong Kong, Japan, Korea, Mexico, the Netherlands, Pakistan, South Africa, Swaziland, Sweden, Taiwan, and Tanzania. From its inception, the honor society has recognized the value of scholarship and excellence in nursing practice. In 1936, the honor society became the first U.S. organization to fund nursing research. Today, the honor society supports these values through numerous professional

501

development products and services that focus on the core areas of education, leadership, career development, evidence-based nursing, research, and scholarship. These products and services advance learning and professional development of members and all nurses who strive to improve the health of the world's people. STTI also produces publications that support the learning and professional development of nurses, and houses in its Indianapolis, Indiana, headquarters the Virginia Henderson International Nursing Library; a premier, online library offering a collection of more than 17,000 nursing research studies; and also researchers' demographic information and study abstracts. The library also contains abstracts from major nursing research conferences, including research events sponsored by the honor society.

The Honor Society of Nursing
Sigma Theta Tau International
550 West North Street
Indianapolis, IN 46202
(888) 634-7575 (Toll-free USA and Canada only)
+1 (317) 634-8171 (International)
stti@stti.iupui.edu

DIANE MANCINO

WEB REFERENCE

Sigma Theta Tau International, http://www.nursingsociety.org

Staff Recruitment

ACCORDING TO THE National Association for Health Care Recruitment staff recruitment for a health care organization can be defined as the search for the "best candidate using a swift, outcome-oriented approach" (National Association for Health Care Recruitment, 2005). The "best candidate" is one who presents as the most qualified, meets basic competency for the position, and is a "fit" for the organization's needs. The search is composed of a number of strategies, processes, and procedures that, when combined and evaluated, will contribute to the operational success of the health care organization. A successful recruitment program begins with knowledge of appropriate employment laws and regulations governing the process, and the development of a recruitment plan that is based on information gathered from various sources.

The recruitment plan should start with a review of the organization's strategic plan for health care program creation, or growth. Questions to be answered in defining the scope of a recruitment plan include: What will the staffing needs for these health care delivery programs look like? Will there be corresponding downsizing of existing services that require redeployment of current staff with needs for additional education and

503

training? Does the organization have educational resources in place to support program change and staff training? What is the available labor market for the specific categories of staff needed? What is the hiring competition within that market? And, last but not least, what is the organization's reputation within the community? Understanding these internal and external influences that impact recruitment of staff is critical to the success of a recruitment plan. Other data necessary for the planning process include measures of vacancy and turnover rates for various health care positions, the number of days on average it takes to fill a vacant position, and the average cost per hire that is expended. These figures should be tracked and trended on an annual basis to determine appropriate allocation of recruitment staff and financial resources. By using the projected numbers of staff needed times the cost per hire, a budget can be determined to support various sourcing and marketing strategies. Vacancy information also can be used to determine where budgeted dollars should be allocated.

A recruitment plan includes diverse sourcing mechanisms, such as use of targeted health care employment and niche Web sites, local and national print advertising, onsite hiring events, and outside career fairs. Another important recruitment source is the organization's employment Web site. The site should be well publicized and easy to navigate. A successful recruitment plan also acknowledges the efforts of current employees in attracting candidates to the organization through an Employee Referral Program (ERP). The message conveyed to prospective candidates through each of these venues should reflect the mission, vision, and values of the health care organization and how it blends with the applicant's own personal philosophy.

To determine the success of the various sourcing strategies, it is important to maintain statistics such as the number of completed applications from qualified applicants, what venues are identified by the applicants, and how many days it took to fill the vacancy. Another aspect of recruitment planning involves how applicants will be screened, interviewed, and selected. "Applicants become candidates when they [are screened] and interviewed for a specific position" (National Association for Health Care Recruitment, 2005). The completed application provides contact information, educational preparation, a detailed outline of the applicant's work experience and history, and the applicant's dated signature acknowledging the accuracy of the information provided. The interview and selection procedures use questions that allow the hiring manager to determine the applicant's specific qualifications for the position and assess the basic competency needed to carry out the associated duties and responsibilities of the job. The questions should be open-ended and focus on the applicant's work experiences and behaviors. By using "behavioral-based" questions, those that seek examples of past experience, the hiring manager can assess future professional or technical competency in a related situation. The interview is also a time when the applicant is assessed for "fit" or how professional conduct and work behaviors in previous positions or roles will translate into the prospective work unit or organizational culture. The goal in this part of the plan is to select the "best candidate" for a position using an outcome-oriented approach. Follow-up and the offer should be done quickly, with the offer of employment contingent upon completion of the postoffer screening process (background/reference information, license and credential verification, health and drug screening, and any other verification of employment documentation). A continuous review of the recruitment plan and the associated information collected and trended provides the opportunity to evaluate the overall success of the organization's staff recruitment program and how it contributes to organizational success over time.

ANN T. BURES

REFERENCE

National Association for Health Care Recruitment. (2005). *Recruiter's handbook.* Orlando, FL: Author.

Staff Retention

S TAFF RETENTION within health care organizations is one of the most important concerns for health care executives today as projections for employment growth opportunities for health care practitioners and technical occupations is expected to rise 30.3% through 2014, while the available labor force during this same period is expected to be reduced by 10% (U.S. Department of Labor, Bureau of Labor Statistics, 2005). There are currently 77 million people in the United States born between 1947 and 1964 (commonly known as Baby Boomers), and only 44 million people born between 1965 and 1977 (Generation X). These statistics have a direct impact on the ability of health care organizations to attract and retain members of a younger generation into the health care workforce, while effectively delivering health care programs to meet the demand of an aging population. To achieve success, health care organizations should assess and implement measures that influence employee engagement. Effective staff retention in a health care organization is rooted in a "sense of community focused on the mission, vision and values of the organization" (National Association for Health Care Recruitment [NAHCR], 2005). This "model of stability" is established by building a "strong, collaborative culture with positive attitudes at all levels within the organization" (NAHCR, 2005).

A successful retention program actually begins with a recruitment process that matches the employee with the job and organizational culture. Important cultural influences in attracting and retaining the "right" employee include, but are not limited to: meaningful work; a clear understanding of work objectives; the quality of relationships with managers and supervisors; the level of trust in the organization; growth and advancement opportunities; compensation and benefits and the ability to balance work/home (NAHCR, 2005).

Meaningful work and a clear understanding of work objectives is provided through a continuous review and update of job descriptions, roles and areas of responsibility, and delivery of regular, timely performance reviews to establish and measure performance expectations. In addition, soliciting feedback and suggestions from current staff on needs for further training and professional development, as well as addressing these suggestions, can directly impact the quality of manager/staff relations as employees recognize the value of their input. Training and development should not be limited to maintaining clinical competency but also should focus on career growth and mastery of new skills. Building an environment of trust and respect means building internal communication tools that keep employees informed. From Intranet sites and Web-based conferencing systems to "town-hall forums" and unit-based staff meetings, the delivery of information to staff should be open, honest, and timely. An open environment also provides the catalyst for collaboration among employees, fostering teamwork and opportunities to contribute to the organization's strategic planning process.

Health care organizations today are continuously challenged to provide fair, market-based pay and benefits to remain competitive in an ever-tightening labor market. In order to avoid violation of federal antitrust laws, use of third-party salary survey data should assure that information collected is valid, reliable, and a fair assessment of the current market. It is equally important to communicate summary findings to current staff related to their pay placement within the community, and to respond as quickly as possible to making pay adjustments to maintain market competitiveness. Again, the message to staff is one of valuing their contributions by assuring fair wages and benefits. Closely tied to offering fair compensation is recognition that at least one-third of a person's life is spent at work. Through programs that monitor the availability of adequate unit supplies, use of adaptive and assistive devices that support workplace ergonomics and safety, support staff that allow those engaged in patient care to focus on patient care, and staff scheduling alternatives that support various employee's needs, the organization is placing emphasis on enhancing the quality of the person's work life. And that internal acknowledgment lends itself to placing emphasis on promoting programs, such as flexible scheduling, job sharing, enhanced time off programs, parking availability and commuter services, on-site services such as child day care, cafeteria "meals-to-go," and dry cleaners to support the employee's "life balance" needs and family considerations.

An effective retention program is "owned" by every staff member in the organization. When those staff members who contribute daily to successful patient outcomes are respected and valued, the organization benefits as a whole by earning trust and achieving credibility to be known in the larger health care community as an "employer of choice."

ANN T. BURES

See Also
Staff Recruitment

REFERENCES

U.S. Department of Labor, Bureau of Labor Statistics. (2005). *BLS releases 2004–14 employment projections*. Retrieved September 30, 2007, from http://www. bls.gov/news.release/ecopro.nr0.htm

National Association for Health Care Recruitment. (2005). *Recruiter's handbook*. Orlando, FL: Author.

WEB REFERENCES

Society for Human Resources Management, http://www.shrm.org
American Hospital Association, http://www.hospitalconnect.org
American Association of Critical Care Nurses, http://www.aacn.org
American College of Healthcare Executives, http://www.ache.org
Nursing Spectrum/NurseWeek, http://www.nursingspectrum.com
Bernard Hodes Group, http://www.hodes.com
Monster.com, http://www.adcomms.tmp.com
Bureau of Health Professions, http://www.bhpr.hrsa.gov

Staffing
Effectiveness

A **N IMPORTANT COMPONENT** of executive nursing practice is the appropriate allocation and utilization of human resources. Whether it is through an annual budgeting process or day-to-day staffing, providing the right number of nurses to meet the care requirements of patients is an art and a science. Accurate definition and quantification of the work of nursing is critical to the identification of appropriate nursing resource requirements. In acute care settings, the most common definition of nursing work is the patient day, and nursing resource requirements are expressed as hours per patient day or, in more recent discussions, as nurse-patient ratios (Graf, Millar, Feilteau, Coakley, & Ives Erickson, 2003). There does not exist, however, a single methodology that is the answer for every health care organization.

Providing the optimal number of nursing personnel with the appropriate mix of registered nurses to unlicensed assistive personnel to meet the needs of patients is based on numerous factors including patient acuity, experience of the nurse, the environment of care, and technology and other staff support systems (Ives Erickson, 2002). Identification of required direct care staffing occurs at three levels: long-term projections for the fiscal year, near-term scheduling for successive time-plan cycles,

509

and daily staffing for shift-to-shift requirements. Commonly, staffing levels are based on volume and acuity of patients (nursing workload) and factored for distribution of workload over various time periods, experience, and mix of staff, as well as logistical and support issues (Ives Erickson, 2002). Each organization must look at structure and process to determine the right approach to staff to effectively meet the patient's requirements for nursing care. Staffing effectiveness involves "defining competencies and expectations for all staff. Staffing includes assessing those defined competencies and allocating the human resources necessary for patient safety and improved patient outcomes" (Joint Commission on Accreditation of Healthcare Organizations, 2006). Staffing projections and total budgeted full-time equivalent (FTE) requirements are developed in conjunction with the overall organizational budgeting process. The budgeting process is based on anticipated volume, admissions, length of stay and procedure volume, and patient acuity. These data are then utilized to develop unit specific staffing budgets. Key target ratios, such as hours per unit of work, staff mix and nonproductive factors, are identified using current and historical data.

One approach to staffing is the implementation of a system that identifies the patient's needs for nursing care. Patient acuity systems or nursing workload measurement systems provide an indication of staffing requirements. Graf et al. (2003) explain that in addition to assisting in day-to-day staffing decisions,

> acuity systems provide an opportunity for storing the raw data from the system at their most basic level provides and opportunities for more extensive analyses and informed, data-driven decision-making related to resource allocation, performance improvement and productivity enhancement." (p. 76)

At a time when many states in the country are considering enacting Nurse Staffing Legislation to establish staffing ratios for hospitals, it is important that everyone understand the issues and challenges of staffing to meet the care requirements of the patient and keep practice safe. Nurse staffing ratio advocates point to the need to mandate minimum staffing. The rationale is that the rates of poor patient outcomes are well known when staffing levels are poor. Several research studies have found significant associations between lower levels of nurse staffing and higher rates of pneumonia, failure to rescue, upper gastrointestinal bleeding, and urinary tract infections (Hickman et al., 2003; Needleman, Buerhaus, Mattke, Stewart, & Zelevinsky, 2002). Other studies found associations between lower staffing levels and pneumonia, lung collapse, falls, pressure ulcers, thrombosis after major surgery, pulmonary compromise after surgery, longer hospital stays, and 30-day mortality rates.

Researchers caution, however, that the research does not advocate for mandated staffing levels. Instead, research indicates that those patient outcomes that are driven primarily by the interventions of the nurse (nursing-sensitive indicators) should be viewed as poor outcomes rather than as measures of the impact of nurse staffing on patient outcomes. Opponents of ratio legislation point out that with staffing ratios, health care organizations run the risk of replacing critical nursing judgment and assessment with fixed numbers. The debate needs to be informed by considering the patient population in need of nursing care. Not all patients are the same. Care needs vary from patient to patient and for the same patient over time (Ives Erickson, 2002). Patient outcomes depend not only on the kind and severity of patients' illnesses but also on human resources factors such as the mix of nurses, doctors, and auxiliary personnel, and on the work environment or culture of the hospital. The key tenet is that no matter what the pressures may be, it is absolutely essential that we be able to provide the right clinician to the right patient at the right time, every time.

JEANETTE IVES ERICKSON

REFERENCES

Graf, C., Millar, S., Feilteau, C., Coakley, P., & Ives Erickson, J. (2003). Patients' needs for nursing care, beyond staffing ratios. *Journal of Nursing Administration, 33*(2), 76–81.

Hickman, D. H., Severance, S., Feldstein, A., Ray, L., Gorman, P., Schuldheis, S., et al. (2003, May). *The effect of health care working conditions on patient safety.* Evidence Report/Technology Assessment Number 74. (Prepared by Oregon Health & Science University under Contract No. 290-97-0018.) AHRQ Publication No. 03-E031. Rockville, MD: Agency for Healthcare Research and Quality.

Ives Erickson, J. (2002, March 7). In the debate over arbitrary staffing ratios, we must be the voice of reason, *Caring Headlines*, 2–3.

Joint Commission on Accreditation of Healthcare Organizations, Department of Publications, Joint Commission Resources. (2006). *2006 hospital accreditation standards.* Oakbrook Terrace, IL: Author.

Needleman, J., Buerhaus, P., Mattke, S., Stewart, M., & Zelevinsky, K. (2002). *Nurse-staffing levels and patient outcomes in hospitals.* Final report for Health Resources and Services Administration. Contract No. 230-99-0021. Harvard.

State and Territorial Health Departments

RESPONSIBILITY FOR THE health of the citizens of the United States is dispersed through a broad array of federal, state, and local governmental, and nongovernmental agencies; however, state and territorial health departments are the agencies that have the ultimate authority and responsibility for the public's health. This authority derives from the sovereign powers reserved for states under the Constitution of the United States. The United States presently has sovereignty over five territories that were ceded as a result of war or treaty. States may and do delegate some of it powers to local units of government. State and territorial health departments have major roles in formulating, implementing, regulating, monitoring, and coordinating public health policies. State and territorial health departments articulate and cooperate with federal agencies, often serving as the conduits for distribution of federal funds to local communities. They initiate action for change, set standards, develop program models, and coordinate program efforts.

Nurses and nursing approaches are key elements in protecting the public's health. There are a number of top leadership positions in state and territorial health departments for which nurses are appropriately credentialed to fill. Among these are heads of departments, bureaus, centers, and institutes such as Chief of the Bureaus of Maternal and Child Health or Chronic Diseases or the Center for Health Promotion. These positions usually require at least a Master's degree in nursing, public health, public administration, or the equivalent plus a minimum of 5 years' public health experience. The chief executive position in state and territorial health departments is that of the Director or Commissioner of Health, also referred to as the state health officer. The first nurses were appointed to the position of state health director in 1983: Barbara J. Sabol in Kansas and Gloria R. Smith in Michigan (Smith, 1990). The appointment is a gubernatorial one with legislature confirmation in majority of the states. Unlike that of many other political appointees, most people appointed to state health director positions have recognized credentials in related fields. Twenty-five states in 2005 still required the state health officer to have a medical degree, with 10 of those requiring in addition a Master of Public Health (MPH) degree or equivalent experience.

Many nurses have appropriate credentials in public health and have creditable experiences in public health practice and administration. Nurses also have demonstrated leadership skills and have experiences in multidisciplinary problem solving and collaboration. The field is fertile for nurses who have an interest in providing leadership in state and territorial health departments. Some settings may be more politically charged than others and there may be expectations for the state health officer to make political contributions of one sort or another. In most settings, these appointees may be more isolated from party politics but always must be aware that they are a part of the government that is temporarily in power. Information about the structure, budgets, salaries, fringe benefits, and characteristics of state and territorial health departments can be accessed at http://www.astho.org (Association of State and Territorial Health Officials, 2005).

GLORIA R. SMITH

REFERENCES

Smith, G. R. (1990). Nursing and political power: The cutting edge of change. In J. C. McCloskey & H. Grace (Eds.), *Current issues in nursing* (3rd ed., p. 444). St. Louis, MO: C. V. Mosby.

Association of State and Territorial Health Officials. (2005). *2005 SHO salary and agency infrastructure study*. Washington, DC: Author. Retrieved September 9, 2006, from http://www.astho.org/pubs/2005SalarySurveyFinal.pdf

Staupers, Mabel Keaton

MABEL KEATON STAUPERS, a courageous nursing leader and black activist, was born in February 1890, in Barbados, West Indies. She died in Washington, DC in 1989 at the age of 99. Staupers was the first executive secretary of the National Association of Colored Graduate Nurses (NACGN). Never known to back down or retreat from an issue, Staupers's life was totally dedicated to the equality and advancement of blacks in general, and to the promotion and greater good of black nurses, in particular (American Nurses Association, 2006). Staupers immigrated to the United States with her parents at age 13. In 1917, she graduated with honors from the Freedmen's Hospital School of Nursing in Washington, DC. Observant of segregated schools of nursing, segregated hospital beds, and rank segregation in organizations that included the National League for Nursing Education and the American Nurses Association, Staupers was resolved to initiate change that would generate and guarantee equal rights for black nurses that would alert the public to disparities in treatment of blacks, and that ultimately would result in improved access to health care services for black Americans everywhere (Carnegie, 1995). In the ANA citation for induction into the Hall of Fame, it is stated (with regard to Staupers's leadership of NACGN), ". . . Staupers

514

increased membership, established a citizens advisory committee, built coalitions with other nursing and non-nursing groups, and effectively tore down the racial barriers that previously kept black nurses out of the military" (American Nurses Association, 2006). Staupers was recipient of numerous awards, including the Mary Mahoney Medal in 1914, the prestigious Springarn Medal from the NAACP in 1931, the Sojourner Truth Medal in 1947, the National Urban League Team Work Award, 1967, and the Medgar Evers Human Rights Award in 1965 (Carnegie, 1995). She was inducted posthumously into the American Nurses Association Hall of Fame in 1996.

M. JANICE NELSON

See Also
American Nurses Association
ANA Hall of Fame
National Black Nurses Association, Inc.
National League for Nursing

REFERENCES

American Nurses Association. (2006). *Mabel Keaton Staupers (1890–1989) 1996 inductee.* Retrieved September 14, 2007, from http://www.nursingworld.org/FunctionalMenuCategories/AboutANA/WhereWeComeFrom_1/HallofFame/19962000Inductees/stauperm5584.aspx

Carnegie, M. E. (1995). *The path we tread: Blacks in nursing worldwide* (3rd ed.). New York: National League for Nursing Press.

Stewart, Isabel Maitland

ISABEL MAITLAND STEWART was born in Canada in 1878 and died in New Jersey at the age of 85. She graduated from the Manitoba Normal School and the Winnipeg Collegiate Institution. She subsequently entered the Nurses Training School at Winnipeg General Hospital and graduated in 1902 (Christy, 1969a). Stewart later attended the nursing program at Teachers College (TC), Columbia University. She earned a 1-year certificate, a 2-year diploma, a Bachelor of Science and a Master of Arts degree, all in that order. She never completed requirements for the doctorate but was awarded three honorary doctorates during the course of her career. Stewart served as Professor of Nursing of the Helen Hartley Foundation, and as Director of the Department of Nursing and Health at TC. Her tenure spanned the years from 1925 until 1947 (Christy, 1969a). Stewart was committed to nursing research and spearheaded a study to delineate between nursing and nonnursing functions. She established, for the first time, university-sponsored studies utilizing a team approach in collaboration with clinical facilities at Lincoln Hospital in Harlem. Stewart (along with Nutting) was often called on for advice and consultation in the development and implementation of nursing education programs. The formation of the National League for Nursing

Education Committee on University Relations emerged from these activities. This committee later became the National Association of Collegiate Schools of Nursing, which was established in 1932. Stewart was deeply involved in setting standards for nursing curricula, establishing guidelines for schools of nursing, and developing of tests and measurements to determine student achievement (Christy, 1969b). In retirement, Stewart served as Chair of the National League for Nursing's Committee on Historical Source Materials. She was inducted posthumously into the ANA Hall of Fame in 1978. Additional information on Stewart and her writings can be accessed on the Web at http://www.teacherscollege.edu/nursing.

M. JANICE NELSON

See Also
ANA Hall of Fame
National League for Nursing

REFERENCES

Christy, T. E. (1969a). Portrait of a leader: Isabel Maitland Stewart. *Nursing Outlook, 17*(10), 88–92.

Christy, T. E. (1969b). *Cornerstone for nursing education: A history of the division of nursing education of Teachers, College, Columbia University: 1899–1947*. New York: Teachers College Press.

Strategic Planning

S TRATEGIC PLANNING is the process of identifying directions and facilitating the alignment of purpose, people, plans, and actions with the aim of serving a cocreated, value driven, desired outcome. Strategic planning is supported by strategic learning. Schwartz (1991) makes a distinction between "strategic" and "tactical" planning. Strategic planning includes attention to the "big picture" of a situation whereas "tactical" planning focuses on detailed local activities. Essential components of strategic planning involve core leadership competencies of anticipation, alignment, and action (Deering, Dilts, & Russell, 2002).

Pietersen (2002) proposes a four-stage strategy for strategic planning: learning, focusing, aligning, and executing. Strategic planning requires an organization and its leadership to ask and answer three key questions (Pietersen, 2002): (1) What is the environment in which our organization must compete and win? (2) What are those few things our organization must do outstandingly well to win and go on winning in this environment? and (3) How will we mobilize our organization to implement these things faster and better than our competitors? The strategic learning cycle involves generating insight into changing environments, making strategic choices, aligning an organization behind a chosen strategic focus and implementing and experimenting with an executed strategy, while concurrently learning throughout the process. Dilts (1996) defines strategic thinking as the ability to identify a relevant desired state, assess the starting state, and then establish and navigate the appropriate path of transition states required to reach the desired state.

A key element of effective strategic thinking is related to discerning which people and processes will most efficiently and effectively influence and change the present state in the direction of the desired state. Robert Dilts (1996) offers a logical-levels model for thinking and acting in terms of learning and planning. There are three levels to consider in the Dilts Model: meta, macro, and micro. Meta level planning involves attention and mindfulness to organizational issues of spirit, vision, and identity. Macro level planning involves attention to path finding, culture building, beliefs, and values that support organizational identity and role-performance configurations. Micro level planning involves attention to environmental variables related to efficiency, task, relationship, and capabilities, as well as behaviors that support or inhibit strategic alignment of purpose, people, plans, and actions that serve a greater good or desired outcome. At each level of learning and planning, a specific leadership skill is called forth. For example, at the meta leadership level, one needs leadership influence that involves the development of a charismatic leadership skill set. This also requires attention to the learning from changes taking place in the environment and developing some insight into the environmental changes. At the level of identity one needs to craft leadership influence with some consideration for individual talents and strengths within an organization and a focus on strategic choices related to the special mission of the organization and its contribution to the environment. At the level of values and beliefs, leaders need to influence and inspire people in the organization, serve as cheerleader and coach, and challenge people to consider how they might rethink their own ideas in light of organizational aspirations and goals.

Leadership for strategic planning is about helping people think through old problems in new ways with intelligence, rationality, and careful outcome specification. As leadership attends to issues of behavior, action, and execution, clear representation of desired goals and evidence for achievement of those goals is essential. Implementing and experimenting with the execution of a strategic plan involves reliance on the capabilities and resources of individuals and the organization to engage in reflective learning processes that contribute to insights and ongoing organizational learning. As the leader's attention turns to specific behaviors, leadership concerns turn attention to contracting rewards for effort and being clear about expectations in exchange for effort and special commendations associated with promotions for good work. Most strategic plans fail because of failure to define end state objectives clearly or because of a poor implementation strategy (Borgesson, 2007).

DANIEL J. PESUT

REFERENCES

Borgesson, M. (2007). *Scenario planning resources*. Retrieved August 13, 2007, from http://www.well.com/~mb/scenario_planning/

Deering, A., Dilts, R., & Russell, J. (2002). *Alpha leadership*. New York: John Wiley.

Dilts, R. (1996). *The new leadership paradigm*. Retrieved September 10, 2006, from http://www.nlpu.com/Articles/article8.htm

Pietersen, W. (2002). *Reinventing strategy: Using strategic learning to create and sustain breakthrough performance*. New York: John Wiley.

Schwartz, P. (1991). *The art of the long view*. New York: Doubleday Currency.

Student Recruitment

ACCORDING TO THE September 2006 fact sheet of the American Association of Colleges of Nursing (AACN; 2001), by the year 2020, the nursing shortage will grow to more than one million nursing vacancies. Recruitment strategies, although varied and innovative, need to start at the academic level, to interest both potential students in the profession and nursing school graduates in furthering their education to facilitate career advancement.

Many recruitment strategies can be utilized at both undergraduate and graduate levels. One example of this is participation in organizational career fairs, such as the state nurse's association and professional journal fairs. Membership in local, state, and national health care recruiter organizations enables the school of nursing to network and affiliate with area hospitals and health care organizations to collaborate on recruitment incentives, such as sign-on bonuses, senior year tuition remission, and participation in mentorship programs that pair the new nurse with an experienced staff nurse.

At the undergraduate level, recruitment starts at an early age, by reaching out to middle school and high school students to increase awareness of the benefits of the nursing profession. "Answers to the question, 'What do I want to be when I grow up?' usually start to gel during the middle and high school years. Savvy college recruiters looking to develop a pool of future nursing students from diverse backgrounds have taken steps to reach this key demographic" (AACN, 2001). With the help of school guidance counselors, information can be disseminated regarding such programs as a Summer Scholars Camp for students to spend a week at a school of nursing with faculty counselors, visits to the local school of nursing to tour and learn and perform hands-on skills, such as assessing vital signs in the school's learning resource lab, and pairing a high school with a nursing school student to shadow for the day. Nursing school recruiters should be a presence at the local middle and high schools by participating in career day sessions to represent the profession with information about health care career options and demonstrations of a basic skill to smaller groups. At the high school level, university enrollment management builds a pool of prospective students by buying lists from organizations, such as the SAT, the ACT, and the Princeton Review. Once the potential student is contacted, invitations to open houses and school tours, and meetings with the nurse recruiter help convert the "contact pool" to an "applicant" pool. Various school "conversion events," such as phonathons, in which nursing faculty and recruiters contact the accepted/undecided students, and "Student for a Day," in which potential students are paired with a nursing student, and scholarship dinners, help convert the applicant pool into an accepted/deposited pool. Another group of potential nursing students is the "second career" group. These are people who are desirous of a career change and have an interest in nursing, or have heard about nursing from a colleague or family member and decided to pursue it. Traditional open houses are not the appropriate venue for this group, so that universities and schools of nursing hold "Information Sessions" in the evening to facilitate attendance for people in the workforce.

There needs to be a great deal of creativity when recruiting graduate nursing students. Because they are already registered nurses, their place of work provides an excellent site for recruitment. This can be done by collaborating with the nursing education or human resources departments of the health care agency to arrange a mutually convenient time and location to set up a table with recruitment materials from the school of nursing or university. Utilizing the World Wide Web is another medium to recruit this population. One example of the use of the Web is delivering e-mail blasts to potential students, informing them of upcoming information sessions and announcements regarding new programs. Another use would be participation in Chat University, where prospective students are invited to participate in a virtual "chat" with nursing school faculty and representatives from enrollment management. A third use of the Internet would be identifying resources for further exploration of nursing programs. Examples of these sites include:

* Allnursingschools.com
* NursingSpectrum.com
* Advanceweb.com
* Minoritynurse.com
* Nursingdigest.com
* Jnj.com
* NAHCR.com

During times when we face enormous nursing shortages, it is vitally important for undergraduate and graduate nursing programs in colleges and universities make a concerted effort to recruit for their respective programs, partnering with health care institutions whenever possible, to facilitate workforce recruitment and retention.

JUDITH DEBLASIO
JANE DOLAN

See Also
Nursing Shortage in the United States
Staff Recruitment
Staff Retention

REFERENCES

American Association of Colleges of Nursing. (2001, December). *Effective strategies for increasing diversity in nursing programs*. Retrieved October 6, 2006, from http://www.aacn.nche.edu/publications/issues/dec01.htm

American Association of Colleges of Nursing. (2006, September). *Nursing shortage*. Retrieved October 10, 2006, from http://www.aacn.nche.edu/media/factsheets/nursingshortage.htm

Center for Nursing Excellence. (n.d.). *Nurse recruitment strategies*. Retrieved October 6, 2006, from http://www.nmnursingexcellence.org/docs/pdf/recruitment_strategies.pdf

Student Retention

MANY FACTORS CONTRIBUTE to the retention of students in nursing programs: student-program fit; program progression policies, opportunities for remediation; financial issues; and cultural and student support issues. Retention strategies need to be planned and implemented long before students are admitted to nursing programs. These strategies need to be consistent with the type of program, philosophy of enrollment, diversity of the student population, and the human and fiscal resources that underpin a successful retention program. Furthermore, the retention of nursing students extends beyond graduation to the successful passing of the NCLEX-RN.

RETENTION AND ADMISSION

ADMISSION policies and criteria vary from program to program, some emphasizing more open access and others using a combination of quantitative measures such as Scholastic Aptitude Test (SAT) scores, high school quintile, and high school grade point average (GPA) to select the highest performing students possible. If the

524

admission of academically disadvantaged students is part of the program's mission, there needs to be a well designed, formal retention plan and program that tracks student progress and provides the necessary supports, such as tutoring, counseling, and other programs that teach study, organizational, cultural adaptation, and stress management skills. Nursing faculty also need support in the form of tools and time to conduct a successful retention program. For example, Arizona State University (ASU) has developed formal retention programs for all of its majors. The ASU retention policy can be viewed at http://www.asu.edu/retention/exemplary/pdf/KA_Nursing.pdf.

CALCULATING NURSING STUDENT ATTRITION/RETENTION

T HERE is no standard formula used by all programs or states to calculate nursing student attrition or retention. The formula used by the North Carolina Center for Nursing calculates the attrition rate using the following formula:

$$\frac{\#\ \text{Students Who Started} - \#\ \text{Students Who Graduated on Time}}{\#\ \text{of Students Who Started}} * 100$$

(http://www.asu.edu/retention/exemplary/pdf/KA_Nursing.pdf)

California defines the retention rate as the percentage of students who complete the program on schedule versus the number who are still enrolled but behind in their cohort (http://www.rn.ca.gov/forms/pdf/schoolrpt04-05.pdf). Nursing programs should have a clearly understood formula that is generally applied across years and cohorts so that the program's retention rate can drive retention strategies.

RETENTION AND PROGRESSION

E VERY accredited nursing program publishes progression criteria so that students understand the performance level they must achieve to move through the program. Because of the clinical nature of nursing programs, nursing progression criteria may be set higher than the overall university policy. It is useful for programs to develop a database that tracks the following: (1) number of "F" and "D" grades that nursing students earn throughout the course of their program; (2) number and demographic profile of students that successfully repeat "F" and "D" grade courses and progress on; and (3) number and demographic profile of students that drop out of the nursing program. The demographic profile can include faculty-selected variables such as overall GPA and SAT on admission; GPA in selected science courses; and admission status, for example, transfer or freshman admit. These cumulative data can provide a predictive success model for faculty to use in their admission process and in improving their retention programs.

RETENTION AND NCLEX-RN SUCCESS

SUCCESS on the NCLEX-RN needs to be part of nursing program retention strategies. It is the responsibility of every nursing program to ensure that the graduate is prepared to attain licensure to practice. There are a variety of strategies that include periodic testing across the nursing curriculum as well as a summative, comprehensive test with predictive values. Any testing program selected by faculty, whether faculty-designed or standardized by a testing service, should be accompanied by a faculty designed remediation policy and program for those students who fall below the passing standard.

SUMMARY

THE EXTENDED U.S. nursing shortage has pushed the nursing student retention issue and NCLEX-RN pass rates increasingly into the spotlight. Retention programs in schools of nursing should be derived from the admission and progression philosophy and policies of the program and should be faculty-designed and -driven.

GLORIA F. DONNELLY

See Also
Licensure

REFERENCES

Arizona State University. (n.d.). *College of nursing exemplary programs for retention.* Retrieved October 7, 2006, from http://www.asu.edu/retention/exemplary/pdf/KA_Nursing.pdf

California Board of Registered Nursing. (2006). *2004–2005 Annual school report.* Retrieved October 10, 2006, from http://www.rn.ca.gov/forms/pdf/schoolrpt04-05.pdf

Student Satisfaction

S TUDENT SATISFACTION may be defined as "a short-term attitude resulting from an evaluation of a student's educational experience. Satisfaction results when actual performance meets or exceeds the student's expectations" (Elliott, 2003). Educational leaders have acknowledged the importance of congruence between what students expect from their educational experience and their satisfaction with what they perceive as the reality of that experience. Research indicates that the greater the congruence, the greater the likelihood for increased student motivation, retention, recruitment, persistence, stability, increased graduation rates and higher overall student success (Bryant & Crockett, 2004).

Student reporting of satisfaction with an institution or specific program includes a combination of academic factors, as well as areas related to student life. Instructional and academic advising effectiveness are reported as being of high importance on the academic scales: Campus climate (belonging), campus life issues (dorms, athletics, policies), campus support (tutoring, library and computer facilities), perceived institutional concern for the individual, recruitment/financial aid effectiveness (availability/access), registration effectiveness (course availability), the

527

institutional response to diversity (ethnic, educational, socioeconomic, gender, gender orientation), safety, service, and the noted level of student centeredness (the extent to which students feel welcomed and valued) also are areas that are addressed when assessing student satisfaction (Bryant & Crockett, 2004).

Student satisfaction assessment should be a systematic process, not an isolated event, with satisfaction shifts tracked and used for ongoing program assessment and evaluation. The measurement of student satisfaction is a significant element of institutional assessment plans. Several instruments have been widely used, most notably the Student Satisfaction Inventory (SSI) and National Survey of Student Engagement (NSSE), both of which yield satisfaction as well as importance ratings data. In addressing student satisfaction, the level of importance that students place on a particular issue indicates the level of expectation and value that a student associates with that issue (Bryant & Crockett, 2004). An institution can use this as a gauge and identify performance gaps when data regarding satisfaction and importance are combined.

Specific to nursing programs, the American Association of Colleges of Nursing (AACN), in partnership with Educational Benchmarking Inc. (EBI), has created nursing education assessments that measure the effectiveness and satisfaction with nursing programs from the student's perspective. Data are collected regarding which learning outcomes and other key dimensions of programs (e.g., nursing labs, clinical placements/partnerships) are the strongest and which areas need to be improved. Other examples of areas addressed are the quality of nursing instruction, workload and class size, course lecture and interaction, professional values, core competencies, technical skills, role development, and overall program effectiveness. The knowledge gained from these assessments can drive and sustain continuous improvement programs and support accreditation efforts (Educational Benchmarking Inc., 2007).

LAUREN M. HUBER

See Also
American Association of Colleges of Nursing
Student Retention

REFERENCES

Beltyukova, S. (2002). Student satisfaction as a measure of student development: Towards a universal metric. *Journal of College Student Development, 43*(2), 161–172.

Bryant, P., & Crockett, D. (2004). *Best practices in student recruitment and retention: What successful institutions are doing to meet their enrollment objectives.* Iowa City, IA: Noel-Levitz, Inc.

Educational Benchmarking Inc. (2007). *Complete assessment solutions: AACN/ EBI nursing education exit assessment.* Retrieved April 13, 2007, from http://www.webebi.com/_AsmtServices/Nursing/exit.aspx

Elliott, K. (2003). Key determinants of student satisfaction. *Journal of College Student Retention, 4*(3), 271–279.

Lau, L. K. (2003). Institutional factors affecting student retention. *Education, 124*(1), 126–138.

WEB REFERENCES

National Survey of Student Engagement, http://nsse.iub.edu/index.cfm

Noel-Levitz, http://www.noellevitz.com

Styles, Margaretta

MARGARETTA [GRETA] STYLES was born on March 13, 1930, in Mount Union, Pennsylvania, and died on November 20, 2005, in Clearwater, Florida. Styles was a leader, visionary, and scholar, both at home and abroad. Styles had an exceptional leadership career. She was a past president of the American Nurses Association, the International Council of Nurses, the California Board of Registered Nursing, and the American Nurses Credentialing Center. Styles held three deanships: one at the University of California at San Francisco, a second at the University of Texas in Austin, and a third at Wayne State University in Detroit. Styles was a pacesetter in credentialing; she was considered the "architect" for the establishing of the American Nurses Credentialing Center which provides specific guidelines for all nursing specialties (Basu, 2005). Styles earned a baccalaureate in biology and chemistry at Juniata College; she earned her master of nursing degree at Yale, and a doctorate in education at the University of Florida. She was a fellow of the American Academy of Nursing and of the National Institute of Medicine. She received numerous awards, including the Nightingale Lamp Award from the American Nurses Foundation, and the Christiane Reimann Prize—the highest international honor—from the International Council of Nurses in recognition of her worldwide contributions to nursing. Styles also held a number of honorary doctorates. Styles will undoubtedly be best remembered for setting standards and credentials for excellence in nursing practice, and for her commitment to the advancement of the profession (American Nurses Association, 2006). She was inducted into the American Nurses Association Hall of Fame in 2000.

M. JANICE NELSON

See Also
American Academy of Nursing
American Nurses Association
ANA Hall of Fame
American Nurses Credentialing Center
American Nurses Foundation

REFERENCES

American Nurses Association. (2006). *Margretta Madden Styles (1930–2005) 2000 inductee*. Retrieved September 14, 2007, from http://www.nursingworld. org/FunctionalMenuCategories/AboutANA/WhereWeComeFrom_1/ HallofFame/20002004Inductees/STYLES5588.aspx

American Nurses Credentialing Center. (2004). *ANCC solicits grant applicants*. Retrieved March 30, 2006, from http://www.nursingworld.org/pressrel/ 2004/pr1007.htm

Basu, J. (2005, December 1). Former UCSF nursing dean Margretta Styles dies. *UCSF Today*. Retrieved September 14, 2007, from http://pub.ucsf.edu/today/ cache/news/200511306.html

Carmen, M. (2004). *A synopsis of the 2003 ANA Convention*. Retrieved March 30, 2006, from http://www.georgianurses.org/president_message_8_04.htm

Fuller, W. (1999). With a little help from our friends. *American Journal of Nursing. Vital Signs, 99*(10). Retrieved March 30, 2006, from http://www. nursingworld.org/AJN/1999/Sep/Vita099a.htm

SWOT Analysis

S TRATEGIC MANAGEMENT is the process through which an organization analyzes the competitive environment to understand threats, opportunities, resources, and capabilities. Based on that understanding, strategies are devised and implemented to neutralize threats and exploit opportunities. A SWOT analysis (*S*trengths, *W*eaknesses, *O*pportunities, and *T*hreats) is a key tool in the strategic management process. A SWOT analysis involves the evaluation of four components: strengths, weaknesses, opportunities, and threats. This method of analysis is used by many organizations to evaluate internal resources and capabilities while also evaluating the external environment to identify opportunities and threats. A SWOT analysis is helpful in identifying how internal and external factors might interact to create advantage for or to increase competitive pressures on a health care academic organization, and it can highlight areas where an organization is vulnerable, where it is constrained, where it should leverage its strengths, and where real problem areas reside.

OPPORTUNITIES AND THREATS

A NALYSES of opportunities and threats are aspects of an external environmental analysis. The external environment has increasingly become a factor in the success of health care organizations, and organizations must anticipate and respond to significant shifts taking place within that environment. Likewise, academic environments have been called on to address shifts in higher education and the marketplace. External factors include technological, social, regulatory, political, economic, and competitive forces. External factors also can include demographic shifts, changes in motivation for workers, and changes in the values, preferences, and expectations of customers. Whether health care or academic environments, organizations must understand and anticipate the impact of these external forces to stay in touch with the needs of the market.

When conducting an *external* environmental analysis, the following goals will help the organization to understand opportunities and threats:

* Identify and analyze current important issues that affect the organization's existing position in the market
* Detect and analyze signals of emerging issues that will affect the organization
* Speculate on future issues that will have significant impact on the organization
* Provide organized information for the development of the organization's mission, vision, values, objectives, internal analysis, and strategy

Several opportunities and threats will be identified as part of the external analysis. Opportunities might include adding to existing product lines or academic offerings, for example, to enter new markets or acquire new technologies. Threats might include new competition, unfavorable government policies, shifting consumer loyalties, or innovations that will radically change care delivery or teaching strategies.

STRENGTHS AND WEAKNESSES

E VALUATING strengths and weaknesses are aspects of an internal organizational assessment within a SWOT analysis, and will inform the organization about internal capabilities. Effective strategic management requires an understanding of internal organizational competencies, capabilities, and resources that lead to a competitive advantage.

When conducting an *internal* analysis, the following goals will help the organization to understand strengths and weaknesses:

* Understand the fit between the external environment and the present internal characteristics of the organization
* Identify which services have attributes that correspond to key preferences and selection criteria of patients, physicians, and staff (i.e., customers) in the target market
* Determine the value of the services provided by the organization versus that of competitors (in the minds of patients, physicians, and staff)
* Gauge the organization's ability to anticipate the future and respond to changing conditions

Several strengths and weaknesses may be identified as a result of an internal analysis. Strengths might include a cost advantage, customer loyalty, attractive physical or service characteristics of the facilities, organizational culture, exclusive contracts, quality outcomes, and high satisfaction levels for employees and consumers. Weaknesses may include a narrow product line, lack of management depth, high-cost operations, or a weak market image.

EFFICIENCY VERSUS EFFECTIVENESS

CREATING and sustaining a competitive advantage requires a balance between the ability to work skillfully with controllable internal factors (strengths and weaknesses) while adapting to factors outside of the organization's direct control (opportunities and threats). SWOT analysis is an effective method within the strategic management process to help organizations become more effective and efficient in their market. Organizational effectiveness can only occur when an organization is well positioned to accomplish its mission, and economies in the use of capital, personnel, or the physical plant will only be realized if an organization operates efficiently. A SWOT analysis helps to understand the strengths and opportunities that must be leveraged, and the weaknesses and threats that must be overcome in order to compete effectively and efficiently in a given market.

NANCY HOLLINGSWORTH

REFERENCES

Barney, J. B. (2001). *Gaining and sustaining competitive advantage* (2nd ed.). Reading, MA: Addison-Wesley.

Ginter, P. M., Swayne, L. M., & Duncan, W. J. (2006). *Strategic management of health care organizations* (5th ed.). Malden, MA: Blackwell.

Internet Center for Management and Business Administration, NetMBA Business Knowledge Center. (2007). *SWOT analysis*. Retrieved September 1, 2007, from http://www.netmba.com/strategy/swot/

T

Teamwork

P ROFESSIONAL NURSES have many roles but all require the skill of working with others. Teamwork involves working collaboratively rather than individually. The nature of nursing work directs us to work collaboratively with other professionals, unlicensed healthcare workers, and most importantly, our patients. Working together with others toward a common goal is a broad definition of teamwork. A team is usually a small group of people with complementary skills who are committed to a common purpose. There is a set of performance goals for which team members hold themselves mutually accountable. The work product of the team is produced through the joint contributions of its members. The work produced by the team is greater than the work that could be produced by each individual. In other words, a team is more than a sum of its parts (Katzenbach & Smith, 2005).

In health care, the nurse might be a member of multiple teams. There are patient care teams responsible for the care of individual patients and families. There are work teams established for a given task that are dissolved when the goal is achieved. There are ongoing teams established to manage and monitor specific outcomes such as patient safety, length of patient hospital stay, or skin care. Regardless of the type of team or its goal there are fundamental underpinnings of all successful teams. They include competent leadership, open communication, a clear purpose and goals, and measurable outcomes.

Leadership of a team is crucial to the team's success. Team leaders motivate and manage members. In health care, the membership of the care giving team is usually made up of several different specialists that are collectively responsible for the care of a patient. The leader is responsible to ensure that members understand their roles and have the opportunity and ability to communicate and participate in the decision making and care planning. The leader must manage the flow of communication and the complementary effect of the individual professional work.

Effective communication is part of a successful team. The leader is responsible for ensuring that all members are heard, remembering that silence may not indicate acceptance. As health care teams have become culturally diverse; therefore, the leader needs to be open to the cultural expectations of the membership. Through effective open communication, all ideas, opinions, and dialogue are valued and encouraged. This reinforces the value of each team member. Active listening, verbally checking your perception of what you heard, is required (Chinn, 2004). Effective communication between team members, especially nurse-physician communication, has been linked to better patient outcomes (Page, 2004).

Conflict and disagreement are part of the life of team-building. With a diverse group of caregivers and professionals from different cultural and educational backgrounds, conflicts sometimes arise as the team develops. An important leadership skill is the ability to deal with conflict and facilitate turning conflict into something positive. Conflict avoidance will result in anxiety and friction and hinder the team process. Addressing conflict while at the same time acknowledging its presence is the first step in leading to resolution.

Team members need to have clear goals with set expectations and definitive timeframes. Whether it is a patient care team or a task team, identifying measurable goals is the first step for a team trying to shape a purpose meaningful to its members. When goals are clear, discussions focus on how to pursue them and are more productive than when goals are ambiguous. Performance goals are symbols of accomplishment that motivate and energize the team (Katzenbach & Smith, 2005). These goals need to be measurable and each member needs to fully understand her or his responsibility in working toward the team's success. To keep members engaged in the work of the team, it is helpful to identify critical measurement points as the team works toward goals. In this way the team can feel success during progress toward reaching the goal. Important to note is at the end of every success, the team should celebrate its accomplishment. Enthusiasm for the work needs to be maintained and reaching a goal is one way to maintain team spirit.

Not all teamwork has successful outcomes. This does not mean the work of the team was a failure. For task teams, time for objective evaluation and reflection needs to be built into the team's schedule. Regardless of its outcomes, opportunities for improvement should be addressed. For patient care teams and ongoing work teams, there should be time set aside for team evaluation. Such evaluation needs to focus on the team-building process as well as the specific outcome measures. Team-building is an ongoing effort and the responsibility of all members.

CHRISTINE COUGHLIN

See Also
Conflict Management for Nurse Leaders
Cultural Diversity
Patient Care Delivery Models

REFERENCES

Chinn, P. (2004). *Peace and power: Creative leadership for building community* (6th ed.). Boston: Jones & Bartlett Publishers.

Katzenbach, J., & Smith, D. (2005). The discipline of teams. *Harvard Business Review, 83*(7/8), 162–171.

Page, A. (2004). *Keeping patients safe: Transforming the work environment of nurses.* Washington DC: National Academies Press.

Technology

TECHNOLOGY HAS TAKEN a prominent role in nursing and health care and has been "inexorably linked" since the late 19th century (Sandelowski, 2000). Technology may serve to define nursing, for example, the IV nurse, and be defined by nursing. Patient care areas have been defined by the technologies used: Hemodialysis units, critical care units, operating rooms. Hoffman (n.d.) categorized technology as "clinical and other information systems and smart medical devices." Technology is used in patient care to assess patients, track and monitor aspects of nursing care and clinical responses (central venous catheters, cardiac monitors, laboratory results), and assist with medication administration, documentation, and patient information. Technology is used in nursing administration for staffing, tracking patient acuity and managing quality improvement; in nursing education it is used to present information, measure skill and knowledge attainment, and validate knowledge and skills; and in nursing research to obtain, analyze, and disseminate information.

Clinical information systems (CIS) integrate information of the patient's medical records, including physician/primary care provider order entry, patient allergies, diagnoses, laboratory results, radiology results, medication administration, and documentation. CIS can provide checks and balances that help prevent repetition of tests and alert caregivers about medication interactions or duplication and patient allergies. Technologies used by nurses in the care of patients vary in complexity and are used wherever nursing care is realized. They include medical devices, such as beds, thermometers, stethoscopes, sphygmomanometers, bedside monitors, IV pumps, and invasive catheters. In addition, nurses utilize information technologies to help them keep abreast of the latest changes impacting patient care, such as personal digital assistants (PDAs) and computers.

New technologies are constantly being introduced. Technologies such as bar code scanning may help to reduce or prevent medication errors but also increase the time needed to provide patient care. Computerized documentation systems provide timely recording of activities provided to the patient and communication with all health care providers. Handheld computers are being evaluated as point-of-care information systems to enhance or change work flow. Telemedicine with videoconferencing has been implemented for palliative and hospice care, cardiac rehabilitation monitoring, patient education, and patient monitoring (Courtney, Demiris, & Alexander, 2005).

Computerized patient classification systems and scheduling systems assist nursing management assign the appropriate level of personnel to provide safe, effective patient care. Information technology skills are used to examine patient records to discover trends in patient care, quality improvement issues, risk management, staffing, and patient acuity. Patient classification system indicators, such as nursing time for teaching, intravenous medications and fluids, suctioning, or frequent turning and assessment, are defined by each institution, as each institution's patient population is unique. The number of nursing hours needed to care for each client is then defined. The scheduling systems assign the appropriate number of staff for daily unit coverage based on the number of nursing care hours needed each day. Although the classification systems help identify the level of nursing care needed and the scheduling systems assure an appropriate number of personnel, the manager must consider staff competency, staff levels, and skill mix (Marquis & Huston, 2006).

The scope of nursing education is changing at a rapid pace. Nurses use technology to help them increase their knowledge base and maintain competence via videos, online courses and discussion and the use of virtual chat rooms. Online courses are offered both for basic nursing education and for continuing education, offering nurses the opportunity to attain degrees, especially if they live a distance from an educational facility. Technology also helps to track the competency of nurses, keeping records of courses the nurse has completed or needs to complete and sending reminders of courses needing to be completed. PDAs are used to assist nurses with the myriad of information needed to provide safe care such as information on medications, diagnostic tests, and calculations (Courtney et al., 2005).

Although technology assists nurses to learn about and provide safe effective patient care, both directly and indirectly, the nurse must remain vigilant about the information provided by the technology and its impact it has on patient care. Technology does not replace good judgment; nurses must rely on their assessment skills to assure accuracy of information provided by the technology. Technology can and does malfunction. Processes and support systems must be in place to provide staff with the resources necessary to address situations when technology malfunctions (Haghenbeck, 2005).

KAREN TOBY HAGHENBECK

See Also
Risk Management in the Health Care Setting
Telehealth

REFERENCES

Courtney, K. L., Demiris, G., & Alexander, G. L. (2005). Information technology. *Nursing Administration Quarterly, 29*(4), 315–322.

Haghenbeck, K. T. (2005 Spring/Summer). Critical care nurses' experience when technology malfunctions. *Journal of New York State Nurses Association*, 13–19.

Hoffman, A. (n.d.). *Technology in nursing.* Retrieved July 31, 2006, from http://healthcare.monster.com/nursing/articles/technology

Marquis, B., & Huston, C. J. (2006). *Leadership roles and management functions in nursing: Theory and application* (5th ed.). Philadelphia: Lippincott, Williams & Wilkins.

Sandelowski, M. (2000). *Devices and desires: Gender, technology, and American nursing.* Chapel Hill: University of North Carolina Press.

Telehealth

THE HEALTH RESOURCES AND SERVICES ADMINISTRATION (HRSA; 2001) defines *telehealth* as "the use of electronic information and telecommunications technologies to support long-distance clinical health care, patient and professional health-related education, public health and health administration." The use of telehealth can provide access to health services for consumers and clinicians by removing the barriers of space and time and make health resources accessible, affordable, and convenient to many consumers and providers who feel empowered by these tools (Englebardt & Nelson, 2002). Using various forms of telehealth, rural clinicians can examine a patient's inner ear from a remote location, a nurse and patient can interact through a video home visit where the nurse can monitor medication compliance and assess vital signs, and a specialist can provide a remote consultation to a local emergency room patient (Thompson & Brailer, 2004). In rural and underserved areas, telehealth can decrease isolation and distance barriers; in school health links, off-site clinicians can provide needed physical exams; in correctional health the risk of escape in patient transfer can be decreased; in emergency care, evaluation and treatment can begin in ambulance transport; and in home care, aging immobile patients can be monitored to decrease emergency visits. Some of the technologies used in telehealth include telephone and faxes paired with an integrated data exchange, computers, interactive video transmissions, direct links to health care instruments, transmission of images, and telecommunications that use audio and video.

KEY ISSUES

THE POTENTIAL BENEFITS of telehealth, however, bring challenges related to reimbursement, cross state licensure, standards, privacy, and the need for guiding principles to direct its use. There is some evidence to support the usability and cost savings for telehealth (HRSA, 2001). Currently to help increase access to in-person care, patients in rural Health Professional Shortage Areas or nonmetropolitan statistical areas (MSA) are eligible for telemedicine reimbursement from Medicare for consultations, office and other outpatient visits, individual psychotherapy, pharmacologic management, the psychiatric diagnostic interview examination, end stage renal disease (ESRD) services included in the monthly capitation payment (except for one visit per month to examine the vascular access site), and individual medical nutritional therapy. In addition, Medicare allows payment for services traditionally not requiring a face-to-face (in-person) encounter with the patient that may be furnished through the use of a telecommunications system (such as the interpretation of an X-ray, electrocardiogram, electroencephalogram, and tissue samples) regardless of geographic area (Craig Dobyski, Health Insurance Specialist, Centers for Medicare and Medicaid Services, personal communication, September 6, 2006).

Fee-sharing challenges exist between primary care clinicians and specialists; and registered nurses and licensed practical nurses are not yet eligible for direct reimbursement under Medicare (Thompson & Brailer, 2004). In addition to reimbursement issues, some states restrict interstate telemedicine practice and challenges regarding cross state licensure. Many states have adopted the Interstate Nurses Licensure Compact, a licensure model based on mutual recognition of licensure for nurses. Safety and standards are becoming increasingly important. Without widely adopted standards and guidelines, interoperability, and interconnection are not possible. Older and newer equipment need to interconnect and different brands of the same equipment need to operate with one another. In addition, clinical protocols and guidelines such as telecommunications transmission specifications are needed. For example, the clinical technical standard for image quality in a video transmission would specify what is needed to correctly diagnose a patient. Regarding privacy, the general principles for the use and disclosure of personally identifiable health information are applicable regardless of the form the information is kept in, methods of transmission, time sequence of its creation and use, or the way it is communicated. Differences between federal and individual state privacy laws, however, make this a challenge for teleheath participants (HRSA, 2001).

TELEHEALTH PRINCIPLES

IN 1999 THE American Nurses Association (ANA) defined 12 core principles to guide the development and use of telehealth. The principles assert that the basic standards of professional conduct and the practitioner's responsibility to provide high-quality and ethical care must not be compromised by telehealth technologies (American Nurses Association, 1999). Telehealth applications can not be used as a vehicle for providing services that are not legally or professionally authorized. Although additional licensure should not be required to use telehealth, these services must adhere to basic assurances of quality. Nurses have a responsibility to examine how telehealth changes the patterns of care delivery and what modifications to standards may be required. The development of guidelines for telehealth needs to be based on empirical evidence; competencies for using such technologies must be ensured. It is important to protect the confidentiality and the integrity of data when using telehealth applications, and documentation requirements for recording telehealth services received need to be developed. When embracing the power of this technology, it is essential that the integrity and therapeutic value of the client/health care practitioner relationship be preserved. To this end, clients must be informed about the process, risks and benefits, and their rights and responsibilities when telehealth applications are used. Client safety needs to be assured through the appropriate use of hardware and software. Finally, the ANA calls for a systematic and comprehensive research agenda for the ongoing assessment and evaluation of telehealth services.

THE FUTURE

IN AN ERA of increased health costs, an aging population for which chronic conditions call for continuous monitoring, and access to providers that is sometimes limited, telehealth has the capacity to provide a vehicle for creative delivery, administration, and education for health care. Nurses are challenged to harness this capacity to create the future of health.

CAROL A. ROMANO

See Also
American Nurses Association
Technology

REFERENCES

American Nurses Association. (1999). *Core principles on telehealth.* Retrieved July 14, 2006, from http://www.nurse.org/acnp/telehealth/th.ana.core.shtml

Englebardt, S. P., & Nelson, R. (2002). *Health care informatics: An interdisciplinary approach.* St. Louis, MO: Mosby.

Health Resources and Services Administration. (2001). *Report to Congress on telemedicine.* Retrieved July 14, 2006, from http://www.hrsa.gov/telehealth/pubs/report2001.htm

Thompson, T. G., & Brailer, D. J. (2004). *The decade of health information technology: Delivering consumer-centric and information-rich health care.* Washington, DC: U.S. Department of Health and Human Services.

Office of the National Coordinator for Health Information Technology (ONCHIT). (n.d.). *Homepage.* Retrieved August 25, 2006, from http://www.hhs.gov/healthit/

Truth, Sojourner

SOJOURNER TRUTH (Isabella Baumfree) was born into slavery in New York State in 1797. As a result of the New York State Emancipation Act of 1827, Sojourner Truth died a free woman in 1883. Although illiterate throughout her life, Truth is remembered as an itinerant preacher, a lecturer on slavery, and a staunch proponent of African-American's rights and women's rights. She was an ardent abolitionist and the mother of 13 children, most of who were sold into slavery. Albeit untrained, Truth performed as a nurse during and after the Civil War. Following the Civil War (1861–1865), the 38th Congress established the Freedman's Bureau to provide for the needs of newly freed slaves and wartime refugees. Sojourner Truth spent much time at "Freedman's Village" in Washington, DC, providing nursing care in the Freedman's Hospital. She personally organized a group of women to clean the hospital, because, as Carnegie quoted her, "the sick can never be made well in dirty surroundings" (Carnegie, 1995, p. 8). She also spent time urging Congress to provide funding to train doctors and nurses. Sojourner Truth is listed in the Women's Hall of Fame in Seneca Falls, New York.

M. JANICE NELSON

REFERENCES

Carnegie, M. E. (1995). *The path we tread: Blacks in nursing worldwide, 1854–1994.* New York: National League for Nursing Press.

New York Life. (2006). *African-American history month: Sojourner Truth.* Retrieved July 28, 2006, from http://www.newyorklife.com/cda/0,3254,13543.html

U

United American Nurses

I N **1946**, the American Nurses Association (ANA) House of Delegates adopted a platform to permit nurses to be involved in collective bargaining.[1] The ANA Economic and General Welfare program has evolved over the years and in 1999, the United American Nurses (UAN) was established. Today, the UAN plays an important role in the challenge for registered nurses to provide high-quality patient care, advocate for the safety of nurses and patients, provide a safe work environment, influence standards of nursing practice, and improve the economic and general welfare of staff nurses. UAN is the collective voice for 102,000 staff nurses working in hospitals and health care agencies in 27 states.

In 2001, the UAN became a chartered affiliate of the AFL-CIO (the American Federation of Labor and Congress of Industrial Organizations). AFL-CIO is a voluntary federation of 53 national and international labor

---

[1] Collective bargaining is a method of negotiation in which authorized union representatives assist employees in contract negotiations. It is a method of mutually determining wages, hours and terms and conditions of employment through negotiations between representatives of the employer and the union. The results of the bargaining are set forth in a collective bargaining agreement. Collective bargaining determines the conditions of employment for all employees holding jobs in a bargaining unit.

unions. High on the UAN agenda is protecting the safety and health of staff nurses. Needle-sticks, spinal cord and musculoskeletal injuries, exposure to infections and chemicals, workplace violence, and stress are addressed in contracts. Through collective bargaining agreements, RNs serve on various health care agency policy committees where their leadership and involvement improve the health and safety of nurses and patients. Collective bargaining also gives nurses a voice in achieving competitive pay and benefits. Through contractual agreements, union representatives negotiate wage and benefit packages for staff nurses. In addition, contracts address issues related to job security. Working for the improvement and availability of affordable, high-quality health care services for all people, the UAN influences public policy affecting registered nurses (RNs) and the delivery of health care services. Through the legislative process at the state and national level, the UAN advocates for safe working conditions and workplaces. Through the collective bargaining program, improvement in the economic and general welfare of nurses has helped to advance the nursing profession and improve the quality of patient care.

United American Nurses
8515 Georgia Ave., Suite 400
Silver Spring, MD 20910
301-628-5118
Web site: www.uannurse.org

DIANE MANCINO

See Also
American Nurses Association
Health Policy

WEB REFERENCES

United American Nurses, www.uannurse.org
American Nurses Association, www.nursingworld.org
AFL-CIO, www.aflcio.org/aboutus/thisistheaflcio
National Labor Relations Board, www.nlrb.gov/nlrb

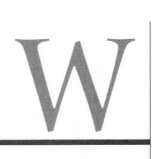

Wald, Lillian

LILLIAN WALD was born on March 10, 1867 in Cincinnati, Ohio, but was raised in Rochester, New York. She died in Westport, Connecticut, in 1940. Wald was a nurse, social worker, reformer, teacher, activist, philanthropist, and humanitarian, who founded The Henry Street Settlement—the forerunner of the Visiting Nurse Service of New York (American Association for the History of Nursing, 2006). A product of a family of scholars, Wald attended the New York Hospital Training School for Nurses. She spent one brief year at the Women's Medical College in New York, but quickly resumed her nursing role when confronted with the poverty and untenable living conditions among the sick poor and immigrants in the lower east side of Manhattan (Christy, 1969). Wald initiated the concept of public health nursing, and was the founder and first president of the National Organization of Public Health Nurses. The Visiting Nurse Program initiated on Henry Street became the national model and eventually a model to the world on public health nursing. Wald's administrative prowess and successful endeavors attracted support, financially and otherwise, from New York philanthropists such as Jacob Schiff and Mrs. Solomon Loeb. Wald is notably responsible for the initiation of the Federal Children's Bureau under President Theodore Roosevelt

(Brody, 2006). Before her death, she was named in the *New York Times* as one of the 12 greatest living American women (1922), and she was a recipient of the Lincoln Medallion and proclaimed the Outstanding Citizen of New York (1936). Wald was inducted into the National Women's Hall of Fame, and she was posthumously inducted into the ANA Hall of Fame in 1976 (American Association for the History of Nursing, 2006).

M. JANICE NELSON

See Also
ANA Hall of Fame

REFERENCES

American Nurses Association. (2006). *ANA Hall of Fame inductee: Lillian D. Wald, 1867–1840*. Retrieved March 23, 2006, from http://www.nursingworld.org/hof/waldld.html

Brody, S. (1996). *Lillian Wald (1867–1940)*. Retrieved March 29, 2006, from http://www.jewishvirtuallibrary.org/jsource/biography/wald.html

Christy, T. E. (1969). *Cornerstone for nursing education: A history of the division of nursing education of Teachers College, Columbia University, 1899–1947*. New York: Teachers College Press.

Christy, T. E. (1970). Portrait of a leader: Lillian D. Wald. *Nursing Outlook. 18*(3), 50–54.

National Association of Home Care. (2006). *Profiles in caring: Lillian D. Wald, 1867–1940*. Retrieved March 29, 2996, from http://www.nahc.org/NAHC/Val/Columns/SCI0-4.html

American Association for the History of Nursing. (2006). *Gravesites of prominent nurses: Lillian D. Wald, 1867–1940*. Retrieved March 29, 2006 from http://www.aahn.org/gravesites/wald.html

Werley, Harriet H.

HARRIET WERLEY was born in Pennsylvania on October 12, 1914. She died on October 14, 2002 (Werley, 2002). Werley earned her nursing diploma from the Jefferson Medical College in Philadelphia. She earned her BS degree in Nursing Education at the University of California at Berkeley, her MA in Nursing Administration at Teachers College, Columbia University, and her PhD in Psychology from the University of Utah. She was a pioneer in the field of nursing informatics (Ozbolt, Zielstorff, & Saba, 1997). Werley began her career with the U.S. Army wherein she served as Chief of the Department of Nursing Research at the Walter Reed Army Institute of Research. She later became director of the Center for Health Research at Wayne State University. She also held the position of Professor of General Nursing and Dean of Research at the University of Illinois, and later, at the University of Missouri, Columbia, she held the position of Associate Dean for Research. From 1983 to 1991, Werley served as Distinguished Professor at the University of Wisconsin at Milwaukee. Werley was a charter member of the American Academy of Nursing, and was founding editor of *Research in Nursing and Health*, and the *Annual Review of Nursing Research*. Werley received numerous citations and awards, among them, the Award for Outstanding

Contributions to Nursing and Psychology from the American Psychological Association and a Distinguished Service Award from the University of Illinois at Chicago, where she had earlier established an endowed chair (Werley, 2002). Werley founded the American Nurses Association Council on Computer Applications in Nursing. She convened the first national conference on nursing information systems, out of which the first book of original papers was published on the topic (Ozbolt et al., 1997). Werley is credited with "...the vision and foresight to create the field of nursing informatics" (Ozbolt et al., 1997).

M. JANICE NELSON

See Also
American Academy of Nursing
American Nurses Association

REFERENCES

Ozbolt, J., Zielstorff, R. D., & Saba, V. K. (1997). Tributes to Harriet H. Werley. *Journal of the American Medical Informatics Association, 4*(2), 161–162. Retrieved March 29, 2006, from http://www.pubmedcentral.nih.gov/articlerender. fcgi?artid=61508

Quirk, K. (2004). *UWM renaming nursing center for research pioneer.* Retrieved March 30, 2006, from http://uwm.edu/News/PR/04.11/Werley.html

Werley, H. H. (2002). *Harriet H. Werley Papers, 1959–2002.* Retrieved March 30, 2006 from http://www.uic.edu/depts/lib/specialcoll/services/lhsc/ead/017-20-04b.html

Whitman, Walt

W**ALTER (WALT) WHITMAN** was born into a family of nine children in Huntington, Long Island, New York, on May 31, 1819. He died and was buried in Camden, New Jersey, on March 26, 1892. Whitman is credited as being among the most influential of American poets along with Emily Dickinson, Hart Crane, Wallace Stevens, and Robert Frost. Although the controversial Whitman is primarily recognized as a poet (*Leaves of Grass*), editor, essayist, and humanist, he was and is closely associated with American transcendentalism and mysticism. Photographs and paintings often depicted a "Christ-figure" mystique about him. Whitman traveled to Virginia in 1862 to search for and visit his brother, Jeff, who was wounded in the Civil War. He was so moved by what he experienced at that hospital that he traveled to Washington, DC, and functioned unofficially and unpaid as a nurse in the army hospital there. He remained at the hospital and spent his own money to purchase supplies and equipment until 1873, when his own health began to fail. Whitman largely renounced the rigidity and metric structures of European poetry in favor of a freestyle verse. This attitude not only pervaded his philosophy and lifestyle, but propelled his role in fulfilling the American destiny as liberator and emancipator of the human spirit (Columbia Encyclopedia, 2004).

M. JANICE NELSON

REFERENCE

Columbia Encyclopedia (6th ed.). (2004). *Whitman, Walt*. New York: Columbia University Press. Retrieved August 8, 2007, from http://www.questia.com/PM.qst?a=o&d=101278089

World Health Organization (WHO)

T HE WORLD HEALTH ORGANIZATION (WHO) was founded April 7, 1948, a day that is celebrated annually as World Health Day. WHO is a component of the United Nations and is an international agency with a sole purpose of monitoring the health issues across the world (WHO, 2006). The World Health Assembly governs this organization and meets in Geneva, Switzerland, on a yearly basis. This meeting is attended by delegates representing the 192 member states. The Executive Board is made up of 34 members who agree to serve for 3-year terms; the Executive Board meets semiannually. The primary functions of the Executive Board are to advise and assist the inner workings of the World Health Assembly. WHO has a primary Director-General who is appointed by the World Health Assembly upon the recommendation of the Executive Board. This position is a 5-year term (http://www.who.int/governance/en/). The top 2006 priority of WHO was the control and prevention of three deadly infectious diseases: HIV/AIDS, tuberculosis, and malaria. Six million people die of these diseases every year and five million people will be newly infected with HIV in 2006 alone. Unfortunately, only one in five will have access to prevention or transmission information and tragically, millions are without antiretroviral medications (WHO, 2006). A second goal in 2006 was to decrease deaths of children under the age of 5, as close to 11 million young children die each year with the largest numbers located in sub-Saharan Africa and south Asia. Ninety percent of these deaths are a result of six medical causes, including diarrhea, HIV/AIDS, malaria, measles, neonatal difficulties, and pneumonia (WHO, 2006). A third priority of WHO in 2006 was to improve the health of new mothers as more than 500,000 women die each year in either pregnancy or childbirth (WHO, 2006). Unfortunately, these deaths are not disease related but, rather, caused by severe lack of prenatal and birthing care. In sub-Saharan Africa alone, 1 in 16 women have a risk of death during pregnancy or childbirth as compared to thriving countries, where the risk is 1 in 2,800 (WHO, 2006).

RONDA MINTZ-BINDER

REFERENCE

World Health Organization. (2006). *Working for health: An introduction to the World Health Organization.* Geneva, Switzerland: WHO Press, World Health Organization. Retrieved July 6, 2006, from http://www.who.int/about/brochure_en.pdf

WEB REFERENCE

WHO Governance, http://www.who.int/governance/en/

Z

Zimmerman, Anne K.

ANNE K. ZIMMERMAN was born in 1914 in Montana and died in Chicago, Illinois, in 2003. She began her nursing career in 1942. Zimmerman was a champion of nurses' rights, better working conditions for nurses, and control over clinical practice. She served as Director of the American Nurses Association's (ANA) Economic and General Welfare Program and later served as a member of the committee (Styles, 2003a). Zimmerman served as executive secretary of the Montana Nurses Association, assistant director of the California Nurses Association, and, for 27 years, served as executive administrator of the Illinois Nurses Association. She also served as chair of the American Journal of Nursing Company (Styles, 2003b). Zimmerman was presented with the Shirley Titus Award by ANA in recognition of her work with the Economic and General Welfare Program; she was designated a "Living Legend" by the American Academy of Nursing in 1997 (Styles, 2003b).

M. JANICE NELSON

See Also
American Academy of Nursing
American Nurses Association

REFERENCES

Styles, M. M. (2003a). *Eulogy: Funeral mass for Anne Zimmerman*. Retrieved July 18, 2006, from http://www.nursingworld.org/about/zimmerman.htm

Styles, M. M. (2003b). *In remembrance of ANA past president Anne Zimmerman*. Retrieved July 18, 2006, from http://nursingworld.org/about/zimmerman.htm

Index